Women's Health

A Guide to Health Promotion and Disorder Management

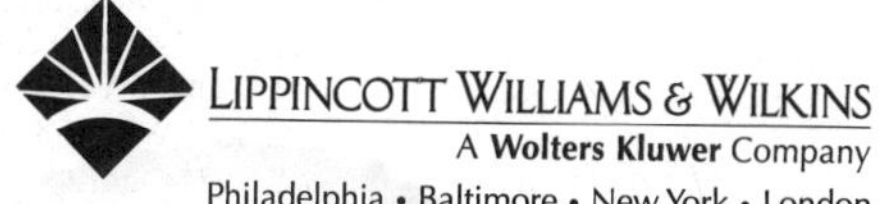

LIPPINCOTT WILLIAMS & WILKINS
A Wolters Kluwer Company
Philadelphia • Baltimore • New York • London
Buenos Aires • Hong Kong • Sydney • Tokyo

Staff

Executive Publisher
Judith A. Schilling McCann, RN, MS

Editorial Director
H. Nancy Holmes

Clinical Director
Joan M. Robinson, RN, MSN

Senior Art Director
Arlene Putterman

Art Director
Mary Ludwicki

Editorial Project Manager
Jennifer Pierce Kowalak

Clinical Project Manager
Minh N. Luu, RN, BSN, JD

Editors
Brenna H. Mayer, Julie Munden

Clinical Editor
Lisa Bonsall, RN, MSN, CCRN

Copy Editors
Kimberly Bilotta (supervisor), Elizabeth Mooney, Dona Hightower Perkins, Dorothy Terry, Pamela Wingrod

Designers
Lynn Foulk

Digital Composition Services
Diane Paluba (manager), Joyce Rossi Biletz, Donna S. Morris

Manufacturing
Patricia K. Dorshaw (director), Beth Janae Orr

Editorial Assistants
Megan L. Aldinger, Tara L. Carter-Bell, Linda K. Ruhf

Librarian
Wani Z. Larsen

Indexer
Barbara Hodgson

WH-D N O S A J J M A M
06 05 04 10 9 8 7 6 5 4 3 2 1

Library of Congress Cataloging-in-Publication Data

Women's health : a guide to health promotion and disorder management.
p. ; cm.
Includes bibliographical references and index.
1. Women—Health and hygiene. 2. Women—Disorders—Prevention. I. Title: Women's health. II. Lippincott Williams & Wilkins.
[DNLM: 1. Women's Health—Nurses' Instruction. 2. Health Promotion—Nurses' Instruction. WA 309 W87115 2004]
RA564.85.W66663 2004
613'.0424—dc22
ISBN 1-58255-282-7 (alk. paper)
2003026096

Contents

Contributors and consultants

Kim L. Armour, MSN,CNP, APN, RDMS
Maternal-Fetal Manager and Nurse Practitioner
Central DuPage Hospital
Winfield, Ill.

Barbara Beacham, RN, MSN
Adjunct Professor
Seton Hall University
South Orange, N.J.

Lisa Morris Bonsall, RN, MSN, CRNP
Clinical Consultant
West Chester, Pa.

Shari A. Regina Cammon, RN, MSN, CCRN
Report Evaluation & Safety Surveillance Associate
Merck & Co., Inc.
West Point, Pa.

Debra C. Davis, RN, DSN
Dean & Professor
University of South Alabama
Mobile

Shelton M. Hisley, RNC, PhD, WHNP
Assistant Professor, School of Nursing
The University of North Carolina at Wilmington

Joyce King, RN, PhD. FNP, CNM
Assistant Professor, Clinical
Emory University School of Nursing
Atlanta

Mary Jo Konkloski, RNC, MSN, ANP-C
Perinatal Clinical Nurse Specialist
Arnot Ogden Medical Center
Elmira, N.Y.

Mary Kostenbauder, MSN, MEd, CNM, ARNP
Professor
Seminole Community College
Sanford, Fla.

Carolyn B. Leach, BSN, CWHNP
Women's Health Nurse Practitioner
Chase City (Va.) Family Practice

Ann S. McQueen, RNC, MSN, CRNP
Nurse Practitioner
Health Link Medical Center
Southampton, Pa.

Jennifer B. Rousseau, RNC, MSN, WHNP
Instructor
Rush University College of Nursing
Chicago

Barbara S. Snyder, PhD, APRN, BC
Assistant Professor
Seton Hall University
South Orange, N.J.

Helen M. Toutkoushian, MSN, CRNP, NP-C
Gerontologist & Certified Adult Nurse Practitioner
Dunwoody Village
Newtown Square, Pa.

Benita J. Walton-Moss, DNS, APRN, BC
Assistant Professor
Johns Hopkins University School of Nursing
Baltimore

Foreword

It's no surprise that women's health has become a driving force in today's health care arena. In the past decade, women have become increasingly knowledgeable and proactive about their own health care, insisting upon the highest level of awareness and requesting evidence-based decisions. In addition, new awareness of differences in disease presentation, new testing techniques, improved diagnostic criteria, and new treatments for a wide range of illnesses affecting women have changed the landscape of health care.

What's more, women will soon make up the larger population with increasing susceptibility to emerging diseases — yet, who will care for this growing group? Many health care providers today have had little specific women's health education and training. Resources that provide knowledge, coupled with current, research-based approaches, for the care of women are desperately needed. *Women's Health: A Guide to Health Promotion and Disorder Management* is just the resource that will give nurse practitioners and practicing nurses the knowledge, skills, and research-base they'll need to care for female patients.

This unique, comprehensive guide to health promotion and disease management focuses on strategies for maintaining health and preventing disease across the lifespan. It clarifies key concepts related to women's health issues using a systematic and practical approach, giving practitioners the tools necessary to provide safe, compassionate, and comprehensive care.

Women's Health: A Guide to Health Promotion and Disorder Management provides an easy-to-access format and a simplified approach, consisting of two parts. Part I contains four chapters, with the first chapter covering an introduction to women's health. The remaining three chapters outline approaches to promoting healthy living and disease prevention across a woman's lifespan — specifically adolescence, adulthood, and older adulthood. They address illness prevention of disorders, such as obesity, heart disease, and diabetes; reproductive issues; screening recommendations for breast cancer, depression, violence, and sexually transmitted diseases; and health maintenance issues, including smoking cessation, stress reduction, and proper nutrition. Part II provides a comprehensive collection of disease monographs, organized A to Z, related specifically to women. Each monograph provides a brief description and offers health care providers a clear and practical approach to causes, signs and symptoms, diagnosis, treatment, and special considerations, along with the framework for effective decision-making. In all, more than 100 diseases are presented, chosen specifically because they're either more prevalent in women, or entail unique issues in women, such as stroke, myocardial infarction, and certain cancers.

Packed with features, such as quick-reference headings, bulleted lists, and a consistent entry format, *Women's Health: A Guide to Health Promotion and Disorder Management* supplies on-the-spot information for solving clinical problems as they arise. More than 50 illustrations, charts, and tables summarize critical facts. Furthermore, special icons alert you to critical information, including:

- *Cutting edge*— summarizes the latest research
- *Alternative therapies*— spotlights alternative treatments, including herbal remedies and natural supplements
- *Prevention pointer*— provides simple tips and strategies for self-care or prevention of diseases or disorders
- *Special needs*— addresses unique issues for special populations including women with disabilities, different races and cultures, and different religions and how these may affect a woman's health.

Because women are living longer than men and, consequently, consuming more health care services, health promotion and disease management should be a major goal in enhancing the health of all women. Information to help practitioners achieve these goals must be easily and readily available. *Women's Health: A Guide to Health Promotion and Disorder Management* offers such a solution. As an educator, speaker, writer, columnist, and women's health practitioner, I find it an essential reference for seasoned and novice practitioners for the management of health issues that affect all women.

Helen A. Carcio, RNC, ANP
President, HC-Institute for Health Professions
Associate Clinical Professor
University of Massachusetts
Amherst
Director, Bladder Health Program
Grace Urological
Brattleboro, Vt.

Part I

Introduction

CHAPTER 1

Introduction to women's health

Overview

Women live an average of 7 years longer than men and their life expectancy is expected to continue to increase. Because women tend to live longer, their health has a greater impact on themselves and everyone around them, including their children, parents, and anyone else for whom they provide care. In addition, despite recent gains in equality in politics and the workplace, women are still typically the primary caregivers when family members become ill. In order for women to continue in this vital caregiving role, they must maintain their own level of health and wellness. To do so, they need accurate and timely health information, access to resources, and support from health professionals so they can understand the significance of health in their own lives and take important steps towards living healthier and longer.

The United Nations Educational, Scientific, and Cultural Organization (UNESCO) reports that the population is getting older as life expectancy nearly doubles. In the 21st century, over 20% of the world population is over age 65, compared with 1% 100 years ago. (See *U.S. female population by age.*) UNESCO projects that by 2030, 1 in 4 women in the United

U.S. FEMALE POPULATION BY AGE

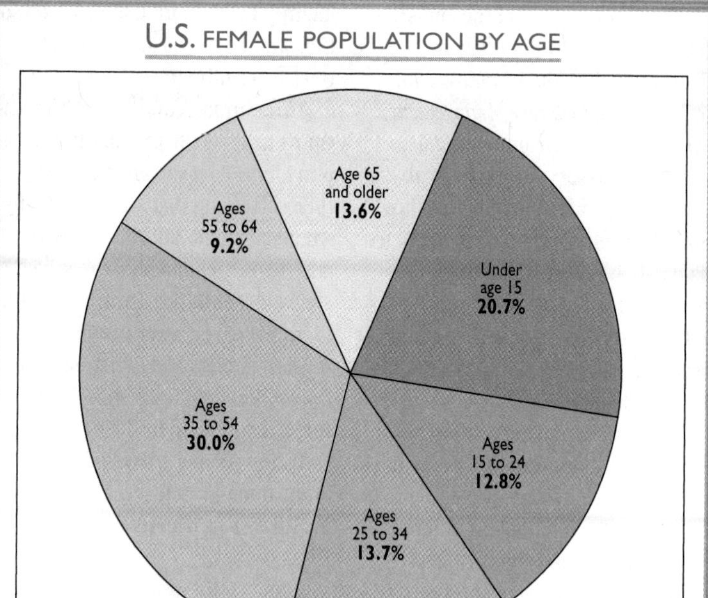

Source: U.S. Department of Health and Human Services, Health Resources and Services Administration, Maternal and Child Health Bureau. Women's Health USA 2003. Rockville, MD: 2003.

States will be over age 65. In addition, 1 in 5 women will be Hispanic, 1 in 11 will be Asian, and the number of Black and Native American women will grow even more steadily. By 2050, White women will make up about half of the adult female population in America. Thus, it's clear that our nation and the world face the challenge of meeting the health needs of an increasingly older, more diverse, more *female* population.

Successful treatment of existing illness is by no means a guarantee and, in some cases, is nonexistent.

The diseases that cause the most deaths in women are heart disease and cancers—particularly lung, breast, and colorectal cancers. The prevalence of these highly preventable diseases in women stresses the need for health promotion, illness prevention, and life-style changes as the essential focus of women's health. Also, with the advancement of medical research and technology, we know that chronic diseases, including osteoporosis, arthritis, diabetes, and other autoimmune disorders, can be prevented or at least delayed. Health care professionals caring for women play an important role not only in informing them about disease prevention, health promotion, and lifestyle changes, but also in reinforcing the message that they must change their health for the better.

Women's Health: A Guide to Illness Prevention and Disease Management provides health care professionals with the necessary information about women, all of which will help to promote the health and lifestyle of the female patient. After discussing women's health in general, this book dedicates separate chapters to the adolescent female, the adult female, and the older female because each period of life has a significantly different focus for health promotion. The second part of *Women's Health* provides information on diseases that are commonly seen in women, primarily affect women more than men, or impact a woman differently than a man. This book will help health care professionals in the field of women's health to understand the nature of a particular disease as well as its causes, signs and symptoms, and treatment options, including special considerations.

The importance of women's health

Why is women's health so important? First, women make up 51% of the population. In addition, women are living longer and are encountering more and more health challenges. In the past, women's health research focused on fertility and reproduction, while research regarding other diseases focused on men. Even now, women are diagnosed and treated based on clinical studies that involved only men. Thus, it's important to identify this inequitable situation so that women can be diagnosed and treated accordingly.

In addition, women have been and continue to be the primary health care providers and decision makers for themselves and their families. Many women perform multiple roles, including caring for elderly relatives and young children. Health education is crucial to empower women to make the best choices and decisions. Also, for women to function in this role, they must remain healthy themselves. Ensuring good health requires cooperation among women, their families, health care providers, employers, and the community.

Financially speaking, women experience significant health care expenditures. In addition to breast and gynecological disorders, other disease processes are now more prevalent or diverse in women — for example, heart disease, stroke, diabetes, asthma, certain cancers, and certain autoimmune disorders. Furthermore, women as a group demonstrate a higher rate of disability than men and report higher numbers of conditions that limit their activity. With women making up 71% of Americans older than age 85, they're experiencing more chronic illness and make up the majority of nursing home residents.

If that wasn't enough, studies have shown that health care providers treat women differently than men. Examples of these differences include:

- Women receive less thorough evaluations for similar complaints.

- Providers minimize a woman's symptoms.
- Providers offer fewer interventions for the same diagnosis.
- Providers prescribe certain medications over others.
- Women receive less detailed explanations to answer their questions.

Populations at risk

Certain groups of women are at greater risk than others for health problems and, thus, may have more health care needs. These groups include adolescent girls, women of color, incarcerated women, older women, and women with disabilities.

Adolescent girls

The leading cause of death among adolescent girls is unintentional injury. One in five suffers from physical abuse, and one in four shows signs of depression. Women in this age-group have increased rates of eating disorders, increased smoking, and frequent binge drinking. A high percentage of this population doesn't wear seat belts regularly. It's also important to note that young female adults under age 24 make up the least medically served population in the country. Increased health education and services are imperative for this group of women.

Women of color

Women of color continue to suffer disproportionately from premature death, disease, and disability. This group demonstrates a greater prevalence of cardiovascular disease, systemic lupus erythematosus (SLE), certain cancers, diabetes, hepatitis, tuberculosis, and acquired immunodeficiency syndrome (AIDS). Infant and maternal mortality rates are also higher in this population than in white women.

Women of color are also more likely to live in poverty, which is associated with a greater frequency and severity of illness and premature death. They experience limited access to health care and utilize lower percentages of preventive health services. Reasons for these issues stem from systemic, cultural, social, and economic barriers to health care.

Incarcerated women

Women make up the fastest growing incarcerated population in the United States. The health care needs of these women are influenced by their:

- status as pregnant women and mothers
- caregiving responsibilities to children who are minors
- growing numbers engaging in high-risk illicit drug behavior
- high rates of human immunodeficiency virus (HIV) infection
- history of physical and sexual abuse.

Older women

Because women live longer, they're at increased risk for developing chronic disorders and disabilities that occur with age. Older women also:

- are more likely to live in poverty than older men

- spend more out-of-pocket dollars for health care expenses
- are less likely to use preventive services such as mammography, due to cost.

Even so, the trend toward women's better use of available health care and screening is promising as women are achieving greater educational and economic independence. We can assume that the older woman of the future will be better able to support and care for herself.

Women with disabilities

The number of American women with disabilities increases as the population is getting older. Nearly 60% of U.S. women age 65 and older are living with a disability. Their varying conditions make their roles as caregiver, mother, wife, coworker, and friend difficult and more challenging because of their physical and mental limitations. A disability may be physical, mental, or psychological. Its severity may be described in terms of how much it limits a person's daily activities. Women are more likely to be limited in the amount or kind of activity they can perform.

Some of the challenges that women with disabilities face include physical barriers, lack of adequate transportation, financial restraints, and a lack of reliable information and services addressing their needs.

Reproductive health

Over 80% of women in the United States have had a child by age 44, underscoring the fact that childbearing and childrearing remain significant factors in women's reproductive health and also shouldn't be discounted as a role in an older woman's reproductive health. However, despite available contraceptive technologies, too many pregnancies are unintended; approximately 20% of women giving birth over age 35 report that their pregnancy was unintended. Therefore, unintended pregnancy isn't just a teenage problem and reflects a lack of awareness of contraceptive options as well as a failure to use appropriate contraceptive methods.

Even so, many advances have already been made in the realm of reproductive health. Use of effective contraception is increasing, including rising use at first intercourse, and rates of unintended pregnancy are decreasing.

The most common contraceptive methods are:

- female sterilization
- hormonal contraceptives
- condoms
- male sterilization.

In addition, more American women than ever are getting prenatal care in their first trimester of pregnancy. Research has repeatedly indicated the correlation between adequate prenatal care and positive pregnancy outcomes. Continued outreach into all, especially poorer, communities is necessary to continue these trends.

Despite advances in contraception, other reproductive health issues continue to need attention. For example, women are more susceptible than men are to becoming infected with sexually transmitted diseases (STDs), and younger women are at greater risk than older women due to age-based differences in cervical anatomy. In addition, women are less likely than men to experience symptoms, making adequate screening vital to reproductive health. The risk of developing pelvic inflammatory disease increases significantly if STDs remain untreated and could, ultimately, lead to infertility.

Other reproductive disorders also require attention. Premenstrual syndrome, dysmenorrhea, and other menstruation-related disorders affect many women; nearly 10% of women experience symptoms severe enough to disrupt their usual activities. In addition, endometriosis and fibroids, which affect 10% to 20% of women, are associated with one-half of the more than 580,000 hysterectomies performed in the United States each year. Finally, increases in infertility rates have occurred, due in part to delayed childbearing. Infertility treatments are costly and psychologically stressful for those involved and can have a negative impact on a woman's health.

Selected disorders

More than 1.2 million women in the United States died in 2000. Heart disease and cancer accounted for more than one-half of those deaths. The other leading causes of death were cerebrovascular disease and chronic lower respiratory diseases. (See *Leading causes of death in females*, page 8.) Black women had the highest death rates in three of the four leading causes: heart disease, cancer, and cerebrovascular disease.

The incidence, characteristics, diagnoses, and treatments of certain disorders — both acute and chronic — have special meaning in women's health. These disorders include cardiovascular disease, cancer, stroke, osteoporosis, asthma, HIV-AIDS, and mental illness. Listed below are important facts regarding each of these disorders.

Cardiovascular disease

- Heart disease is the number one killer of women.
- More women die of heart disease each year than men.
- Women present with atypical symptoms and are less likely to have adequate primary prevention.
- Women develop heart disease later in life than men.
- Women are more likely to have other coexisting chronic conditions that may mask their symptoms.
- Women who recover from a heart attack are more likely to have another heart attack or a stroke.
- Compared to 24% of men, 42% of women die within a year after myocardial infarction.

Cancer

- Cancer is the second leading killer of women and lung cancer is the leading cause of cancer death.
- Although more women die of lung cancer, more women are diagnosed

Leading Causes of Death in Females

The leading cause of death in women in the year 2000 was heart disease followed by cancer and stroke. Black women had the highest death rates for diseases of the heart, malignant neoplasms, and cerebrovascular diseases.

Accidents (unintentional injuries) **2.8%**

Alzheimer's disease **2.9%**

Influenza and pneumonia **3.0%**

Diabetes mellitus **3.1%**

Chronic lower respiratory diseases **5.1%**

Cerebrovascular diseases (stroke) **8.4%**

Malignant neoplasms (cancer) **21.8%**

Diseases of the heart **29.9%**

All other causes **23%**

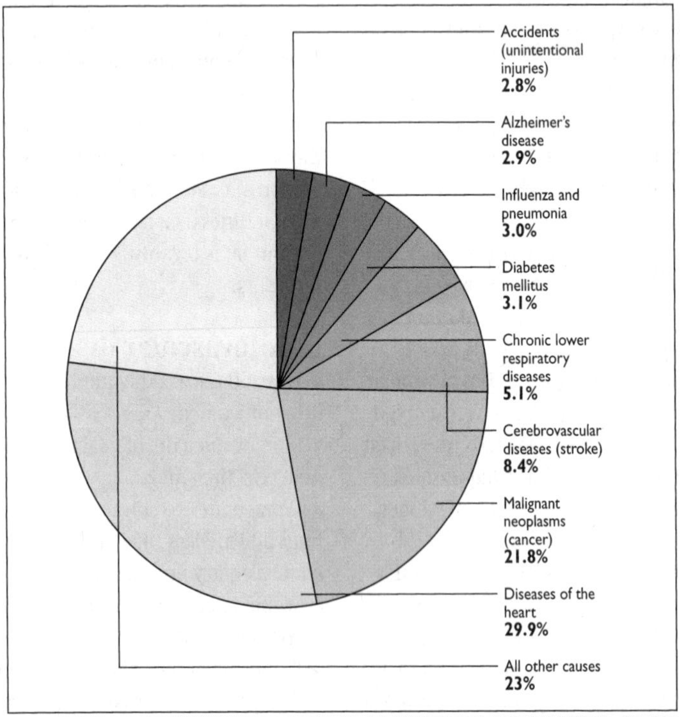

Source: U.S. Department of Health and Human Services, Health Resources and Services Administration, Maternal and Child Health Bureau. Women's Health USA 2003. Rockville, MD: 2003.

with breast cancer each year than any other cancer. In 2001, the National Cancer Institute reported that 67,300 females died of lung and bronchus cancer, compared with 40,200 deaths from breast cancer.

- Lung cancer deaths continue to rise in women, which is considered to be almost exclusively due to increased cigarette smoking in women.
- Breast cancer death rates are declining due to earlier detection using mammography and improved treatment.

SPECIAL NEEDS

Black women have the highest lung cancer death rates, White women have the highest breast cancer death rates.

- Colon cancer is the second leading cause of cancer deaths in women.
- Screening for colon cancer, exercise, low-fat diet, increased diet of fruits, vegetables, and whole-grain foods are methods to prevent this disease.
- Although once considered a "man's disease", it's now known that colon cancer affects men and women equally.
- Early detection and prevention of cervical cancer has improved due to Papanicolaou (Pap) tests. However, cervical cancer still occurs in many elderly, low-income, and rural women due to lack of adequate screening. Other risk factors for cervical cancer include smoking and human papilloma virus infection.
- Endometrial and ovarian cancer rates are lower but these forms of cancer are more deadly — especially ovarian cancer because symptoms don't appear until late in the disease.
- Women under age 40 make up the fastest growing group of skin cancer patients. The rate of melanoma, the most serious form of skin cancer, is increasing in women.

Stroke

- Stroke kills more than twice as many women each year as breast cancer.
- Women account for 43% of the 550,000 strokes that occur each year and 61% of stroke deaths.

SPECIAL NEEDS

Stroke occurs at a higher rate among Black and Hispanic women than White women.

Osteoporosis

- Nearly 90% of patients with osteoporosis are women.
- Osteoporosis is especially common in women over age 65 and commonly goes undiagnosed.
- One out of two women will be affected by osteoporosis at some point in their lifetime.
- In 2002, there were 8 million women with osteoporosis with an estimated 30 million women having low bone density, therefore placing them at risk for the disease. These figures are expected to rise as the nation ages.
- Osteoporosis is considered a major public health threat costing the U.S. health care system $17 billion dollars annually.
- Routine screening for osteoporosis is now recommended for women age 65 and older.

HIV-AIDS

- In 2000, 10,459 cases of AIDS were diagnosed in females age 13 and older.
- HIV and AIDS are becoming more prevalent among Black and Hispanic women.
- Due to barriers to treatment and decreased adherence to prescribed regimens, different treatment approaches are needed in women.
- Gender differences in $CD4^+$ counts and viral load may warrant revisions

of current treatment standards for women. Current guidelines were originally developed for men.

- The most common mode of HIV infection in women is heterosexual contact; the second most common mode is I.V. drug use.
- Women experience significant differences from men in the course of HIV-AIDS illness and modes of transmission, impacting diagnosis and treatment in women.

Autoimmune disorders

- More than 85% of patient's with SLE are women.

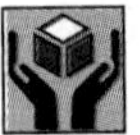

SPECIAL NEEDS

SLE is three times more common in Black women than White women and also more common in women of Hispanic, Asian, and Native American descent.

- Nearly 75% of all autoimmune diseases occur in women, including SLE, Sjögren's syndrome, rheumatoid arthritis, scleroderma, type 1 diabetes, multiple sclerosis, and autoimmune thyroid disease.
- Autoimmune diseases represent the fourth largest cause of disability among women in the United States.

Mental illness

- Major depression affects twice as many women as men.
- Women are two to three times more likely to have certain types of anxiety disorders, including anxiety, panic attacks, and phobias.
- Women account for 90% of all cases of eating disorders.
- Women are more likely to attempt suicide than men (although more men are successful).

Emerging issues in women's health

Women's health in the 21st century focuses on many of the topics discussed previously. However, more attention is being focused on several other issues affecting women's health. These issues include hormone replacement therapy, poverty, violence, and preventive health care.

Hormone replacement therapy

The Women's Health Initiative was a medical trial that, in part, studied the use of combined hormone replacement therapy (HRT) as a treatment for cardiovascular disease and osteoporosis. The NIH stopped the trial early because researchers detected a greater risk of breast cancer, heart attacks, strokes, and thromboembolism among the women taking HRT. Consequently, women are increasingly uncomfortable using HRT for conditions related to menopause. In addition, manufacturers of the drugs are stopping production due to fear of lawsuits in the wake of the latest findings as well as the existing challenges of pharmacologic treatment of the complex, changeable conditions of menopause. As a result, consumers and providers are looking to alternative and complementary treatments to manage menopausal symptoms. However, data is limited regarding the efficacy and safety of such treatments.

Poverty

Poverty continues to be a problem in the United States, with 12.8 million women living below the federal poverty level. Many women are sole providers with multiple children, which adds to the increasing rate of poverty among women. Of these women, those between ages 18 and 24 have the highest poverty rate; however, the poverty rate among elderly women is increasing. Women age 65 and older make up 11.2% of women living in poverty and those age 75 and older account for 13.6%. Furthermore, older women lack access to affordable health care. (See *Women living below the poverty level.*)

Violence

Violence is a major public health problem for American women. More than 4.5 million women are victims of violence each year. In addition, violence causing maternal mortality is increasing. Violence during pregnancy ranges from 4% to 8% of cases and could become a more common problem for pregnant women than preeclampsia, gestational diabetes, or placenta previa.

Preventive health care

Preventive health care can help to promote good health throughout a woman's life span. Overall, women

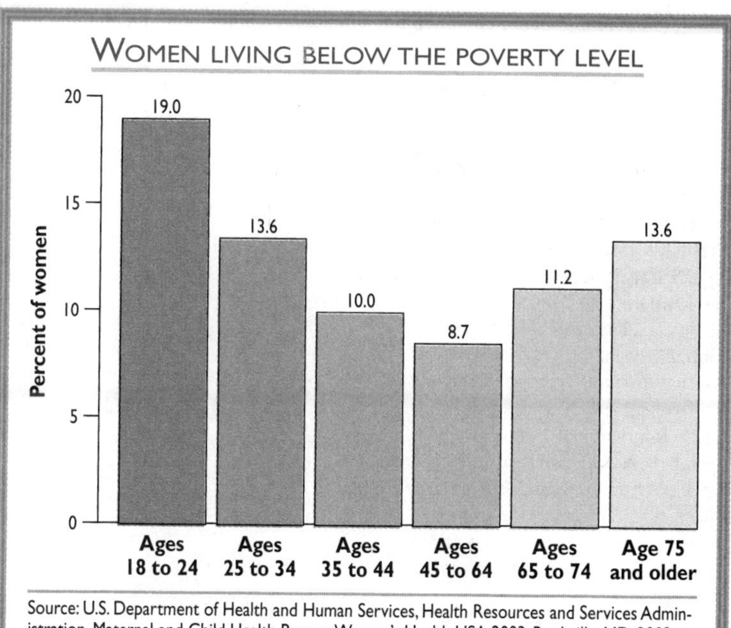

Source: U.S. Department of Health and Human Services, Health Resources and Services Administration, Maternal and Child Health Bureau. Women's Health USA 2003. Rockville, MD: 2003.

are more likely than men to seek preventive care as Pap tests and mammograms but are less likely to engage in leisure time physical activity. They're also less likely to eat the recommended servings of fruits and vegetables and less likely to stop smoking. The percentage of women who smoke has remained steady at just above 20% of the adult female population. Connections between lifestyle choices and chronic illnesses are being drawn but it's clearly evident that education and activities to promote healthful behaviors are essential.

Selected references

Anderson, J., and Kessenich, C.R. "Women and Coronary Heart Disease," *The Nurse Practitioner: The American Journal of Primary Health Care* 26(8):12, 18, 21-23, August 2001.

Cohn, S.E. "Women with HIV/AIDS: Treating the Fastest-growing Population," *The AIDS Reader* 13(5):241-44, May 2003.

DiPalma, J.A. "Women's Colonic Digestive Health," *Gastroenterology Nursing* 25 (1):3-9, January-February 2002.

4women.gov – The National Women's Health Information Center. A project of the U.S. Department of Health and Human Services' Office on Women's Health. "The History and Future of Women's Health" [Online]. Available: *www.4woman.gov/owh/pub/History/* [accessed 2003, July 7].

4woman.gov – The National Women's Health Information Center. A project of the U.S. Department of Health and Human Services' Office on Women's Health. "Women's Health Issues: An overview" [Online]. Available: *www.4woman.gov/owh/pub/womhealth%20issues/index.htm* [accessed 2003, July 7].

Moore, A. "After HRT: What now?" *Nursing Management* 34(7 Suppl):13-15, June 2003.

"National Women's Health Report: Women and Osteoporosis." (2003). A Guide to Women's Health, supplement to *Nursing2003*.

U.S. Department of Health and Human Services, Health Resources and Services Administration, Maternal and Child Health Bureau. "Women's Health USA 2002" [Online]. Available: *www.mchb.hrsa.gov/data/women. htm* [accessed 2003, July 7].

Women's Health Initiative Participant Web Site. "WHI Findings Summary" [Online]. Available: *www.whi.org/findings/summary_bc.asp* [accessed 2003, July 7].

CHAPTER 2

Health promotion and illness prevention in the adolescent female

Overview

Adolescence is the period between childhood and adulthood, typically between ages 10 and 21. It's marked by tremendous growth and development in all areas. The adolescent phase is commonly broken into three major stages:

- early adolescence from ages 10 to 13
- middle adolescence from ages 14 to 16
- late adolescence from ages 17 to 21.

Each stage has its own unique growth tasks that must be achieved for the individual to develop into a healthy, functioning adult. It's important for the health care provider as well as the parents to remember that every individual has her own unique pattern and time frame for these stages and comparisons with peers should be avoided. It's also important to stress to the adolescent girl that, although physical, social, emotional, and intellectual changes occur in their own time, they will occur.

The physical changes the adolescent girl experiences result in a final growth spurt to full adult height as well as the development of secondary sexual characteristics and the ability to conceive. These changes usually occur during the early stage of adolescence. Girls usually experience this final growth spurt about 2 years before boys but are typically shorter than their male counterparts at its conclusion.

Defining one's self and separating from one's parents are important developmental goals of adolescence. During early adolescence, the separation from parental guidance begins and the adolescent prefers friends to family. During the middle-adolescent phase, the individual may feel ambivalent about separating from family and works on resolving these issues during late adolescence. Body image is also important for the adolescent, and the female must become comfortable with her changing and developing body. Issues involving sexual roles and sexuality also become apparent during this period. It isn't uncommon for girls who reach sexual maturity early to be conflicted regarding their sexual role and develop high-risk behaviors as a way of coping with their new body. Early adolescence is a time when sexual curiosity begins, and occasional masturbation is common. Middle adolescence may begin sexual experimentation and the opposite sex may be viewed as a sex object. Late adolescence marks the beginning of intimacy and the ability to have a caring, sexual relationship.

Relationships are important during the adolescent period. In early adolescence, a girl's peer group is commonly all female and group activities are the norm. During the middle-adolescent period, heterosexual peer groups are formed and adult role models are commonly sought. During late adolescence, individual relationships begin to take on more importance than the peer group. This shift corresponds with developing intimacy skills within the realm of developing sexuality.

Cognition continues to develop during adolescence. Concrete thinking dominates during early adolescence; as the adolescent mind develops, it enables the girl to think more abstractly. The adolescent girl may become fascinated by her ability to think about thinking. This progression also allows her to consider career plans. Although the early adolescent may have vague and unrealistic career goals, by late adolescence her career plans become specific and connected to a system for achieving goals.

Due to the magnitude and diversity of the changes that occur during the adolescent years, problem behaviors aren't uncommon. The separation from parents during the early years can lead to tension and unrest in the home environment as parents may feel they're losing control over their child (and so they are). The adolescent, trying to spread her wings, may react to parental concern by rebelling and striving even harder to exert her independence. Experimentation in such high-risk behaviors as smoking, alcohol, and drugs may begin during this age. As the trials of adolescence, separation, individuality, and independence are met with success or failure, the adolescent attempts to cope with the changes. Antisocial behavior, violence, depression, and "acting out" may be seen in the adolescent female as she attempts to integrate her new abilities and desires with the world she's experiencing.

Health promotion

Adolescence is a time of striving for independence. It's also a time when teens begin to develop health patterns and engage in risk taking, both of which will influence their future health. High-risk behaviors common to the adolescent include using tobacco, alcohol, and illegal substances; engaging in unprotected sexual activities; and carrying weapons.

Morbidity and mortality

Because adolescents are more likely to engage in risky behaviors, their mortality and morbidity rate continues to rise. (See *Leading causes of death.*) Accidents are the leading cause of death among those between ages 15 and 24 and account for 38.5 deaths per 100,000 females. Accidental deaths include:

- motor vehicle accidents, at 16 deaths per 100,000 persons
- drowning accidents, at 0.4 deaths per 100,000 persons
- firearm accidents, at 0.3 deaths per 100,000 persons
- poisoning accidents, at 0.3 deaths per 100,000 persons.

Alcohol use has been implicated in a high percentage of motor vehicle accidents involving teenagers. Another risk factor increasing mortality rates among teens involved in motor vehicle accidents is the failure to use seatbelts. Teenagers rarely report using seatbelts when riding in a vehicle driven by someone else. Not knowing how to swim, choosing an unsafe place to swim, and swimming alone accounted for a high number of drowning deaths.

Homicide accounts for 20.3 deaths per 100,000 persons. Most homicides of adolescent girls also involve friends or gangs, and firearms were involved in a high percentage of these deaths.

Suicide accounts for 13.3 deaths per 100,000 females. Although males commit suicide at a higher rate than females, attempted suicide is more commonly reported in females than completed suicide. Factors that place teens at risk for death by suicide include mental disorders such as depression; substance abuse (drugs and

Leading causes of death

The leading causes of death between ages 15 and 24 are:

1. accidents
2. homicide
3. suicide
4. HIV infection.

alcohol); family history of substance abuse, mental disorders, or suicide; the presence of family violence; previous suicide attempts; and accessibility to firearms in the place of residence.

Human immunodeficiency virus (HIV) infection is responsible for 1.7 deaths per 100,000 females. The Centers for Disease Control and Prevention (CDC) (2000) states that one-quarter of all new HIV infections in the United States are believed to occur in young people under the age of 22. In 2000, almost 2,000 new cases of acquired immunodeficiency syndrome among adolescents ages 13 to 19 were reported to the CDC. Male and female black adolescents have the highest reported number of HIV infections when compared with other groups. An increasing number of females are among reported adolescent cases of HIV infection, most of which occurred from unprotected sexual behavior. Areas of concern related to sexual risk-taking behavior in adolescent females include:

- increasingly younger age at first sexual encounter
- older sexual partners who may already be infected with the virus
- spread of HIV through adolescents who are infected but have no symptoms and engage in unprotected sexual activity
- common adolescent perception that they aren't at risk for acquiring the infection.

Exercise and fitness

In the U.S., only about one-half of the young people in the United States between ages 12 and 21 regularly participate in vigorous physical activity. As the age and the grade of the child increases, physical activity decreases. The CDC found that only 64% of all high school students reported that they had participated in vigorous physical activity for at least 20 minutes during 3 or more days of a 7-day period, with males being more likely than females to do so. More than 60% of women in the United States don't engage in the recommended amount of physical activity and more than 25% aren't physically active at all. In addition, another study found that Blacks have lower levels of physical activity as compared with other Americans. By encouraging physical activity early in life, teens are more likely to continue physical activity as they grow older.

A 2003 study looked at factors influencing physical activity levels among females ages 12 to 24 and found that an absence of social support (parents and peers) and depression were significant predisposing factors that influenced females to avoid physical activity. Females who engaged in a regular program of physical activity usually had the support of family members and friends.

The benefits of physical activity include building and maintaining healthy bones and muscles, controlling weight, reducing body fat, and preventing or delaying the development of hypertension and diabetes. A documented link exists between regular exercise as an adolescent and a reduced risk of cardiovascular disease during adulthood. Physical inactivity places the adolescent girl at risk for developing various diseases as an adult. Early changes that later lead to these health consequences become apparent in childhood and adolescence.

In addition to the physiologic benefits of physical activity, research abounds about the positive aspects of being involved in activities that support physical activity. In 2003, a study demonstrated that middle and high school students who were involved in sports, engaged in exercise, and had a healthy self-image were significantly less distressed emotionally and demonstrated less suicidal behavior than students who weren't involved in sports.

The CDC recommends that health care providers talk to their female patients on a regular basis about the importance of physical activity as part of their lifestyles. The basics of physical activity counseling that the health care provider should address at every office visit include:

- inquiring about the physical activity habits of the adolescent
- encouraging involvement in physical activities that could be enjoyed into adulthood (such as walking, running, swimming, basketball, tennis, golf, dancing, and bicycling)
- emphasizing the need for appropriate use of safety equipment (such as helmets, safety pads for elbows and knees, and mouth guards to protect teeth)
- counseling that the use of cigarettes, alcohol, and other drugs impairs performance and may lead to an increased risk of injury
- advising adolescents of the dangers of eating disorders.

Exercise and physical disability

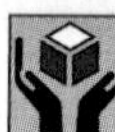

SPECIAL NEEDS

The adolescent female with a physical disability should be encouraged to participate in a program of physical activity or a sport commensurate with her interests and physical capabilities. Physical inactivity should be discouraged to ensure that the adolescent performs needed exercise. Because most people with physical disabilities tend to live a less active lifestyle, the benefits of exercise are even more important to them. Regular exercise and physical activity may increase heart and lung function, control weight gain, improve performance in activities of daily living, protect against the development of chronic disorders, decrease anxiety and depression, and enhance feeling of well-being and self-esteem. Recommendations to support the young female with disabilities in physical activity include:

- encouraging activities that are compatible with her disability
- helping the adolescent assess her own strengths and assets
- assisting the adolescent to set realistic goals for physical activity
- introducing the adolescent to other females with similar disabilities who engage in physical activity
- suggesting involvement with special groups and facilities for adolescents with similar physical disabilities

Safety considerations for exercise

The National Center on Physical Activity and Disability (NCPAD) encourages everyone—especially those with physical disabilities—to exercise. The NCPAD established some general guidelines for those with disabilities before and during physical activity and exercise:

Before you begin

1. Obtain physician consent.
2. Participate in a graded test to determine your current level of fitness, if possible.
3. Find out the effects of your medication on exercise and make sure they don't pose a hazard.
4. If possible, consult a trained exercise professional for an individualized exercise prescription.
5. Set realistic short- and long-term goals.
6. Find and follow an exercise program that meets your specific goals.
7. Engage in physical activity or exercise with a partner.

During exercise

1. Stop exercising if you have pain, discomfort, nausea, dizziness, light-headedness, chest pain, irregular heart beat, shortness of breath, or clammy hands.
2. Drink plenty of water and fluids.
3. Wear appropriate clothing, based on type of activity, weather, and personal safety.

- pointing out the positive aspects of physical activity, such as improved appearance
- teaching safety considerations about a chosen physical activity to decrease the risk of unintentional injury. (See *Safety considerations for exercise.*)

Nutrition

A balanced diet is essential during the adolescent period of accelerated physical development to ensure growth and sexual maturation. (See *RDA for the adolescent female.*) The typical adolescent diet is deficient in calcium, iron, zinc, folic acid, vitamin C, and vitamin A. Teenage girls of low socioeconomic status also intake inadequate levels of folic acid, vitamin B_6, vitamin A, iron, calcium, and zinc. Low levels of fruit and vegetable consumption have been associated with female adolescents, American-Indian adolescents, and Black adolescents. Excess intake of calories, sugar, fat, cholesterol, and sodium is evident in both genders in all racial and ethnic groups.

Poor nutrition problems

Poor eating habits common to adolescents place young females at risk for such immediate health problems as iron-deficiency anemia, eating disorders, obesity, and dental caries as well as long-term health problems that include heart disease, diabetes, and osteoporosis. The incidence of osteoporosis can be significantly reduced if

RDA FOR THE ADOLESCENT FEMALE

The chart below outlines the recommended daily allowance (RDA) of various nutrients that should be included in the female adolescent's diet.

Nutrient	RDA	Nutrient	RDA
Calcium	1,500 mg/day	Vitamin C	65 mg/day
Phosphorous	1,250 mg/day	Vitamin E	15 ug/day
Magnesium	360 mg/day	Calories	220 cal/day
Vitamin D	200 IU/day	Total fat	73 g/day
Niacin	14 mg/day	Saturated fat	< 24 g/day
Riboflavin	1 mg/day	Protein	44 g/day
Thiamin	1 mg/day	Vitamin A	800 mcg/day
Vitamin B_6	1.2 mg/day	Iron	15 mg/day
Folate	400 mcg/day	Zinc	12 mg/day
Vitamin B_{12}	2.4 mcg/day	Iodine	150 ug/day

Sources: Institute of Medicine, Food and Nutrition Board (1997 and 2000) and National Research Council, Food, and Nutrition Board (1989).

children — especially adolescents — include an adequate amount of calcium in their daily diet. The need for calcium increases in and around puberty because growth accelerates at this time. A study identified a lack of adequate calcium-enriched foods in the typical adolescent diet. Because peak bone mass in the femoral and lumbar spine is achieved by age 18, a diet rich in calcium is imperative for adolescents girls to prevent osteopenia and osteoporosis later in life.

Diet influences

As adolescents spend more time away from home, irregular eating habits, skipping meals, snacking, and eating at fast-food restaurants can result in a poor diet. Fast-food restaurants provided approximately 32% of meals eaten away from home for adolescents in 2002. These meals are notoriously high in calories, fat, saturated fat, and sodium, not to mention low in iron, calcium, vitamin A, and fiber.

Snacking is actually a major source of nutrition for the adolescent female. Study after study estimates that 30% of the adolescent diet is based on snacking. Two major sources of snack items include vending machines and convenience stores. Typical snack item purchases for the adolescent include beverages (soft drinks), candy, gum, salty snacks (potato chips, pretzels, tortilla chips), and bakery items (cookies and cakes). A recent study hypothesized that the constant marketing and accessibility of these foods in vending machines and convenience stores make them extremely appealing to adolescent consumers.

Another influence on an adolescent girl's diet may be peer pressure; wanting to fit in can lead to fad dieting. Especially for the adolescent female, concern for physical appearance and attractiveness has a profound impact on diet. Many adolescent girls consider themselves to be too heavy and want to lose weight. Especially during adolescence, females tend to become fixated with their body size and shape. This fixation can lead to the development of eating disorders, including anorexia nervosa and bulimia. Adolescents' perceptions of healthy foods can influence their food selections. According to another study, adolescents commonly use words such as "boring" and "expensive" to describe healthy foods.

Parental monitoring can also influence the dietary habits of adolescents. A recent study found that careful parental monitoring of an adolescent's diet resulted in high fruit and vegetable intake and a consistent intake of healthy breakfasts and lunches.

Nutritional counseling

Health care providers can also make a positive impact on the eating behaviors of the adolescent female. Those who work with adolescents need to be proactive in promoting healthy nutritional practices among members of this group. Adolescents need to make informed choices regarding their diet, a practice that starts with education. Health care providers should strategize with the adolescent to find convenient and realistic ways of incorporating highly palatable, healthy foods into her diet. Because families also influence the dietary practices of their adolescent children, every effort should be made to include family members in nutritional counseling.

School nurses play a crucial role in influencing the eating behaviors of adolescents. A study found that nutrition education programs can have a positive impact on the dietary practices of adolescents. Therefore, school nurses must be at the forefront by teaching students proper nutrition in school. The school nurse should teach students that soft drinks should be replaced with water and pure fruit juices and high-fat, high-calorie snack foods should be replaced with low-fat, low-calorie alternatives such as fruit.

Dietitians also play an important role in the types of messages that teenagers receive about nutrition by influencing the media to project more positive messages about food and body image. In addition, dietitians can contribute with effective menu planning for the school cafeteria. Highly nutritious and tasteful foods should be made available. The availability of good tasting, low-fat food items is an important factor in influencing adolescents to select healthier foods.

The National Health and Medical Research Council provides these guidelines for healthy eating in the adolescent:

- Enjoy a wide variety of foods.
- Eat plenty of breads, cereals, vegetables, and fruits.
- Maintain a diet low in saturated fat.
- Drink water as the beverage of choice.
- Only eat sugar or those foods containing sugar in moderate amounts.
- Choose low-fat foods.
- Eat foods containing calcium.
- Eat foods containing iron.

All adolescents need a balanced diet that incorporates a wide variety of foods. Adolescents should choose a diet that's low in total fat (30% or less of total calories), saturated fat (less than 10% of total calories), and cholesterol. Sugar and salt should be used only in moderation (choose foods low in salt and with reduced sugar content). Encourage adolescent females to eat foods rich in calcium (milk and milk products), iron (lean red meats, dry legumes, fortified cereals, whole-grain products), and folic acid (dry beans, leafy green vegetables, citrus fruits).

The adolescent vegetarian

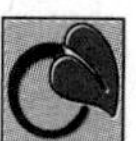

ALTERNATIVE THERAPIES

Vegetarians differ in the make-up of their diets:

- vegans eat no animal products
- lacto vegetarians include milk products in their diets
- ovovegetarians eat eggs
- semivegetarians may eat some meat in the form of fish or chicken.

Vegetarian diets are popular among adolescent females. In the past, these diets have been associated with nutritional deficiencies (protein-energy malnutrition, iron deficiency, and vitamin B_{12} and D deficiencies). However, a recent study found adolescent vegetarians more likely to meet Healthy People 2010 dietary recommendations than adolescents who didn't adopt a vegetarian diet. The researchers also concluded that, contrary to previous impressions, adolescent vegetarians consumed more iron, vitamin A, folate, and fiber than adolescent nonvegetarians.

The key to a nutritionally sound vegetarian diet is variety: fruits, leafy green vegetables, whole grain products, nuts, seeds, and legumes. Different types of vegetarians also include dairy products and eggs. Protein sources in the vegetarian diet include cow's milk, cheese, yogurt, beans, bread, cereals, nuts, peanut butter, tofu, and soy milk. Calcium content of the vegetarian diet can be maintained at adequate levels through ingesting cow's milk, cheese, yogurt, tofu processed with calcium sulfate, green leafy vegetables (collard greens, mustard greens, kale), calcium-fortified soy milk, and calcium-fortified orange juice. The vegetarian can meet iron requirements by eating such foods as broccoli, raisins, watermelon, spinach, black-eyed peas, blackstrap molasses, chickpeas, and pinto beans. To increase the amount of iron absorbed from a meal containing these food items, the addition of a citrus fruit that contains vitamin C is encouraged. Oranges, tomatoes, and broccoli are good sources of vitamin C. Nutritionally sound snack food items for teenage vegetarians might include apples, oranges, bananas, grapes, peaches, plums, dried fruits, bagels with peanut butter, carrot or celery sticks, popcorn, rice cakes, and frozen juice bars.

Immunizations and vaccinations

According to a report in 2000 from the U.S. Department of Health and Human Services, vaccine-preventable diseases are responsible for significant medical costs, morbidity, and mortality in the adolescent. As stated by the American Academy of Pediatrics (1997), adolescents are susceptible to vaccine-preventable diseases because:

- they haven't received the recommended vaccines throughout childhood
- incorrect timing of immunizations
- failure to complete the entire series for a particular immunization.

The CDC's recommendations published in 2002, advise that adolescents receive the tetanus-diphtheria vaccine, hepatitis B vaccines, measles-mumps-rubella vaccine, and varicella vaccine. (See *Recommended immunizations*, pages 24 to 27, and *Does MMR cause autism?* page 28.)

SPECIAL NEEDS

Additional vaccines recommended for teenagers include the meningococcal vaccine for college students and the influenza and pneumococcal vaccines for those individuals with chronic illnesses that are associated with an increased risk of pneumococcal disease or its complications.

Travel immunization

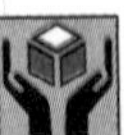

SPECIAL NEEDS

Americans who travel oversees are at increased risk for contracting infectious diseases. The risk of acquiring an infectious disease while traveling abroad depends on several factors, including:

- destination
- length of stay
- health status at the time of departure
- prophylactic measures taken prior to travel.

The type of immunizations recommended or required for foreign travel depends on the area visited, length of stay, and status of current disease outbreaks. When someone is traveling overseas, immunization is common for such diseases as hepatitis A and B, polio, meningococcal meningitis, yellow fever, typhoid fever, and rabies. Specific guidelines for recommended and required immunization are available from the CDC Web site (*www.cdc.gov*). The CDC also has an automated International Traveler's Voice Information Service (404-332-4559).

Provider's role

Regardless of the setting in which the adolescent patient is seen, health care providers should routinely discuss issues related to immunization. Areas that must be addressed include the adolescent's current health status, immunization history, and previous reaction to immunization. Adolescent patients should be encouraged to begin keeping a record of receiving vaccinations.

Sexuality

One aspect of an adolescent girl's growth and development is the emergence of sexuality. Several factors affect her sexual development, including changes in:

- hormonal state
- outward physical appearance
- social environment.

Sexuality is first influenced by physical changes in the body, brought on by surges in reproductive hormones. Breast development and the appearance of pubic hair are the first visible changes experienced by the adolescent female. Adolescents typically progress through a series of behaviors related to the development of their sexuality. Progression through these behaviors is greatly influenced by the teen's value system, beliefs regarding sex, and culture. These behaviors include:

- engaging in self-exploration and fantasy play
- dating members of their peer group
- establishing intimate relationships.

Menarche

The onset of menstruation, or *menarche*, is a definitive measure of puberty in females. The median age of menarche for all girls in the United States is 12.43 years, with 10% of girls menstruating at 11.11 years and 90% menstruating by 13.75 years. However, a female may begin menstruating any time between ages 8 and 16.

Race and weight have been found to influence sexual maturation in females. According one study, the age at menarche depends on a female's race. The age at menarche for non-Hispanic Black girls (median age 12.06 years) was significantly earlier than the age of non-Hispanic White girls (median age 12.55 years) with Mexican-American girls assuming an intermediate position (median age 12.25 years). A large body of literature exists that demonstrates a relationship between obesity and early maturation in females, with early-maturing females more likely to be obese than average- or late-maturing females. Another study found that girls with a higher percent of body fat at age 5 were more likely to show signs of pubertal development at an earlier age.

Promotion of healthy sexuality

The health care provider, during any health encounter with an adolescent girl, should discuss issues related to sexuality. Education and counseling opportunities should focus on responsible sexual behavior that will prevent unplanned pregnancy and transmis-

(Text continues on page 26.)

Recommended immunizations

This chart lists immunizations recommended for the adolescent female, along with appropriate timing, additional considerations, and possible adverse reactions.

Immunization	Timing
Tetanus-diphtheria (Td)	If the recommended schedule of childhood immunizations has been received, a booster is needed at age 14 to 16.
Hepatitis B	Individuals who are at increased risk for hepatitis B virus (HBV) infection should be vaccinated with the hepatitis B vaccine. These high-risk individuals include: ▪ heterosexual individuals who have had more than one sex partner in the previous 6 months or those with a sexually transmitted disease ▪ sexually active homosexual or bisexual males ▪ illicit injectable drug users ▪ household contacts and sex partners of persons who have tested positive for hepatitis B surface antigen (HBsAg) ▪ international travelers who spend more than 6 months in areas with high HBV infection rates and have close contact with the local population (Inuit, Indochinese, Haitian, and sub-Saharan refugees).
Measles-mumps-rubella (MMR)	Immunization should take place between ages 11 and 12.
Varicella virus	Immunization should take place between ages 11 and 12.

Additional considerations	Adverse reactions
▪ Booster vaccination is needed every 10 years.	▪ Local reactions, such as erythema and induration, can occur at the injection site. ▪ Arthus-type reactions, such as fever and malaise, can occur if the tetanus booster is given more frequently than recommended. ▪ Anaphylaxis has been reported (rare) with tetanus booster administration.
▪ If not previously immunized, children age 7 through age 20 should receive a series of three doses, with the first dose at the current visit, the second dose 2 months later, and the third dose 6 months after the second dose. ▪ Maximum antibody response occurs at approximately 6 weeks following the third dose of the vaccine.	▪ Local reactions, such as erythema and induration, can occur at the injection site. ▪ Although rare, hepatitis B vaccine may cause anaphylaxis.
▪ Make sure that the child didn't receive a second dose of MMR after her second birthday. If the child received MMR at that time, immunization shouldn't be administered at ages 11 to 12.	▪ The vaccine may cause a mild burning at the injection site. ▪ The vaccine may cause symptoms of measles, mumps, and rubella, including mild fever, swelling of salivary glands, and joint pain and swelling, respectively.
▪ Unvaccinated adolescents who lack a reliable history of chickenpox should receive the vaccine. ▪ The vaccine is contraindicated in pregnancy. Pregnancy should be ruled out in sexually active adolescent females prior to administering the vaccine. ▪ Salicylates shouldn't be taken for 6 weeks following receipt of the vaccine to avoid the possibility of developing Reye's syndrome.	▪ The vaccine is usually well tolerated with only pain and redness reported at the site of injection. ▪ Some individuals may develop a mild varicelliform rash following vaccination. ▪ Administration of the vaccine should be encouraged to protect individuals who come in contact with immunocompromised individuals.

(continued)

RECOMMENDED IMMUNIZATIONS *(continued)*

Immunization	Timing
Pneumococcal polysaccharide	1 or 2 doses should be given 6 to 8 weeks apart at any time in the adolescent period with revaccination every 6 years for those at highest risk for fatal pneumococcal disease.
Influenza	Immunization should take place annually.
Meningococcal	The adolescent female will most likely receive this vaccine prior to entering college.

sion of sexually transmitted diseases (STDs) and HIV. Abstinence should be at the forefront of any discussion related to sexual behavior. If the teen chooses to engage in sexual activity, the use of latex condoms should be encouraged.

Sexuality and disability

Even though females with mental and physical disabilities have fewer opportunities to establish sexual relationships compared to their nondisabled counterparts, the health care provider should counsel parents that their teenage daughter still has the same sexual needs and concerns as any other teenager. Many times, parents and medical professionals overlook the sexuality of a disabled person. Parents should be told to watch for cues that signal their teen's readiness for information on sexuality. Parents and health care providers must be prepared to recognize factors that limit a healthy outlook on sexuality and sex-

Additional considerations	Adverse reactions
▪ Additional immunization should be administered every 6 years in cases of chronic illness or disease associated with an increased risk of pneumococcal disease or its complications, including cardiovascular disease, pulmonary disease, diabetes mellitus, alcoholism, cirrhosis, splenic dysfunction, human immunodeficiency virus infection, and acquired immunodeficiency syndrome.	▪ Mild local reactions, such as erythema and pain, can occur at the injection site. ▪ Fever, myalgia, and severe local reactions have been reported with administration of the vaccine. ▪ Anaphylactic reactions are rare with this vaccine.
▪ The vaccine should be administered in patients with chronic illness or disease associated with an increased risk of influenza or its complications, including diabetes mellitus, renal dysfunction, hemoglobinopathies, and immunosuppression. In addition, persons ages 6 months to 18 years who are receiving long-term aspirin therapy should receive the vaccine annually because of the risk of developing Reye's syndrome following influenza.	▪ Because the influenza vaccine contains only noninfectious virus particles, it can't cause influenza. Respiratory illness following vaccination is merely coincidental. ▪ The most common adverse reaction to the influenza virus vaccine is soreness at the injection site that may persist for up to 2 days. ▪ Fever, malaise, and myalgia occur infrequently.
▪ Immunization is recommended for those at high risk for the disease, including those in the armed forces, boarding schools, travelers to endemic areas, and those with asplenia or inherited immunological deficiencies.	▪ Mild local reactions, such as erythema and slight pain, can occur at the injection site. ▪ Fever greater than 101.3° F (38.5° C) occur in a small percentage of patients.

Source: Centers for Disease Control and Prevention (2002)

ual issues in a girl with disabilities in order to discuss those issues. (See *Sexuality and disability*, page 29.)

Illness prevention

Preventing illness in the adolescent female involves dealing with physical changes in the body as well as changes in body image (menarche, obesity, weight loss, physical disability). In addition, initiation of self-destructive behaviors (smoking, alcohol and drug abuse, sexual promiscuity) is more prevalent in this age-group and bears watching.

Changing adolescent body

As a young girl begins the onset of puberty, the physical changes that she experiences are varied. Breast development, pubic hair growth, and the onset of menarche all contribute to a girl's changing body during adolescence. The Tanner scale, which rates breast development and pubic hair

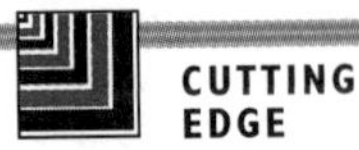

Does MMR cause autism?

Although many benefits of immunization are apparent, some concern has arisen over the measles-mumps-rubella (MMR) vaccine and a suspected link to autistic spectrum disorders (ASD), also known as *autism*. Parents and researchers are concerned about the linkage between administration of the MMR vaccine and the emergence of ASD in the child's 2nd year of life.

First link

The hypothesis first appeared in a 1988 issue of *The Lancet*, where researchers described the emergence of behavioral problems in 12 children following vaccination with MMR. Following publication of these findings, the Centers for Disease Control and Prevention and National Institutes of Health encouraged the Institute of Medicine (IOM) to assess this public health concern.

IOM findings

The Immunization Safety Review Committee appointed by the IOM issued *Immunization Safety Review: Measles-Mumps-Rubella Vaccine and Autism*, a report summarizing the committee's assessment of this issue. In 2001, the committee rejected any causal relationship between MMR vaccine and ASD based on a lack of epidemiologic evidence to support the association. Its members also couldn't find any biological mechanism to explain the hypothesized relationship.

Additional findings

Following this report, other leading medical groups, including the American Academy of Pediatrics and the World Health Organization, arrived at similar conclusions. Thus, no change has occurred in the current United States MMR administration policy. The vaccine still remains a prerequisite for entry into school or day care in all 50 states.

patterns, is commonly used to assess where along the sexual development curve an individual female lies. It's important to note that menarche doesn't signal achievement of adult height; on average, the height gain after menarche is approximately 3″ (7.5 cm) and growth may continue for 4½ years after menarche. When assessing growth patterns, it's important to measure the adolescent yearly and note growth trends over time. Growth charts may be obtained from the CDC's Web site *(www.cdc.gov)*. The site also provides a self-study module with instruction on accurate measurement and interpretation of the growth measures and body mass index (BMI).

Body image

Because an adolescent girl is increasingly concerned with fitting in with her peers, negative signals she might receive from them regarding her body may lead to efforts to change her appearance. She may try several different styles during this period in an attempt to define her self-image. In the extreme, these attempts could lead to

Sexuality and Disability

Although sexuality is commonly overlooked in females with mental or physical disabilities, it's an important issue to any adolescent female. Interpersonal relationships in general and sexual relations in particular greatly impact a person's self-esteem and support network. The same is true for a person with a mental or physical disability. Even so, various factors must be addressed to help a disabled person feel comfortable with herself and her sexuality, including:

- assurance that sexual responses are normal
- help with communication of her needs and her feelings concerning sexual issues
- discussions with the mentally disabled teen about the mental maturity and responsibility required for a sexual relationship
- discussions with the physically disabled teen about her sexual behavior prior to the disability or, if the disability predates sexual development, discussions about her physical limitations and possible options as well as information on how she may have a healthy sexual relationship
- recognition and intervention if signs of depression develop
- recognition and intervention if signs of an altered body image develop
- discussions with the physically disabled teen about overcoming social isolation and meeting new people
- discussions with the disabled teen about her fears of rejection, inadequacy, and pain that attempt to allay anxiety
- discussions about contraception and pregnancy
- discussions about sexually transmitted diseases and safer sex.

an eating disorder. One study found that individuals with above average weights were found to have more negative feelings regarding their bodies than their below-average-weight counterparts. They also found that below-average-weight girls tend to perceive themselves as larger while average- to above-average-weight girls tend to perceive themselves as smaller than they truly are.

During the adolescent period it's important to assess her comfort with the changes that she's going through. Addressing any concerns she may have regarding these changes and her body allows the health care provider to reinforce positive behaviors. Anticipatory guidance also aids the adolescent in dealing with these changes and lets her know that she's experiencing something that other girls also experience.

Acne

In addition to sexual maturation, acne is another physical change that can affect body image. It's important to make the adolescent girl aware of good hygiene habits and, if necessary, prescribe appropriate medication. Decreasing acne flare-ups and amounts will help bolster her self-image.

Obesity

Obesity has reached epidemic proportions in this country. Regardless of race, ethnicity, or gender, the prevalence of obesity in adolescents is higher today than 20 years ago. The rate of increase in obesity in children and adolescents is up 7% in the past 10 years. One-fourth of all children under age 21 are obese and one study estimates that over 30% of children or adolescents are overweight. The number of children and adolescents who are overweight (with a BMI greater than the 95th percentile for age and gender) has tripled in the past three decades. In response to this alarming trend, the U.S. Department of Health and Human Services launched its latest program, Healthy People 2010, to reduce the number of overweight and obese children between ages 6 and 19 and reduce chronic diseases associated with diet and weight.

Obesity has physical, psychological, and social consequences. Increased body weight has been found to predispose adolescents to many medical complications. Diseases associated with obesity include impaired glucose tolerance, type 2 diabetes mellitus, hypertension, hyperlipidemia, cardiovascular disease, sleep apnea, osteoarthritis, and stroke. (See *Morbid obesity in youth.*) Psychological consequences associated with obesity include depression and low self-esteem. A social stigma is also attached to obesity. Obese individuals suffer from chronic embarrassment and shame about their size and guilt about their inability to be thin. Many obese people are the subjects of others' hostility and rejection. Obese adolescent females will become adults who are known to earn lower wages and live in poverty compared with their nonobese counterparts.

Obesity is a complex, chronic condition with multiple factors. Primary contributors to obesity include genetic predisposition, poor nutrition, sedentary lifestyle, and depressed mood. Parental obesity is an important predictor of childhood obesity. Statistics show that the offspring of two obese parents have an 80% chance of developing obesity in their lifetime with the chances dropping to 40% if only one parent is obese.

Environmental factors, such as increased intake of calories (especially fat and sugar), irregular patterns of eating, excessive snacking, and sedentary activities (playing video games, watching television, and using the computer) contribute as much as 80% to childhood obesity. Teens who watched 5 or more hours of television per day were 4.6 times more likely to be obese than those teens who spent 2 hours or less per day engaged in television viewing.

Some researchers have implicated various "western lifestyle habits" as significant contributors to this ever-growing problem. Such factors at play in the United States include lack of physical activity, over-reliance on sedentary modes of transportation rather than walking or bicycling, increased television viewing, increased use of the computer for entertainment, and lack of time spent out of

Morbid obesity in youth

This list includes the many complications of morbid obesity in youth organized by body system.

Cardiovascular
- Accelerated atherosclerosis
- Dyslipidemia (increased triglycerides, low high-density lipoprotein level, increased low-density lipoprotein level)
- Hypertension
- Increased left ventricular mass

Respiratory
- Hypoventilation (Pickwickian syndrome)
- Frequent respiratory infections
- Sleep apnea

Endocrine
- Hyperinsulinemia
- Insulin resistance
- Early puberty (accelerated linear growth and bone age)
- Polycystic ovaries and dysmenorrhea

Musculoskeletal
- Coxa vara
- Slipped capital femoral epiphyses
- Blount's disease
- Legg-Calvé-Perthes disease

doors engaged in physical activity. Factors that have contributed to the fattening of America include aggressive television advertising of fast-food products, larger portions served by restaurants, the presence of snack and soft drink machines in elementary and high schools, and the increased number of meals that Americans consume outside the home.

One study determined through a longitudinal analysis that depressed mood may be a harbinger of obesity during adolescence. The neurobiological mechanisms that may explain this relationship could involve serotonin and the chronic excretion of cortisol.

Provider's role

Health care providers should target those individuals at risk for developing obesity. Targeting these adolescents is extremely important because 70% of overweight 10- to 13-year-olds will become obese adults. Intervention begins with screening. Routine nutritional screening should assess meal patterns, dieting behaviors, and recent weight changes. In addition, the health care provider needs to perform an assessment of exercise and activity patterns. Determining the types and amounts of both physical and sedentary activities that the adolescent engages in will help the health care provider determine how to counsel these adolescents. (See *Preventing obesity in children*, page 32.)

Education plays a critical role in the prevention and treatment of obesity in young persons. Unhealthy eating and exercise patterns need to be replaced with healthier lifestyles. Educational efforts must begin in the home environment because children are strongly influenced by the behav-

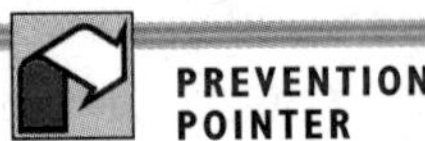

Preventing obesity in children

Use these guidelines to help identify children at risk for obesity and help them achieve and maintain an ideal weight.

Who's at risk?

Childhood obesity has many causes. However, heredity plays a large part. Typically, one or both parents of an obese child are seriously overweight themselves. Inactivity is a major cause and a result of obesity; overweight children may be too embarrassed to wear swimsuits or shorts or to be seen exercising. Childhood obesity may also be associated with overfeeding in infancy, introducing solid foods too early, poor parent-child relationships, feeding problems, and poor eating habits of the family as a whole.

Prevention rather than treatment

Emphasize that preventing childhood obesity is easier than treating it. Encourage parents to begin teaching about the importance of good nutrition and exercise when their child is age 5 or 6—an age when most children are eager to learn.

Instruct parents to monitor their child's weight. Children between ages 6 and 12 typically gain weight slowly and steadily—about ½ lb (0.23 kg) per month, or 6 to 7 lb (2.5 to 3 kg) per year. Growth spurts occur in preschoolers and adolescents.

Cutting back

If the child's' weight is significantly above normal, encourage her parents to try to modify her eating habits. Advise them to talk to her about her food habits and to discuss her feelings about food. They could mention that she'll look and feel better if she loses weight. Suggest that they try to help her resist peer pressure to eat junk foods. Explain that reducing serving size, refusing second helpings, and avoiding fattening snacks may be the key to losing weight and keeping it off. Suggest that they keep raw vegetables and fresh fruits handy for snacking.

Parents could also appoint their child the family food expert by teaching her about the five basic food groups and nutrition. This should help improve her self-esteem as well as her compliance with a weight-loss program. Tell her parents to give her choices, teach her how to recognize an average-size serving, and praise her when she selects healthy food and loses weight.

Advise the parents to involve their child in menu planning, grocery shopping, and meal preparation to help her feel more committed to losing weight.

Urge them to limit television watching and encourage exercise. Suggest activities that the family can do together, such as walking or playing ball. Emphasize that the best way to teach their child is to limit their own intake of high-calorie foods.

Finally, tell the parents never to use food as a threat ("No dessert for you!") or as a reward ("If you take out the garbage, we'll go for ice cream").

iors and social practices of their parents. A home environment where parents lead a sedentary lifestyle and practice poor nutrition will only rein-

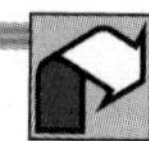

PREVENTION POINTER

Seven simple changes for healthy eating

These seven simple changes can make a great difference in eating healthier:

1. Choose water as the beverage of choice.
2. Eliminate drinks that are high in sugar.
3. Eat all meals at the kitchen or dining room table.
4. Don't eat while driving in the car, watching television, or reading.
5. Minimize unnecessary snacking by preparing snacks ahead of time and making sure they're of the healthy variety.
6. Increase the amount of fruits and vegetables consumed in the diet.
7. Pack children's lunches, rather than allowing them to purchase meals and snacks at school.

force these same behaviors in their children. Health care providers need to make parents aware of their own unhealthy lifestyle choices so that changes can be implemented. When parents adopt healthier patterns of nutrition and exercise, they can be good role models for their children.

Nutritional information should involve helping adolescents select healthy foods at home and school that appeal to their taste. Health care providers should stress the importance of balanced nutritional intake that will provide the needed components to ensure adequate growth and development. Teenagers need to eat a variety of foods that will meet their recommended daily requirements for such important nutrients as calcium, vitamin D, iron, and folate. Foods that are high in fat, sugar, and salt should be eaten in limited quantities. (See *Seven simple changes for healthy eating.*)

Health care providers should discuss the role that a sedentary lifestyle plays in the development of obesity. Time spent watching television, using the computer, and playing video games should be replaced with leisure activities that involve physical activity. Running, walking, and bicycling are just a few activities that families can enjoy together as a means of increasing daily physical activity.

Weight loss

In girls, peak weight commonly occurs before peak height. Many adolescents and their parents become concerned about weight and try weight loss programs. Attempts to lose weight loss during adolescence may affect the girl's adult height. Developing a healthy regimen of physical activity is more helpful during adolescence than dieting.

Most people can lose weight safely. Losing weight takes a commitment on the part of the person to change behavioral patterns that influence nutrition and exercise. Only 5% of U.S. residents who lose weight will keep it off

Finding the right weight-loss program

Health care providers should encourage those interested in joining a weight-loss program to ask these questions:
- Are there any health risks associated with the diet program?
- What data are available that can demonstrate that the program actually works?
- Do customers keep the weight off that's lost through participation in the program, or do they regain the weight when they leave the program?
- What are the costs?
- What are the qualifications of the personnel who work at the weight-loss center?
- How time-consuming is the regimen?
- How time-consuming is food preparation?
- Do many customers find the program too difficult to follow?

in the long-term. One of the reasons for relapse is that many people who want to lose weight look for a quick and easy solution to weight loss.

Americans spend 30 billion dollars every year on pills, potions, gadgets, and programs that promise a slimmer and happier future for the overweight and obese. Individuals who want to lose weight need to know three important facts:
- Products or programs that claim effortless weight loss aren't truthful. The only way that people can lose weight is to reduce the number of calories they eat or increase the number of calories that they burn off.
- Very low calorie diets (below 1,200 calories/day) are risky and can lead to serious health consequences (such as gallstones).
- Most diet experts recommend a slow, gradual weight loss. To lose 1 lb/week would require a reduction in 500 calories per day because 1 lb of body fat is equal to 3,500 calories.

Several thousand diet centers are operating across the country. LA Weight Loss, Jenny Craig, and Weight Watchers are three of the most popular diet programs in the United States. If a patient is interested in participating in a program offered by one of these commercial diet centers, health care providers should encourage her to perform research regarding the program and ask other people who have tried the program what they thought of it. (See *Finding the right weight-loss program.*)

Provider's role

Warn patients to be wary of programs that use words like "easy," "effortless," "guaranteed," "miraculous," "magical," or "breakthrough." Only those individuals who make modest changes and avoid quick-fix schemes will achieve long-term success. Successful long-term weight management requires practicing good nutrition, understanding what triggers unhealthy eating, engaging in healthy exercise, and seeking support from family, friends, self-help groups and, possibly, trained weight-loss counselors. Discourage teens from joining fad diets, such as the Atkins and South Beach diet (which stress no or low carbohydrates) as well as the Zone and Pritikin diets, among others. Because teens' bodies are still developing, they need to maintain adequate intake of all basic food groups. Although fad diets may be effective for some, long-term studies can't support their safety or effectiveness. In addition, those who use fad diets commonly regain the weight they lost — and sometimes gain even more weight. By subjecting the body to "yo-yo" diets, these teens risk undermining the full potential of their bodies' development and affecting their metabolism.

Body image and disability

SPECIAL NEEDS

Not only does the disabled teen have to cope with the normal physical changes associated with puberty, but she must also confront an increased sense of difference from her peers. In addition, the adolescent who has a physical disability must also accept that she may be less able to compete with peers regarding physical appearance and skills.

Provider's role

SPECIAL NEEDS

Recommendations for the health care provider that will help the disabled adolescent girl deal with body image issues include:

- Encourage socialization with peers, including those with and without special needs.
- Emphasize ways in which the disabled teen can improve her appearance.
- Point out positive aspects related to the teen's appearance.
- Reinforce positive coping behaviors.
- Encourage exercise and physical activity to control weight gain and enhance self-esteem.

Self-destructive behaviors

Risk taking and self-destructive behaviors seem to be almost a right of passage through the adolescent period. The self-centered nature of the adolescent — especially the mid-adolescent — leads to decisions based on what "feels good." Consequences of such behaviors often aren't fully understood or considered. With more freedom to make her own decisions and simultaneously explore a variety of new behaviors, the adolescent female may choose to participate in activities that increase her risk of injury or illness. Smoking, use of illicit drugs and alcohol, and exploration with sexual encounters are some of the high-risk activities to which adolescents may be exposed. Driving under the influence or with someone who's under the influence and failure to use a seatbelt or wear safety gear (such as a helmet when biking) are other behaviors that can lead to serious and, sometimes, fatal injury. One study measured self-reported health risk behaviors, including smoking, drinking, failure to use seatbelts, bullying, excess time with friends, alienation at school and from parents, truancy, and an unusually poor diet. They found that the risk of reported injury increased in direct association with increasing frequency of reported high-risk behaviors. Therefore it's extremely important for the health care provider to be aware of these behaviors when assessing the adolescent female and counsel against such activities.

Provider's role

When caring for the adolescent patient, it's important to establish a trusting relationship before asking about high-risk behaviors, which the teen may consider "prying." Beginning with questions about access to drugs, alcohol, and cigarettes in her school and then moving on to questions about activities her friends may participate in, may smooth the way to discussion about the adolescent's participation in high-risk behaviors. The health care provider should ask specific questions regarding these behaviors as the adolescent may not attribute the same risk to a certain activity as adults do.

Cigarette smoking

Recent data has shown a decrease in cigarette smoking among 8th, 10th, and 12th graders, with the peak of smoking among these grade levels occurring in 1996 and 1997. Even with this reduction, the University of Michigan Monitoring the Future study in 2001 reported 12% of 8th graders, 21% of 10th graders, and 30% of 12th graders stated they had smoked during the 30 days prior to the survey. Although the trend is promising, recent research shows that smoking remains a high-risk behavior that many adolescents experiment with daily.

Researchers found that adolescent females who had tried to control their weight within the prior 12 months had increased odds of being smokers. In addition, working part-time was associated with cigarette use. Teens ages 13 to 16 working moderate (11 to 20 hours/week) or long (21 or more hours/week) hours were found to have an increased probability of being smokers. One study found that teens who experienced moderate to high levels of anxiety were two to three times more likely to smoke than their peers with lower levels of anxiety. Another study linked increased television viewing to increased likelihood of smoking initiation, while a third study found that some young women use smoking as a coping mechanism. Other studies found that, in adults, nicotine acts as a stimulant and reduces symptoms of attention deficit hyperactivity disorder (ADHD), that adults with ADHD were more likely to smoke and less likely to quit, and that adolescents with ADHD who reported symptoms of inattention were more likely to begin smoking and be current smokers than those who didn't suffer the symptom of inattention.

One researcher questions the efforts of targeting antismoking campaigns toward adolescents by suggesting that delaying smoking initiation doesn't necessarily result in decreased prevalence rates through adulthood. Although delaying smoking initiation doesn't guarantee avoidance as an adult, the adolescent may not have the capacity to make a rational decision regarding the long-term effects of smoking. Therefore, preventing teens from initiating smoking is acceptable.

Given the long-term risks surrounding smoking, it's important to understand and assess for the risk factors that may increase the likelihood of smoking. Prevention is much easier than quitting and health promotion strategies aimed at preventing the adolescent from starting a smoking habit are preferred. Assessment of a teen's risk for smoking initiation requires evaluation of risk factors for smoking as well as the adolescent's personal views regarding smoking.

Although girls are more likely to experiment with smoking than boys, researchers report that females respond better to cessation programs that incorporate social support. In a study of 1,081 students from four middle schools, Results showed that parents who were more involved in the adolescent's life had a strong impact on whether the teen would begin smoking. This was especially true with the young adolescent, who seemed more reluctant to experiment with smoking behaviors. Therefore, the health care provider should counsel the parents regarding the impact they can have on their daughter's behavior. It has also been noted that adolescents are more likely to smoke when one or both parents smoke.

Provider's role

The Office of the Surgeon General's tobacco cessation guidelines for the adolescent recommend that all adolescent patients and their parents be screened for tobacco use. (See *Surgeon General's tobacco cessation guidelines*, page 38.) The health care provider should also strongly counsel his patients regarding the importance of refraining from tobacco use. For the adolescent who smokes, counseling and behavioral interventions that are developmentally appropriate should be initiated. Health care providers may consider prescriptions for the adolescent to aid in smoking cessation when there's evidence of nicotine dependence and the adolescent expresses a desire to quit. It's also important for the health care provider to tell the patient about available community resources regarding smoking cessation and support for the adolescent who's attempting to quit.

The National Center for Chronic Disease Prevention and Health Promotion has a pamphlet *I Quit!* which is targeted toward the adolescent who wants to quite smoking. It gives recommendations regarding how to prepare to quit, what actually may occur during the first couple of days after quitting, and how the adolescent may handle the effects of withdrawal and the temptations that occur. It provides suggestions regarding alternative activities that may replace smoking when the urge to smoke occurs.

Surgeon General's Tobacco Cessation Guidelines

For those who wish to stop smoking, the U.S. Surgeon General provides guidelines in the form of a "You Can Quit Smoking 5-Day Countdown," which outlines steps to follow each of the 5 days, counting down to a scheduled "quit date."

5 days before quit date
- Think about your reasons for quitting.
- Tell your friends and family that you're planning to quit.
- Stop buying cigarettes.

4 days before quit date
- Pay attention to when and why you smoke.
- Think of other things to hold in your hand instead of a cigarette.
- Think of habits or routines to change.

3 days before quit date
- Think about what you'll do with the extra money when you stop buying cigarettes.
- Think of who to reach out to when you need help.

2 days before quit date
- Buy the nicotine patch or nicotine gum.
- Alternatively, see your doctor to get the nicotine inhaler, nasal spray, or the non-nicotine pill.

1 day before quit date
- Put away lighters and ashtrays.
- Throw away all cigarettes and matches.
- Clean your clothes to get rid of the smell of cigarette smoke.

Quit day
- Keep very busy.
- Remind family and friends that this is your quit day.
- Stay away from alcohol.
- Give yourself a treat or do something special.

First smoke-free day
- *Congratulations!!!* If you "slip" and smoke, don't give up. Set a new date to get back on track.
- Call a friend or "quit smoking" support group.*
- Eat healthy food and get exercise.

*To find out where to get help in your area, call The American Cancer Society: 1-800-ACS-2345 (toll-free).

Source: U.S. Department of Health and Human Services, Public Health Service.

Substance abuse

Experimentation with alcohol and illicit drugs is common in adolescence. In 1999, the Maternal and Child Health Bureau estimated that 1.4 million U.S. residents age 18 and younger were first-time users of marijuana. This figure shows a decline of 15% from 1998 but a considerable increase from 1990's figures. The same report estimated that 34,000 persons age 18 and younger smoked, sniffed, or snorted heroin for the first time in 1999. In 2001, 20.5% of females ages 12 to 17 reported using an illicit drug in the previous year, with marijuana and hashish as the most commonly used drugs. Teens also had the

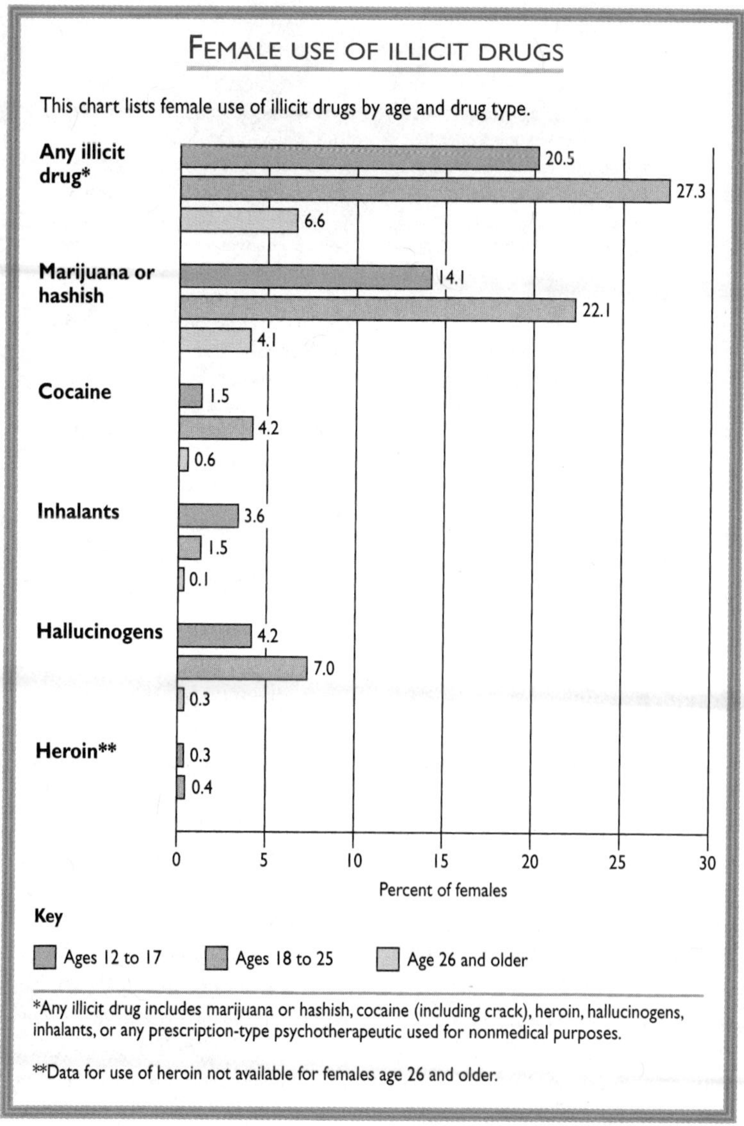

highest use of inhalants. (See *Female use of illicit drugs.*) In addition, 54% of adolescents reported that marijuana is easy to obtain, and approximately 16% reported being approached by someone selling drugs in the month prior to the survey. In 2001, approximately 10% of adolescents ages 12 to 17 participated in binge drinking and about 2% reported heavy alcohol use.

CRAFFT SCREENING

The CRAFFT screening method is designed specifically for adolescents. It draws on adult screening instruments, covers alcohol and other drugs, and discusses situations that are suited to adolescent experience. The list below outlines the *CRAFFT* method. Two or more positive responses indicate the need for further assessment.

1. **C**AR—Have you ever ridden in a *car* driven by someone (including yourself) who was high or had been using alcohol or drugs?
2. **R**elax—Do you ever use alcohol or drugs to *relax*, feel better about yourself, or fit in?
3. **A**lone—Do you ever use alcohol or drugs while you are *alone?*
4. **F**orget—Do you ever *forget* things you did while using alcohol or drugs?
5. **F**amily—Do your *family* or friends ever tell you that you should cut down on your drinking or drug use?
6. **T**rouble—Have you ever gotten into *trouble* while you were using alcohol or drugs?
7. Does your alcohol or drug use ever make you do something that you wouldn't normally do—like breaking rules, missing curfew, breaking the law or having sex with someone?

Adapted with permission from Knight, J.R., et al. "Validity of the CRAFFT substance abuse screening test among adolescent clinic patients," *Archives of Pediatrics & Adolescent Medicine* 156(6):607-14, 2002.

Provider's role

Because experimentation with drugs and alcohol is so common in adolescents, primary care providers should screen for alcohol and drug use during each office visit. As with tobacco, begin with questions about peer group use of drugs and alcohol and then transition to questions specifically directed at the behavior of the adolescent. There are several screening tools available, such as the CRAFFT screen, which was developed in a 2003 study and is specifically designed for the adolescent client. (See *CRAFFT screening.*)

The study also recommends positive reinforcement when the screen proves negative. This feedback praises the teen for her current behavior and may help her resist peer pressure in the future. If the adolescent screens positive for substance abuse, refer her to a detoxification clinic and for psychological counseling, where they may develop a plan or safety net for her when she finds herself in a situation where things are getting out of control. Also essential to the safety net is parental support and understanding. The parents must promise to pick up the teen when she calls, and defer discussing or lecturing about the behavior at that time. Teens commonly find themselves in situations they hadn't previously considered and helping them think about potential consequences and workable solutions can decrease additional risks.

Questions regarding certain behaviors may alert the health care provider to warning signs of potential substance abuse. The Focus Adolescent Services Web site identifies several warning sings of teen abuse, including:

- fatiguc
- red, glazed eyes
- persistent cough
- personality change
- sudden mood changes
- irritability
- irresponsible behavior
- low self-esteem
- poor judgment
- depression
- general lack of interest.

The teen may also withdraw from the family, begin breaking rules, start arguments, show a decreased interest in or negative attitude toward school, experience a drop in grades, have many absences, and become a discipline problem. New friends may appear who have less interest in home and school activities. These friends may also have problems with the law and reflect less conventional styles in dress and music. Although some of these behaviors may be attributed to the adolescent trying to develop her own sense of self-identity, substance abuse should be considered if the parent expresses concern regarding any of the above behaviors.

Another consideration for the health care provider when counseling female adolescents regarding drug use is to stress the importance of not sharing medications. One survey found that girls are more likely to share medications than boys. The survey reported that 20.1% of girls never borrow medication or share medication, 15.7% report borrowing prescription medications from others, and 14.5% report sharing their prescription medication with someone else. Sharing medication was acceptable when the individual had already been prescribed the same medication, had an emergency, or needed the medication but was unable to afford it. Girls will also share medication when the individual has a complaint similar to the one the prescription was written for. The hazards of sharing a prescription with someone else should be reviewed when prescribing a medication to the adolescent as well as reinforcing with the adolescent why she shouldn't accept medication from her friends.

Sexually transmitted diseases

Adolescent females become sexually active for many reasons:

- succumbing to peer pressure
- engaging in sexual experimentation
- needing to feel close to their partner
- establishing maturity
- seeking pleasure.

Even though contraceptive devices are readily available to adolescents, many teens fail to use them to avoid unplanned pregnancy and STDs. Adolescents are more likely to approach a health care professional regarding contraception if they feel that the encounter will remain confidential, that their privacy will be respected, and that the health care provider possesses a nonjudgmental attitude.

STDs are diseases that spread from one individual to another through sexual contact. In the United States, the most commonly diagnosed and treated STDs include gonorrhea, chlamydia, syphilis, genital herpes, human papilloma virus (HPV), and HIV. STDs are among the major causes of morbidity among adolescents and young adults, and more than 15 million new cases of STDs occur in the United States annually. The consequences of STDs are extremely serious for female adolescents. STDs can cause cervical cancer, infertility, damage to multiple organ systems, and even death. (See *STD diagnosis and management,* pages 44 to 47.)

Adolescents who are at highest risk for contracting an STD include those who:

- engage in sexual activity and fail to use a barrier method of contraception (latex condoms)
- engage in sexual activity with persons who have a documented history of STDs or I.V. drug use
- have a past medical history that includes STDs.

Several identifiable factors predispose teenagers to STDs. First, because of the histology of the female adolescent's cervical tissue (columnar epithelium cells), she's more susceptible to chlamydia and HPV than older women. Second, developmentally, teenagers don't equate current behavior with implications for future health status and, therefore, commonly don't protect themselves adequately against acquiring an STD. Third, adolescents lack sufficient knowledge regarding the commonly subtle signs and symptoms of STDs and don't recognize them when they occur. This puts them at risk for spreading the disease to future sexual partners.

Provider's role

Health care professionals must make every effort to prevent the acquisition and spread of STDs. (See *Sexual behavior interview,* page 48.) As part of routine care, the provider should ask the adolescent girl about sexual behavior and counsel her regarding sexual practices (partner selection, use of barrier methods of contraception, and abstinence) and STDs. All sexually active teens should be screened for gonorrhea and chlamydia. Health care professionals may also want to consider screening for syphilis and HIV with adolescents who are assessed to be at high risk for STDs. Education and screening efforts must be carried out by health care professionals who are sensitive to an adolescent's developmental needs in order to promote health and prevent the spread of disease.

Pregnancy

Each year, 1 million females under the age of 20 will become pregnant. Of this 1 million, 42% will give birth, 40% will choose elective abortion, 13% will miscarry, and 3% will place the baby for adoption. In 1999, teens between ages 15 and 19 had 49.6 births per 1,000 females in the United States. Of these young mothers, 19% were Black, 13% were Hispanic, and 8% were White. There are many factors involved in teenage pregnancy. Some possible explanations include:

- Teens engage in sexual activity at an earlier age than a decade ago.
- Few teens consistently use a reliable method of contraception.
- Teens possess an unrealistic expectation of motherhood.

Provider's role

The primary responsibility of the health care provider is to give information regarding the options available to the pregnant teen. The health care provider should encourage the teen not to make the decision alone. Her family as well as her partner should be involved in making a decision to continue or terminate the pregnancy. The American Academy of Pediatrics strongly supports parental participation in this decision.

The teen who decides to terminate the pregnancy should be referred to a clinic or private physician with experience caring for pregnant adolescents. In addition, follow-up counseling, which is an essential component of postabortion care, should be arranged. The teen who decides to continue the pregnancy should be referred to a competent health care provider who can provide sensitive and developmentally appropriate prenatal care.

Various physical risks are associated with teenage pregnancy. Many of these risks can be reduced with good prenatal care. Early, consistent prenatal care is essential for good outcomes for the mother and infant. Inadequate prenatal care places the adolescent at risk for:

- premature labor
- low birth weight infants
- increased neonatal mortality.

Several studies provide reasons why adolescents receive inadequate prenatal care:

- The teen doesn't realize that she's pregnant because her menstrual cycle can be extremely irregular.
- The teen is in denial about the pregnancy until late in the second or early in the third trimester.
- The teen doesn't understand the importance of prenatal care and, therefore, doesn't seek such care.

Abortion

Of the 1 million females age 20 and younger who become pregnant each year, 40% terminate their pregnancy through elective abortion. When performed by a skilled, experienced health care provider, abortion is a safe gynecologic procedure. Second trimester surgical abortions (mostly dilatation and evacuation procedures) are more complicated to perform than first trimester abortions and are associated with a greater risk for complications, especially hemorrhage. First trimester abortions (performed at 12 weeks or sooner, mainly by suction curettage) have complication rates of less than 1%. The complications associated with them include:

- endometriosis
- hemorrhage
- retained fetal material
- pulmonary embolism
- death.

(Text continues on page 46.)

STD DIAGNOSIS AND MANAGEMENT

This chart lists methods of diagnosis and management of various sexually transmitted diseases (STDs) along with their causative organisms and clinical manifestations.

STD	Causative organism	Clinical manifestations
Chlamydia	*Chlamydia trachomatis*	▪ Incubation period of 8 to 21 days ▪ Patient may be asymptomatic or infection may be one involving mucopurulent cervicitis, nongonococcal urethritis, or pelvic inflammatory disease (PID)
Genital herpes	Herpes simplex virus	▪ Prodromal symptoms, including intense burning or itching at the site of the outbreak ▪ First lesions appearing as painful, clear, raised vesicles ▪ Recurrent lesions becoming less painful and resolving more quickly than first lesions
Gonorrhea	*Neisseria gonorrhoeae*	▪ Symptoms possibly appearing as early as 1 day or as late as 2 weeks after sexual contact ▪ Patient may be asymptomatic or infection may be one involving mucopurulent cervicitis, urethritis, or PID
Human immunodeficiency virus (HIV)	Retrovirus	▪ Patient is commonly asymptomatic ▪ Common complaints of a flulike syndrome that include headache, malaise, myalgia, fever, and sore throat 2 to 6 weeks after viral exposure
Human papilloma virus (HPV)	Over 70 virus types identified	▪ Incubation period of 4 to 8 months ▪ Possible manifestation as genital warts (condyloma acuminata), cervical dysplasia (low-grade squamous intraepithelial lesion/high-grade squamous epithelial lesion), or cervical cancer ▪ Genital warts that appear as soft, moist, pink-red swellings on the vulva, anus, vagina, groin, or thighs

Diagnosis	Management
▪ Cell culture is the gold standard for diagnosing chlamydia. ▪ Staining techniques have low sensitivity and aren't useful in diagnosis. ▪ Rapid, inexpensive diagnostic tests are available, including leukocyte esterase test, ligase chain reaction (LCR) swab, and polymerase chain reactor (PCR) swab.	▪ Doxycycline ▪ Azithromycin ▪ Erythromycin ▪ Single-dose therapy is ideal ▪ Treat presumptively for gonococcal infection
▪ History and physical examination should indicate appropriate diagnostic testing. ▪ Diagnosis is confirmed with the Tzanck test (smear) of scrapings from lesions.	▪ Acyclovir ▪ Famciclovir ▪ Valacyclovir ▪ Medications don't cure genital herpes, they only shorten the duration of symptoms and prophylactically help to reduce the number of subsequent outbreaks
▪ Microscopic examination of gram-stained specimens or culture from sites of exposure is the most sensitive and specific method of diagnosing gonorrhea. ▪ LCR and PCR swabs are also useful for diagnosis.	▪ Cefixime ▪ Ceftriaxone ▪ Treat presumptively for chlamydial infection
▪ Testing can be done using various fluids (whole blood, serum, plasma, oral fluid, urine). ▪ Informed consent is required prior to initiating HIV testing. ▪ Enzyme immunoassay is used to detect the presence of antibodies to HIV-1. ▪ The Western blot assay confirms HIV infection.	▪ Treatment to prevent various complications associated with HIV illness trajectory ▪ No cure for HIV
▪ Viral deoxyribonucleic acid (DNA) or ribonucleic acid sampling detects HPV DNA in tissues and can show whether the infection is active or latent.	▪ External warts on females may be treated with a topical application of podophyllin or trichloroacetic acid ▪ Cryotherapy can effectively treat low-level dysplastic lesions of cervix

(continued)

STD DIAGNOSIS AND MANAGEMENT *(continued)*

STD	Causative organism	Clinical manifestations
Primary syphilis	*Treponema pallidum*	▪ Incubation period of 10 to 90 days with an average of 21 days after sexual contact ▪ Site of infection showing ulcer or chancre that's a hard, nontender lesion with sharply defined borders ▪ Possible erosion on the surface of the lesion ▪ Possible presence of a slight amount of yellow discharge

The administration of mifepristone (Mifeprex) followed by misoprostol (Cytotec) offers a nonsurgical therapeutic abortion method to females in the United States. This safe alternative to surgical abortions demonstrates a 95% effectiveness. A drawback to this approach is that it can only be used with females who are no more than 7 weeks pregnant.

Provider's role

Unless otherwise specified by state law, federal law mandates that minors have the right to obtain abortions without parental consent. When the diagnosis of pregnancy is confirmed, the health care provider must make the appropriate referral to a freestanding clinic or private physician with experience performing abortions on adolescents. The referral should be initiated as quickly as possible because pregnancy termination is safest when performed early in gestation.

Prior to the procedure, the adolescent should be educated about what she should expect during and after the procedure. This education is best accomplished with a combination of verbal and written instructions. Following the procedure, the health care provider should initiate a discussion about the subsequent use of contraception to avoid the potential for future unplanned pregnancies.

Contraception

Between 60% and 67% of adolescents report using some form of contraception to avoid unplanned pregnancy, yet the rate of unplanned pregnancies in the United States remains high. The contraceptive method chosen by the adolescent female must be safe, effective, and suited to her needs. The two methods used most commonly by ado-

Diagnosis	Management
▪ Darkfield microscopy is used to demonstrate actively moving *T. pallidum* in material from lesions or lymph nodes. ▪ Initial screening involves nontreponemal tests (rapid plasma reagin and Venereal Disease Research Laboratory). These tests measure antibody to nonspecific cardiolipin lecithin antigen. They are moderately specific for syphilis, but highly sensitive. The tests are easy to perform and also may be useful in monitoring the patient's response to therapy. ▪ Diagnosis of syphilis is confirmed using treponemal tests (micro-hemagglutination-*T. pallidum* and fluorescent treponemal antibody-absorption). These tests measure antibody specific to *T. pallidum* and are highly specific and sensitive.	▪ Penicillin G benzathine ▪ Doxycycline in patients allergic to penicillin

lescents are hormonal contraceptive pills and male condoms. Other protective barrier methods are also available and hormonal contraceptive options are vast. (See *Barrier methods for teens,* pages 50 and 51, and *Hormonal contraceptives for teens,* pages 52 and 53.)

Several contraceptive methods aren't recommended for teens, including:

- sterilization
- intrauterine device (IUD)
- fertility awareness methods (FAMs)
- withdrawal.

Because male and female sterilization must be considered permanent and irreversible, they shouldn't be recommended to anyone who may want to have a child in the future. Teenagers are too young to make this type of life-altering decision and shouldn't be presented with this option. Even though the IUD is an extremely effective means of contraception (97.4% to 99.2% of women reported effectiveness against pregnancy), this device isn't recommended for teens because the young female's uterus may be too small to adequately and safely contain an IUD. Also, IUDs can make women more susceptible to pelvic inflammatory disease that, in turn, can lead to infertility. FAMs only work well for a woman with regular menses who's in a relationship with a partner who wishes to cooperate with this contraceptive method. Adolescent girls commonly experience very irregular cycles and many aren't involved in the type of trusting, committed relationship necessary for success with this method. Teenagers shouldn't consider withdrawal an effective means of birth control because young men commonly lack the experience and self-control to withdraw their penis in time to avoid ejaculating into the vagina. The pre-ejaculatory fluid

Sexual behavior interview

Key points for an interview that focuses on sexual behavior include:

- Conduct the interview alone with the adolescent, without the parent or guardian present.
- Inform the adolescent about the positive role abstinence plays in preventing sexually transmitted diseases (STDs).
- Educate the sexually active adolescent about proper use of latex condoms as a means of preventing the transmission of STDs.
- Encourage the adolescent to find out her potential partner's sexual and drug-use history prior to engaging in sex with this person.
- Provide the adolescent with explicit information about the risk behaviors that can lead to the transmission of STDs.

that's released can contain viable sperm.

In addition to considering a method's effectiveness for preventing unplanned pregnancy, it's also extremely important to consider its ability to prevent the spread of STDs. Only abstinence and the male latex condom (used with a spermicidal foam or gel) provide protection against STDs. Therefore, teenagers who use other recommended methods to avoid unplanned pregnancy (diaphragm, the pill, the patch, Depo-Provera, or Norplant) should be counseled regarding concurrent use of a latex male condom and spermicide to protect themselves against STDs.

Adolescents offer varied reasons for their failure to use contraception. Common reasons given by adolescents included:

- perception that birth control devices or methods are dangerous
- fear that parents will discover that they're using birth control
- fear of the examination required to obtain birth control
- becoming sexually active unexpectedly
- objection to chosen method by partner.

Two other important factors that influence adolescent use of contraception are lack of information and anxiety. Most teenagers lack basic information regarding reproductive anatomy and physiology, contraception, and fertility. In addition, teenagers possess a great deal of anxiety related to contraception. Their anxiety stems from fear about being discovered by their parents and the many adverse effects associated with contraceptive methods.

According to Planned Parenthood, a common way that many teenagers avoid pregnancy is to engage in what's termed "outercourse." Outercourse, by definition, is sexual play without penetrative vaginal intercourse and can include oral and anal sex, mutual masturbation, erotic massage, and fantasy play. Teens find this method of birth control acceptable because of the sexual satisfaction that can be experienced without the threat of pregnancy.

However, this method also presents potential dangers because, even though outercourse can be a way to preserve "virginity," STDs can be transmitted if bodily fluids (semen or vaginal fluid) are exchanged between partners.

Provider's role

A health care provider who cares for adolescents should routinely counsel them in the prevention of unintended pregnancy and STDs. Counseling begins with a thorough assessment of the adolescent's sexual experiences and current use of contraceptives. It should be aimed at discussing the benefits as well as the disadvantages of all available methods and those recommended for teenage use. Having the partner present during the counseling can help the adolescent female make an informed choice as well as one that will be acceptable to her partner. Information should be presented using a matter-of-fact approach that addresses instructions on proper use, explains the percentage of failure (pregnancy rate) associated with the particular method, and dispels commonly held misconceptions. The health care provider should also stress that, to be effective, all methods of contraception must be used consistently. To ensure that the teenager continues to use the contraceptive method correctly and consistently, follow-up is usually necessary. Information should be provided to the adolescent both verbally and in the form of written instructions.

Postcoital contraceptive regimens are available for women who have experienced a single episode of unprotected intercourse in a given menstrual cycle. Emergency contraception, or the "morning after pill," works by preventing the implantation of the fertilized ovum into the uterus. All regimens must be taken within 72 hours of unprotected vaginal intercourse. Currently, two medications approved by the U.S. Food and Drug Administration, norgestrel/ethinyl estradiol (Ovral) and levonorgestrel/ethinyl estradiol (Preven), are available in the United States. Common adverse effects of these medications include nausea, vomiting, breast tenderness, and abdominal pain.

Planned Parenthood

Planned Parenthood Federation of America, Inc., founded by Margaret Sanger in 1916, is the world's largest voluntary reproductive health care organization. Planned Parenthood provides comprehensive reproductive health care services to women in 49 of the 50 United States and the District of Columbia through 855 health care centers. Locations for health care centers can be found by accessing the Planned Parenthood Web site (*www.plannedparenthood.org*) or by calling 1-800-230-PLAN.

Violence

Violence has become a critical health issue for adolescents in the United States. The Maternal and Child Health Bureau reports that, in the year 2000,

(Text continues on page 54.)

BARRIER METHODS FOR TEENS

This chart lists possible barrier methods to prevent pregnancy and spread of sexually transmitted diseases (STDs) along with their rate of effectiveness in pregnancy prevention, overall advantages and advantages specific to adolescent females, and disadvantages.

Contraceptive method	Effective pregnancy prevention	Overall advantages
Abstinence	100%	▪ Prevents pregnancy and STDs.
Male latex condom	86% to 98%	▪ Latex condoms offer very good protection against STDs. ▪ Condoms are inexpensive (about 50¢ each). ▪ Condoms are easily accessible in supermarkets and drug stores.
Diaphragm	80% to 94%	▪ A diaphragm can be inserted 4 to 6 hours prior to vaginal intercourse to avoid stopping sex to initiate use.
Female condom	79% to 95%	▪ Easily accessible in supermarkets and drugstores ▪ Female condoms are inexpensive (about $2.50 each) ▪ People who are allergic to latex can use female condoms.
Spermicide	72% to 94%	▪ Spermicide is easily accessible in supermarkets and drugstores. ▪ Spermicide is inexpensive (about $8 for a gel, foam, or suppository applicator kit and $4 for refills).

Advantages for the adolescent female	Disadvantages
Abstinence is a good way for teens to postpone taking the risks inherent in a sexual relationship.	▪ People find it difficult to abstain from sexual intercourse for long periods of time. ▪ Abstinence is commonly ended without a readily available alternative method of contraception.
The use of the latex condom is the best way to protect both males and females against contracting STDs.	▪ Partners may resist the use of latex condoms. ▪ Latex allergies can occur. ▪ Some may complain of loss of sensation and interference with spontaneity.
With the use of the diaphragm, teens who engage in occasional vaginal intercourse can avoid the adverse effects commonly associated with hormonal contraceptives.	▪ A diaphragm isn't effective against STDs. ▪ It requires a fitting by a health care professional, which may be considered inconvenient as well as expensive ($13 to $25 for the diaphragm plus $50 to $125 for the examination). ▪ Correct insertion requires the female to have an adequate comfort level with touching intimate parts of her body. ▪ Women who use diaphragms are at increased risk for urinary tract infection.
With the use of the female condom, teens who engage in occasional vaginal intercourse can avoid the adverse effects commonly associated with hormonal contraceptives.	▪ Female condoms may produce noise during intercourse. ▪ The lip may inadvertently slip into the vagina during intercourse. ▪ Women have difficulty inserting female condoms.
With the use of a spermicide, teens who engage in occasional vaginal intercourse can avoid the adverse effects commonly associated with hormonal contraceptives.	▪ Spermicide doesn't offer protection against STDs when used alone. ▪ Spermicide should be used in combination with a condom to increase the effectiveness of this method. ▪ Spermicide may be irritating to the vagina. ▪ Some consider spermicide to be messy to use.

Adapted with permission from Planned Parenthood Federation of America, Inc. (2001).

Hormonal contraceptives for teens

This chart lists hormonal contraceptives that can be used to prevent pregnancy along with their rate of effectiveness, overall advantages, advantages specific to adolescent females, and disadvantages.

Contraceptive method	Effective pregnancy prevention	Overall advantages
Oral contraceptive pill (combination and progestin-only)	95% to 99.9%	▪ Nothing to insert or apply prior to vaginal intercourse
Contraceptive patch (Ortho Evra Transdermal System)	95% to 99.9%	▪ No daily pill to remember ▪ Nothing to insert or apply prior to vaginal intercourse
Norplant (levonorgestrel)	99.95%	▪ Slow release of hormones into circulation for up to 5 years ▪ No daily pill to remember ▪ Nothing to insert or apply prior to vaginal intercourse
Depo-Provera (medroxyprogesterone acetate)	99.7%	▪ No daily pill to remember ▪ Nothing to insert or apply prior to vaginal intercourse

Advantages for the adolescent female	Disadvantages
▪ Reduces menstrual cramping and improves cycle regularity ▪ Allows continuous use without a placebo to avoid a monthly period ▪ Helps reduce occurrence of acne	▪ The pill must be taken daily. ▪ Serious health problems (such as myocardial infarction [MI], blood clots, and stroke) have been associated with the use of the pill, especially in women who smoke. ▪ The pill can cause such adverse effects as weight gain or loss, breast tenderness, mood swings, and nausea. ▪ The pill provides no protection against STDs. ▪ The pill requires a prescription, which may be considered inconvenient and expensive ($15 to $25 per month).
▪ No daily pill to remember ▪ Reduces menstrual cramping and improves cycle regularity ▪ Allows continuous use without a placebo to avoid monthly period ▪ Helps reduce occurrence of acne	▪ Serious health problems (such as MI, blood clots, and stroke) have been associated with the use of hormonal contraception, especially in women who smoke. ▪ The patch can cause such adverse effects as weight gain or loss, breast tenderness, mood swings, and nausea. ▪ The patch provides no protection against STDs. ▪ The patch requires a prescription, which may be considered inconvenient and expensive ($15 to $25). ▪ Some experience irritation at the application site.
▪ No daily pill to remember	▪ Norplant requires a surgical procedure for insertion and removal. ▪ Norplant can be expensive ($500 to $700 for the examination, implants, and insertion, plus $100 to $200 for removal). ▪ Norplant provides no protection against STDs. ▪ The implants are sometimes visible. ▪ Norplant can cause such adverse effects as irregular vaginal bleeding, headaches, depression, and weight gain or loss.
▪ No daily pill to remember ▪ May reduce menstrual cramps ▪ Most private form of contraception available	▪ Depo-Provera provides no protection against STDs. ▪ Common adverse effects include irregular periods, weight gain, headaches, depression, and abdominal discomfort. ▪ Depo-Provera requires an injection every 12 weeks. ▪ Depo-Provera can significantly decrease bone mass density in normal adolescents up to age 21.

Adapted with permission from Planned Parenthood Federation of America, Inc. (2001).

homicide was the second leading cause of death among persons ages 15 to 24. In addition, more adolescents are carrying weapons such as knives, clubs, and even guns to school in order to protect themselves from the threat of violence.

Rape

Adolescents have the highest rates of rape and other sexual assaults of any age-group, with female victims exceeding males by a ratio of 13.5:1 The female adolescent typically knows her assailant; an acquaintance or relative commits an estimated two-thirds to three-quarters of all adolescent sexual assaults. The younger adolescent is more commonly victimized by a member of her extended family, whereas older adolescents are more likely victimized during a social encounter. The American Academy of Pediatrics reports that adolescents are more likely to have used alcohol or drugs before being raped. They're also more likely to delay seeking medical attention and less likely to press charges than their adult counterparts.

Date rape is a term applied to situations where the assailant and the victim know each other. The drug flunitrazepam (Rohypnol), also know as *the date rape drug*, is a benzodiazepine sedative-hypnotic. It can be added to a drink without detection by the victim, increasing the risk of successful sexual assault. The effects of the drug begin after 30 minutes, peak within 2 hours, and may last for as long as 8 to 12 hours. It produces somnolence, decreased anxiety, muscular relaxation, and profound sedation as well as an amnesic effect.

Provider's role

The victim of a rape or sexual assault must be managed by a health care provider trained in the forensic procedures required for proper documentation and collection of evidence. Referral to an emergency department or rape crisis center with access to these trained individuals is recommended. A pregnancy test is done immediately to rule out pregnancy prior to the assault. Pregnancy prevention and postcoital contraception should be addressed with every adolescent female rape and sexual assault victim.

The effects of a rape are both physical and psychological. Post-traumatic stress disorder occurs in up to 80% of rape victims. For the adolescent patient, attention should be given to the psychological impact of the experience and appropriate contacts with community services should be pursued. Reactions to rape include disbelief, anxiety, fear, emotional lability, and guilt. These reactions lead to feelings of self-blame and diminished self-concept, alcohol abuse, a younger age of first voluntary sexual activity, poor use of contraception, STDs, and a greater number of abortions and pregnancies. The adolescent female may feel that her actions contributed to the act of rape and have confusion as to whether the incident was forced or consensual.

Recent research has found that physical and sexual violence were associated with high-risk behaviors

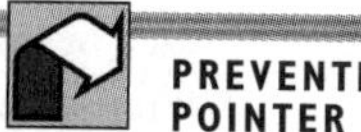

PREVENTION POINTER

Rape prevention recommendations

The American Academy of Pediatrics (AAP) provides the following recommendations for preventing rape. According to the AAP, pediatricians should:

- be knowledgeable about the epidemiology of sexual assault in adolescence
- be knowledgeable about the current reporting requirements for sexual assault in their communities
- be knowledgeable about sexual assault and rape evaluation services available in their communities and when to refer adolescents for a forensic examination
- screen adolescents for a history of sexual assault and potential sequelae
- be prepared to offer psychological support or a counseling referral and should be aware of the services in the community that provide management, examination, and counseling for the adolescent patient who has been sexually assaulted
- provide preventive counseling to their adolescent patients regarding avoidance of high-risk situations that could lead to sexual assault.

Adapted with permission from American Academy of Pediatrics. "Care of the Adolescent Sexual Assault Victim," *Pediatrics* 107(6):1476-79, June 2001.

such as smoking, diet and laxative use, binge drinking, cocaine use, early sexual intercourse (before age 15), pregnancy, and suicidal ideation. Although they didn't determine whether these behaviors precipitated the violence or resulted from the violence, screening for interpersonal violence and sexual victimization is important and should be part of a routine history. (See *Rape prevention recommendations.*) Further research notes that girls who experience early sexual maturation may not have the ability to protect themselves from victimizing forces. Preventive counseling for the adolescent regarding the avoidance of high-risk situations that may lead to sexual assault must be reviewed, strategies to prevent rape should be discussed, and appropriate educational materials should be distributed.

Domestic violence

Research has revealed that girls who are exposed to domestic violence are more likely to participate in violent acts themselves. Exposure to violence appears to be a much stronger predictor of violent behavior in girls than in boys. Being a victim of violence appears to be the single most important factor in predicting violence in girls. She suggests that violence in girls is influenced by social context and environmental variables that impact their perception of their ability to make sound behavioral choices. The violent behavior is commonly used by the adolescent girl to protect herself from further violence or abuse.

Research also found that family support (parent communication), school connectedness, and physical and emotional well-being were buffers against the negative effects that instigate violent behavior in girls. Family and school bonds seem to have a strong influence on the competence of girls. In addition, having older friends increases the adolescent's tendency toward violence.

Provider's role

Screening for domestic violence or abuse in the home is essential for accurate assessment of the adolescent female patient. To reduce the incidence of violence in girls, the health care provider should pursue efforts directed toward building competence, strengthening decision-making skills, and developing supportive relationships that encourage responsible decision-making.

Every state has a standard for reporting child abuse; however, they differ from state to state. It's the responsibility of the health care provider to know and follow the standard set in her state. The health care provider should be aware of the standard for reporting, what conditions constitute abuse in her state, to whom the report is made, and how the report must be made. Standards of reporting range from knowledge or suspicion and reasonable cause to suspect belief, knowing, or having knowledge or reasonable suspicion. What to report might include child abuse or neglect; harm as a result of child abuse or neglect; injury; commercial sexual exploitation of a minor; incest; child prostitution; abuse, or nonaccidental physical neglect; child maltreatment; or conditions that will reasonably result in child maltreatment and abandonment.

The government agency to which the provider should report the abuse or neglect may also differ from state to state. Again, the health care provider must be aware of the procedures defined by her state and abide by them. Some states require that the report be verbal, others require a written report, and some may require both. Regardless, screening the adolescent for abuse or exposure to abuse should be considered at every visit and, when suspected, it must be reported.

Comprehensive health care services

Health care providers are encouraged to provide comprehensive services to adolescent patients annually. These services should incorporate risk factor screening and anticipatory guidance at all wellness visits. Primary health care services specific to the adolescent female should integrate assessment, counseling, and interventions that address:

- lifestyle
- risk-taking behaviors
- psychological health
- potential for abuse.

In addition, fostering communication and trust and possessing a full understanding of legal issues are essential for successful comprehensive care of the adolescent female.

Lifestyle

Lifestyle assessment and care should focus on exercise and activity patterns, nutritional intake, body measurement, and unhealthy weight control.

Exercise and activity patterns

Health care providers should become actively involved in promoting physical fitness in their adolescent patients. An assessment of activity patterns should include questions regarding the type, frequency, and duration of physical activity. The teen that engages in regular physical activity should be praised for her efforts. For the teen that doesn't exercise, the health care provider can encourage her to incorporate regular exercise that's fun, varied, and moderately intense. Exercises that are easily incorporated into a daily routine include walking, aerobic dancing, running, and bicycling. The health care provider must be aware that even children are at risk for cardiovascular disease and health promotion is the key to fighting against morbidity and mortality of heart disease. (See *Promoting cardiovascular health in children*, page 58.)

Nutritional intake

The health care provider should incorporate routine nutritional screening into the wellness visit. Questions that address nutrition include:

- What do you typically eat during the course of a day?
- Are you currently dieting to lose weight?
- Do you take any vitamin or mineral supplements (calcium and folic acid)?

Body measurement

All adolescents should have their weight and height measured annually. An electronic or balance beam scale is the most accurate way to measure weight. A stadiometer is the preferred method for measuring height. BMI (weight [kg]/height [m^2]) values from the 5th to the 95th percentile for age and gender are considered healthy. The health care provider should perform an in-depth dietary assessment if the teen's BMI is above the 95th percentile or has increased by 2 or more percentiles in the previous 12 months.

Unhealthy weight control

The health care provider should screen for such eating disorders as anorexia nervosa and bulimia nervosa. If an eating disorder is diagnosed, the health care provider should refer the teen for treatment and management. Key findings in the health history that should alert the health care provider to disordered eating include the adolescent who:

- maintains an extremely strict diet
- participates in excessive exercise
- uses laxatives, enemas, or diuretics
- induces deliberate vomiting
- develops a distorted body image
- engages in binge eating
- is amenorrheic.

Risk-taking behaviors

Assessment and care regarding risk-taking behaviors should focus on to-

PREVENTION POINTER

Promoting Cardiovascular Health in Children

This chart lists goals for promoting cardiovascular health in children along with recommendations for ways to achieve those goals.

Health promotion goals	Recommendations
Diet	
▪ Overall healthy eating pattern ▪ Appropriate body weight ▪ Desirable lipid profile ▪ Desirable blood pressure	▪ Assess diet at every visit. ▪ Match nutritional intake with energy needs for normal growth and development. ▪ Encourage appropriate changes to maintain a healthy weight and achieve weight loss when indicated. ▪ Advocate consumption of a variety of fruits, vegetables, whole grains, dairy products, fish, legumes, poultry, and lean meat. ▪ Fat intake is unrestricted prior to age 2. After age 2, emphasize importance of limiting foods high in saturated fats (< 10% of cal/day), cholesterol (< 300 mg/day), and trans-fatty acids. ▪ Encourage limiting salt intake to 2,400 mg/day (about 1 teaspoon). ▪ Emphasize importance of limiting sugar intake as much as possible.
Smoking	
▪ No new initiation of cigarette smoking ▪ No exposure to environmental tobacco smoke ▪ Complete cessation for those who smoke	▪ Question tobacco use by parents at every visit. ▪ Question tobacco use by children at every visit starting at age 10. ▪ Provide clear, strong, informed, and personalized counseling against initiation of smoking. ▪ Advise avoidance of second-hand smoke at home, with friends, at school, or at work.
Physical activity	
▪ Being physically active every day ▪ Reducing sedentary time (such as television watching, computer use, playing video games, and talking on the phone)	▪ Assess physical activity at every visit. ▪ Advise young people to participate in at least 60 minutes of moderate to vigorous physical activity every day. ▪ Suggest ways to make physical activity fun for children and adolescents. ▪ For adolescents, resistance training (10 to 15 repetitions at moderate intensity) can be combined with aerobic activity in an overall activity program. ▪ Encourage limitations on sedentary time—for example, limiting time watching television to no more than 2 hours per day.

bacco use, alcohol and drug use, and sexual activity.

Tobacco use

The health care provider should inquire about the adolescent's use of tobacco. A smoking assessment should include:

- length of time the patient has smoked cigarettes
- number of cigarettes smoked per day
- time of day that the first cigarette is smoked
- patient's interest in smoking cessation.

The health care provider should strongly advise the current smoker to stop as well as offer her assistance with an individualized smoking-cessation program that may include medication (such as nicotine replacement therapy and bupropion [Zyban]).

Alcohol and drug use

Alcohol and substance abuse can be explored through the use of the mnemonic CAGE:

- Cut down — Have you ever felt the need to *cut down* on your use of alcohol or drugs?
- Annoyed — Have you ever been *annoyed* by someone's criticism of your drug or alcohol use?
- Guilty — Do you ever feel *guilty* about your alcohol or drug use?
- Ever need a drink or drugs — Do you *ever need a drink or drugs* in the morning before going to school?

An answer of "yes" to two or more questions is considered a strong indication that alcohol or drug abuse exists. The health care provider should consider referral to community treatment services (peer counseling, support groups, in-patient treatment) if alcohol or substance abuse is diagnosed.

Sexual activity

The most important concept to remember regarding speaking to teens about sexual behaviors is *atmosphere.* Teens require a comfortable atmosphere where they can feel at ease discussing sex. Exploration of the patient's risk factors and needs should begin any discussion. All patients who are determined at risk for STDs and HIV should be offered the opportunity to be tested.

An open dialogue with the adolescent patient regarding responsible sexual behavior that will prevent STDs, HIV, and unplanned pregnancy should follow the assessment. Subjects on which the health care provider should provide explicit education include:

- abstinence
- consistent and proper use of latex condoms
- avoidance of sexual contact with high-risk individuals (I.V. drug users and persons with a history of multiple sex partners).

Psychological health

Assessment and care of an adolescent's psychological health should focus on depression and suicide risk and violent behavior.

Depression and suicide risk

All adolescents should be screened for signs and symptoms of depression. The health care provider should pay particular attention to the adolescent who:

- performs poorly in school
- uses alcohol or drugs
- has been physically or sexually abused
- has deteriorating relationships with family members and friends.

Referral for an in-depth psychiatric evaluation and subsequent treatment may be necessary. The adolescent female who suffers from depression may complain of:

- irritable mood
- diminished interest in previously pleasurable activities
- lack of energy
- feelings of worthlessness
- significant weight loss
- hypersomnia or insomnia.

All teens should be questioned about the presence of suicidal thoughts in a straightforward manner. The health care professional should ask those patients with suicidal thoughts about the extent and specificity of their plans. Suicidal ideation requires an immediate referral to a mental health care professional. Teens at risk for suicide include those who:

- have experienced recent loss of a close friend or family member
- are socially isolated
- have a personal or family history of depression or suicide
- lack coping skills
- have a chronic or terminal illness
- have a history of alcohol or drug abuse
- have been sexually or physically abused.

Violent behavior

Adolescent violence is widespread in the United States. Adolescent females aren't only the victims of violence, but they're the perpetrators as well. The health care provider should question the adolescent about her tendency to engage in fighting, carrying a weapon, and watching violent television shows or movies. The health care provider should carefully monitor the teen that demonstrates aggressiveness, anger, impulsivity, and acting-out behaviors such as fighting, lying, or destructiveness.

Potential for abuse

Assessment of the potential for abuse of an adolescent should focus on indications of sexual, physical, or emotional abuse. Female patients should be screened for these indications at every health care encounter. One approach that the health care provider can use for this assessment is to ask the teen the SAFE questions. (See *SAFE questions.*)

For additional areas for assessment of the adolescent female, see *Additional preventive services guidelines for adolescents*, page 62.

Communication

One of the most important aspects of providing health care services to the adolescent patient is fostering communication and trust. The adolescent

SAFE QUESTIONS

This list outlines questions the health care provider can ask an adolescent about abuse using the acronym *SAFE*. If any of these questions are answered affirmatively, the clinician should inquire further about how the mistreatment occurs, when it occurs, and who the perpetrator is. Also, remember that laws in all 50 states require health care professionals to report any suspected abuse involving minors.

Stress and safety

- What *stresses* do you have in your current relationships with family members and friends?
- Do you feel *safe* in your current relationships with family members and friends?
- Should I as your health care provider be concerned about your *safety* regarding your current relationships with family members and friends?

Afraid and abuse

- Are there situations in your current relationships with family members and friends where you feel *afraid*?
- Has anyone ever tried to physically, sexually, or emotionally *abuse* you?

Friends and family

- Are your *friends* or *family* members aware that you're being abused?
- If your *friends* or *family* members were aware that you were being abused would they try to help you?

Emergency plan

- Do you have a safe place to go in case of an *emergency* situation?
- Would you like to talk to someone who could assist you in developing an *emergency plan* in case your safety is ever jeopardized?

patient should come to trust the health care provider for maintaining patient confidentiality and acting in her best interest. Adolescents will be more receptive to care and open to discussing issues if they feel welcome and comfortable in the health care environment.

Parents

At some point during the health care encounter, parents and guardians should be asked to leave the room so that the health care provider can speak with the adolescent privately. Without a parent present, the adolescent is more likely to provide the health care provider with an accurate picture of such activities as sexuality; alcohol, drug, and tobacco use; and abuse.

Rebellious adolescent

An adolescent will usually respond in a positive way to a health care provider who demonstrates a genuine interest in them as a person. The rebellious adolescent will usually open up to the health care provider when the focus of the interview is on her rather than on any specific problem areas. Rapport is best established when the health care provider opens the interview with conversational topics that focus on nonthreatening

Additional preventive services guidelines for adolescents

These lists include guidelines for illness prevention in adolescents at various stages of assessment and care.

Physical examination

- Blood pressure measurement annually
- Scoliosis evaluation annually
- Examination of teeth for presence of dental caries, malocclusion, and gingivitis at each visit

Laboratory evaluation

- Cholesterol testing as needed on teens who have a positive family history of cardiovascular disease or hyperlipidemia
- Anemia testing as needed on girls who report heavy menses, weight loss, disordered eating, or extreme athleticism

Screening

- Vision and hearing testing at ages 12, 15, and 18 or more often depending on history
- Tuberculosis (TB) testing with purified protein derivative for adolescents considered at high risk (homeless, immigrant, incarcerated, positive for human immunodeficiency virus, or living with persons infected with TB)
- Pelvic examination with Papanicolaou smear annually for all girls who are sexually active or age 18 and older

Immunizations

- Verification of up-to-date immunizations at every clinical encounter

Anticipatory guidance

- Inquiring about presence of working smoke and carbon monoxide detectors at each visit
- Assessment of helmet use during bicycling or motorcycling at each visit
- Determining correct and consistent seat belt use at each visit

Social issues

- Assessment of school performance at each visit
- Discussions about career planning annually, starting at age 15
- Assessment of peer influences on behavior

subjects, such as friendships, hobbies, and school.

Occasionally, the rebellious adolescent may direct anger and hostility toward the health care provider. The health care provider should accept negative feelings without taking them personally and try not to overreact. Negative feelings should be expressed by the teen and validated by the health care provider.

To facilitate the interview process with a rebellious adolescent patient, the health care provider should avoid:

- expressing value judgments about behaviors because the teen to become defensive.
- interrupting the patient and allowing the teen to complete her thoughts.
- being paternalistic by never approaching the adolescent patient with an “I know best” attitude.
- asking “why” questions, which have a tendency to place the adolescent on the defensive.

Overly shy adolescent

The overly shy adolescent can present another type of challenge to the health care provider. Shy teens tend not to talk very much during interviews, and the silence can be awkward. The tendency of most health care providers is to want to break the silence with a comment or a question. Rather than interrupt the silence, the health care provider should try to evaluate why there may be silence. Is the subject matter sensitive and difficult to discuss? Is the patient ready to discuss such a topic? During periods of silence the health care provider should be alert to nonverbal cues or messages. In addition, the health care provider should be alert for signals that indicate that the teen is ready to talk. Some suggested guidelines for communicating with the shy adolescent include:

- spending extra time with the patient to allow rapport to be established
- praising the teen when she responds appropriately to questioning
- giving the teen your undivided attention
- being courteous
- listening closely to what's being said
- avoiding putting the teen on the spot by continuous questioning.

Legal issues

Legal issues are always a part of clinical practice. Some legal issues that relate specifically to adolescent patients include confidentiality and consent.

Confidentiality

The American Medical Association supports the policy that health care providers should offer care to adolescents that maintains the same standards of patient confidentiality that are afforded to adults. Health care providers should develop teen confidentiality policies that are setting-specific, adhere to the recent Health Information Patient Privacy Act guidelines, and meet the needs of their particular patient population. All policies should be clearly articulated to parents and patients at the beginning of each visit. The health care provider should delineate the situations in which confidentiality may be breached. These situations may include:

- if the health care provider learns of adolescent behaviors that may lead to the harm of self or others
- if the health care provider suspects that the adolescent is a victim of physical, emotional, or sexual abuse
- if the health care provider discovers that the adolescent has an infectious disease that must be reported as mandated by state health departments.

Consent

In certain circumstances, an adolescent younger than age 18 may consent for the diagnosis and treatment of a medical condition without the knowledge or approval of a parent or guardian. Laws vary from state to state and health care providers should be aware of the laws specific to the state where they practice. In most states, adolescents under the age of 18 may consent to medical care if they're:

- on active duty in the armed forces
- considered an emancipated minor
- pregnant
- legally married
- seeking care for an STD, substance abuse or dependence, or a mental health problem.

Selected references

American Academy of Pediatrics. "Care of the Adolescent Sexual Assault Victim," *Pediatrics* 107(6):1476-79, June 2001.

American Academy of Pediatrics Committee on Adolescence. "Counseling the Adolescent About Pregnancy Options," *Pediatrics* 83(1):135-37, January 1989.

Barkley Burnett, L. and Adler, J. "Domestic violence" *emedicine* 7/10/2001. *www.emedicine.com/emerg/topic153.htm* [accessed 12/18/03].

Breslin, F.C., and Adlaf, E.M. "Part-time Work and Cigarette use Among Teenagers," *Canadian Journal of Public Health* 93(5):356-61, September/ October 2002.

Centers for Disease Control and Prevention (1996a). "Youth Risk Behavior Surveillance — United States, 2001," *MMWR* 515(SS04), 8-9, June 2002.

Centers for Disease Control and Prevention (2002). *National immunization program. Vaccines for teenagers.* [On-line] *www.cdc.gov/nip/recs/teen-schedule.htm.*

Daniel, K. L., et al. "Sharing Prescription Medication Among Teenage Girls: Potential Danger to Unplanned/Undiagnosed Pregnancies," *Pediatrics* 111:1167-70, May 2003.

DiNapoli, P.P. "Guns and Dolls: An Exploration of Violent Behavior in Girls," *Advances in Nursing Science* 26:140-48, April-June 2003.

Elster, A., and Kuntz, N. (eds.) *AMA Guidelines for Adolescent Preventive Services (GAPS).* Baltimore: Williams & Wilkins, 1994.

Gaffney, K.F., et al. "Smoking Among Female College Students: A Time for Change," *Journal of Obstetric, Gynecologic, and Neonataal Nursing* 31(5):502-07, September-October 2002.

Gidwani, P. P., et al. "Television Viewing and Initiation of Smoking Among Youth," *Pediatrics* 110(3):505-08, September 2002.

Goodman, E., and Whitaker, R. "A Prospective Study of the Role of Depression in the Development and Persistence of Adolescent Obesity," *Pediatrics* 110(3): 497-504, September 2002.

Harrison, P., and Narayan, G. "Differences in Behavior, Psychological Factors, and Environmental Factors Associated with Participation in School Sports," *The Journal of School Health* 73(3):113-20, March 2003.

Higgins, J., et al. "Factors Influencing Physical Activity Levels Among Canadian Youth," *Canadian Journal of Public Health* 94(1):45-51, January/February 2003.

Hoelscher, D., et al. "Designing Effective Nutrition Interventions for Adolescents. *Journal of the American Dietetic Association. (Supplement: Adolescent Nutrition: A Springboard for Health)* S52-S63, March 2002.

Institute of Medicine, Food and Nutrition Board (2000). "Dietary Reference Intakes for Thiamin, Riboflavin, Niacin, Vitamin B_6, Folate, Vitamin B_{12}, Pantothenic acid, Biotin and Choline," *Report of the subcommittee on calcium and related nutrients* Washington, D.C.: National Academy Press [On-line] *www.nap.edu/catalog/6015.html.*

Institute of Medicine, Food and Nutrition Board (1997). "Dietary Reference Intakes for Calcium, Phosphorous, Magnesium, Vitamin D, and Fluoride. *Report of the subcommittee on calcium and related nutrients.* Washington, D.C.: National Academy Press [On-line] *www.nap.edu/catalog/5776.html.*

Mangels, R. (2001). "Vegetarian Nutrition for Teenagers," *The Vegetarian Resource*

Group [on-line] *www.vrg.org/nutrition/teennutrition.htm.*

Maternal and Child Health Bureau. (2002). *Child Health USA 2002: Health Status- Adolescent: Cigarette Smoking.* Retrieved July 3, 2003, from U.S. Department of Health and Human Services: Health Resources and Services Administration Web Site: *www.mchb.hrsa.gov/chusa02/main_pages/page_44.htm.*

Maternal and Child Health Bureau. (2002). *Child Health USA 2002: Health status–Adolescent: Substance Abuse.* Retrieved July 3, 2003, from U.S. Department of Health and Human Services Web Site: *www.mchb.hrsa.gov/chusa02/main_pages/page_45.htm.*

Monroe, K., and Hook, E. "Presentation and Management of Common Sexually Transmitted Diseases," *Emergency Medicine* 34(8):17, 2002.

Morantz, C., and Torrey, B. (2003). Surgeon General's report on women and smoking. *American Family Physician, 67,* 649.

Office of the Surgeon General. (n.d.). *Tobacco Cessation Guidelines: Children and Adolescents.* Retrieved July 6, 2003, from National Library of Medicine Web Site: *www.hstat.nlm.nih.gov.hq/Hquest/screen/TextBrowse/t/1057519354483/s/62202.*

National Academy of Sciences (2001). *Immunization and safety review: Measles-mumps-rubella vaccine and autism* [Online] *www.iom.edu/IOM/IOMHome.nsf/Pages/MMR+Autism+Summary.*

National Health and Medical Research Council (2002). *Dietary guidelines for children, and adolescents* [On-line] *www.nhmrc.gov.au/publications/synopses/n1syn.htm.*

National Research Council, Food and Nutrition Board. *Recommended Dietary Allowances,* 10th ed. Washington, D.C.: National Academy Press, 1989.

Perry, C., et al. "Adolescent Vegetarians: How Well do Their Dietary Patterns Meet the Healthy People 2010 Objectives?" *Archives of Pediatrics & Adolescent Medicine* 56(5):431, May 2002.

Pickett, W., et al. "Multiple Risk Behavior and Injury: An International Analysis of Young People," *Archives of Pediatrics & Adolescent Medicine* 156(8):786-93, August 2002.

Planned Parenthood Federation of America, Inc. (2001). "Birth Control Choices for Teens." [On-line] *www.plannedparenthood.org/bc/030205_bc4teens.htm.*

Public Health. "Teen Anxiety, Chances of Harmful Smoking and Eating Behavior Higher than Expected," *Medical Letter on the CDC & FDA* 6, October 2002.

Root, A.W. "Bone Strength and the Adolescent," *Adolescent Medicine* 13(1):53-72, February 2002.

Spear, B.A. "Adolescent Growth and Development," *Journal of the American Dietetic Association* 102(3 suppl):s23-s29, March 2002.

Story, M., et al. "Individual and Environmental Influences on Adolescent Eating Behaviors," *Journal of the American Dietetic Association (Supplement: Adolescent Nutrition: A Springboard for Health)* 102(3 suppl):S40-S51, March 2002.

Tercyak, K.P., et al. "Association of Attention Deficit/Hyperactivity Disorder with Levels of Cigarette Smoking in a Community Sample of Adolescents," *Journal of the American Academy of Child and Adolescent Psychiatry* 41(7):799-805, July 2002.

U.S. Food and Drug Administration (2000). "The Facts About Weight Loss Products and Programs," [On-line] www.*vm.cfsan.fda.gov/~dms/wgtloss.html.*

Winter, A. L., et al. "The Relationship Between Body Weight Perceptions, Weight Control Behaviours and Smoking Status Among Adolescents," *Canadian Journal of Public Health* 93(5):362-65, September-October 2002.

Yanoski, J., and Yanoski, S. "Treatment of Pediatric and Adolescent Obesity," *JAMA* 289(14):1851, April 2003.

CHAPTER 3

Health promotion and illness prevention in the adult female

Overview

Throughout her life, a woman may experience many uniquely female milestones, including menstruation, pregnancy, lactation, motherhood, and menopause. Her understanding of these experiences influences her identity, self-concept, self-worth, and the development of her value system.

Another influence on a woman's self-identity comes from the culture in which she lives. From birth, a female receives messages about what it means to be female in her particular culture. Unfortunately, these messages are commonly negative and restricting, resulting in a diminished sense of self-worth. Many cultures continue to further stereotypes of women as weaker, less intellectual, and centered on domestic matters, all of which place limitations on her complete development. These cultural norms also impact her ability to make good choices about her health.

This chapter discusses the major health issues a woman faces in her lifetime. Areas of interest include health promotion, illness prevention, reproductive issues, and recommended screening. These areas help to shape the female as a whole, yet all rely on her ability to remain healthy in this process.

Health promotion

Good health isn't just the absence of disease. Rather, it depends on a wide spectrum of lifestyle habits that enable the individual to feel better physically and mentally. These habits may also help increase longevity. It has been said, "Wellness isn't a destination but a process."

Morbidity and mortality

Causes of morbidity and mortality in women vary depending on age and race. For instance, young women (ages 15 to 24) are at greatest risk for death from accidents and violence. In contrast, heart disease is the leading cause of death in women ages 25 to 44. As much as 36% of all deaths in women (500,000 American women each year) are attributed to heart disease, and the incidence of its major causes rises continuously from middle age through old age. The incidence of cancer also increases with age. Significantly, lung cancer became the leading cause of cancer among white women in the late 1980s as women's smoking reached an all-time high. Smoking now contributes to 25% of all cancer deaths in women. The third-highest cause of death for women ages 15 to 44 is human immunodeficiency virus and acquired immunodeficiency syndrome (HIV/AIDS). (See *AIDS and the adult female*, page 68.)

In addition to the three leading causes of death in women, many chronic conditions, including hypertension, diabetes mellitus, arthritis, and osteoporosis, impact a woman's overall health and well-being as well as her quality of life. For example, osteoporosis is considered a leading cause of disability in women after age 45. However, measures taken by the time the woman reaches age 30 may prevent or delay onset of osteoporosis.

Exercise and fitness

The benefits of exercise have become increasingly clear as technological advances have made exercise an option, rather than a daily requirement for normal functioning. Exercise can dramatically reduce the risk of coronary artery disease, lower cholesterol levels and high blood pressure, aid in weight control, delay or prevent osteoporosis, and generally improve a person's sense of well-being.

Conversely, a lack of exercise, according to the American Heart Association, is a major risk factor for the development of cardiovascular disease. The relative risk of coronary heart disease associated with physical inactivity ranges from 2.5 to 2.4, an increase in risk comparable with that observed for high cholesterol, high blood pressure, and cigarette smoking. In fact, the Centers for Disease Control and Prevention (CDC) estimate that as many as 250,000 deaths per year are indirectly related to a lack of regular exercise. Americans are among the most sedentary people in the world. Only about one in four exercises enough to be considered physically active, and American women are less physically active than American men.

There are no age limitations on increasing physical activity. Moreover, staying physically active appears to

AIDS AND THE ADULT FEMALE

As of December 2001, a total of 141,048 cases of acquired immunodeficiency syndrome (AIDS) had been reported in adolescent and adult women in the United States. The following graph shows what the Centers for Disease Control and Prevention reported for adult female AIDS cases by age of diagnosis and race and ethnicity.

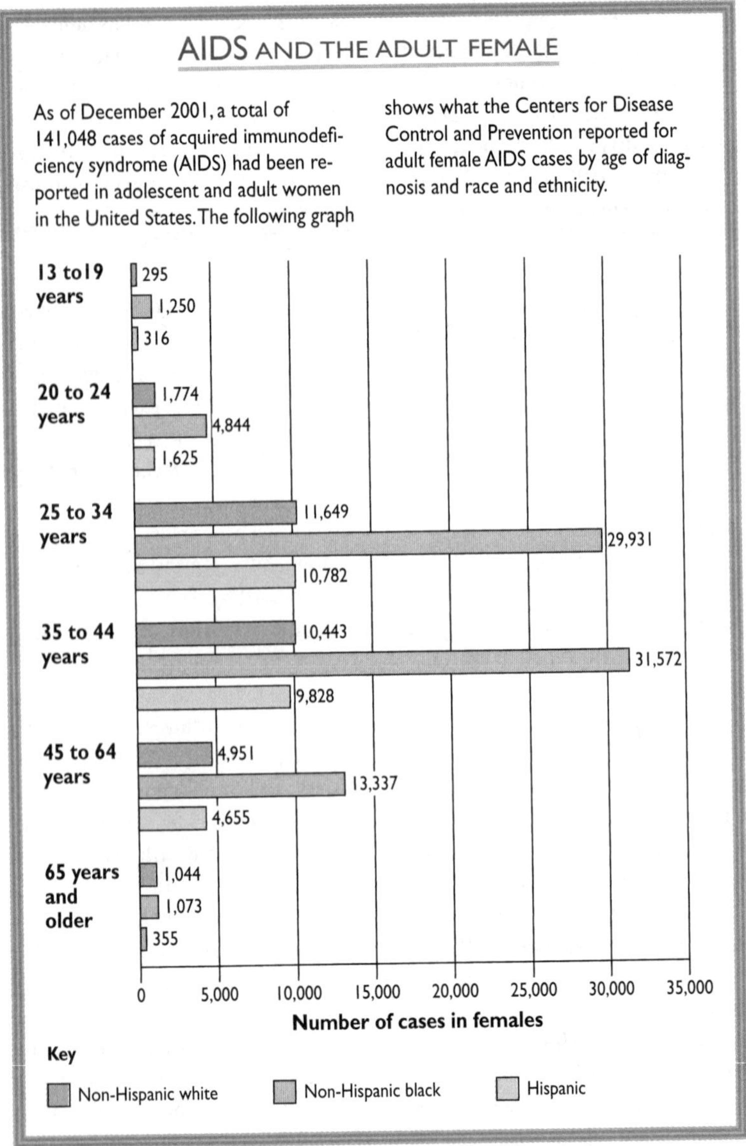

become more important as a person ages. Many of the problems commonly associated with aging — increased body fat, decreased muscle strength and flexibility, loss of bone mass, and lower metabolism — can be minimized or even prevented by exercise.

A well-rounded exercise program that includes both aerobic exercise and strength training is recommended

PREVENTION POINTER

Physical activities for adult women

It's important to teach your female patients to exercise for at least 30 minutes most days of the week, preferably daily, or to participate in any one, or combination, of the activities listed below. Encourage her to look for additional opportunities among other activities that she enjoys.

Routine activities

- Walk up stairs instead of taking an elevator
- Get off the bus a few stops early and walk or jog the remaining distance
- Mow the lawn with a push mower
- Rake leaves
- Garden
- Push a stroller
- Clean the house
- Do exercises or pedal a stationary bike while watching television
- Take a brisk 10-minute walk or jog in the morning, at lunch, and after dinner

Recreational routine activities

- Walk, roller blade, or jog
- Bicycle or use an arm pedal bicycle
- Swim or do water aerobics
- Golf (pull cart or carry clubs)
- Canoe
- Cross-country ski
- Play basketball
- Dance
- Take part in an exercise program at work, home, or school, or at a gym

by the American College of Sports Medicine. Stretching to maintain flexibility is also important for preventing injuries to muscles, tendons, and ligaments. Variety is the key to a workable fitness program. Anything from fitness walking to swimming to ballroom dancing can help a person become and stay physically fit. (See *Physical activities for adult women.*)

In addition to variety in exercise, frequency is also important. The American Heart Association recommends exercising aerobically for at least 30 minutes on most days to improve heart and lung health. This exercise could include brisk walking, running, swimming, bicycling, roller skating, or jumping rope. Even low- to moderate-intensity activities, when done for 30 minutes per day, can bring benefits. These activities include pleasure walking, climbing stairs, gardening, yard work, moderate to heavy housework, dancing, and home exercise, such as walking on a treadmill or lifting weights. Of course, many people may not be able to do 30 minutes of exercise at first, but it's a goal to strive for in order to improve cardiovascular fitness. In addition, exercising at a level of intensity called your target heart rate helps a person more readily achieve fitness. (See *Healthy heart rate target zones by age*, page 70.)

When developing a fitness program, it's also important to include muscle-strengthening exercises. Well-conditioned muscles and joints help

Healthy heart rate target zones by age

Age	Target heart rate zone
20 years	100 to 150 beats/minute
25 years	98 to 146 beats/minute
30 years	95 to 142 beats/minute
35 years	93 to 138 beats/minute
40 years	90 to 135 beats/minute
45 years	88 to 127 beats/minute
50 years	85 to 127 beats/minute
55 years	83 to 123 beats/minute
60 years	80 to 120 beats/minute
65 years	78 to 116 beats/minute
70 years	75 to 113 beats/minute

an individual perform better physically, maintain good posture and, possibly, prevent injuries and chronic lower back pain. It's best to start a weight-training program with an exercise specialist, who can demonstrate proper positioning and lifting techniques to prevent strain or injury, explain which weights or machines to use, and recommend the number of sets and repetitions.

Exercise and pregnancy

In general, it isn't necessary for pregnant women to limit exercise. It's recommended, however, that a woman not become excessively fatigued or participate in activities where she may risk injury to herself or her fetus. In addition, such exercises as abdominal "crunches" from the supine position should be avoided. After the first trimester, undue pressure from the uterus on the vena cava can cause reduced cardiac output and lead to orthostatic hypotension. Women should also be aware that, as pregnancy progresses, their sense of balance will change and that some activities should be modified or discontinued until after delivery. In addition, studies have shown that exercise doesn't increase the incidence of spontaneous abortions. Moreover, well-conditioned women who perform aerobics or run regularly were found to have shorter active labors, fewer cesarean deliveries, and less fetal distress in labor. Several studies, however, did show that continuation of severe exercise regimens resulted in reduced birth weight (average 310 g). Another study observed that continuing regular exercise throughout pregnancy had a positive effect on early neonatal behavior. The American College of Obstetricians and Gynecologists states that women who are accustomed to aerobic exercise before pregnancy can continue to exercise during pregnancy; however, they caution against starting new aerobic exercise programs during this time. With some pregnancy complications, such as hypertensive disorders, exercise is commonly discouraged. Women with multiple fetuses or women suspected of having a growth-restricted fetus may also be advised to live a more sedentary lifestyle during pregnancy.

Nutrition

Eating is one of life's greatest pleasures; however, what a person eats directly impacts her health. A healthy diet will help prevent many chronic diseases, including heart disease, hypertension, stroke, certain types of cancer, and type 2 diabetes mellitus. The U.S. Department of Agriculture's Food Guide Pyramid provides the recommended daily servings from the basic food groups to constitute a nutritious daily food plan. Each food group in the pyramid provides some, but not all, of the nutrients a female needs. (See *The Food Guide Pyramid and RDA*, page 72.) In addition, the U.S. Department of Health and Human Services and the Department of Agriculture publish guidelines for good dietary habits to promote health. (See *Dietary guidelines for Americans*, pages 73 and 74.)

Nutrition and pregnancy

Good nutrition before and during pregnancy is a proven way to decrease the risks of significant fetal and infant health problems, such as premature birth, low birth weight, and malformations. Women who are underweight or who gain little weight during pregnancy are more likely to have low–birth weight babies, while women who are obese or who gain excessive weight during their pregnancy are at risk for pregnancy-induced hypertension and diabetes. Since 1990, the Institute of Medicine has recommended a weight gain of 25 to 35 lb (11.5 to 16 kg) for women with normal prepregnancy body mass index.

Many of the dietary recommendations for pregnant women are similar to those for nonpregnant women, with the exception of the number of calories and amount of folic acid. The National Research Council recommends a daily caloric increase of 300 kcal throughout pregnancy (2,500 calories versus 2,200 calories). Calories are necessary for energy production, and whenever caloric intake is inadequate, protein is metabolized for energy rather than utilized for its vital role in fetal growth and development. It's also recommended to increase the intake of folic acid from 180 mcg to 400 mcg daily. It's estimated that over 50% of the approxi-

(Text continues on page 74.)

The Food Guide Pyramid and RDA

Vitamin A

- Recommended daily allowance (RDA): 800 mcg retinol equivalents
- Night vision
- Growth and tissue healing

Vegetarian source:
Beta-carotene in yellow, orange, and dark green leafy vegetables is converted to vitamin A during the day.

Animal sources:
Cheese, eggs, chicken, liver

Vitamin B_{12}

- RDA: 2.4 mcg
- DNA metabolism
- Red blood cell (RBC) formation
- Central nervous system maintenance

Vegetarian sources:
Fortified cereals, fermented miso

Animal sources:
Milk, eggs, yogurt, fish, crab, oysters, liver, kidney, muscle meats

Vitamin D

- RDA: 5 mcg/day
- Maintenance of bones and teeth

Vegetarian source:
Sunlight (30 minutes per week; mild exposure)

Animal sources:
Fortified milk, fish-liver oil, egg yolks, butter, liver

Calcium

- RDA: 1,000 mg
- Maintenance of bones and teeth

Vegetarian sources:
Broccoli, kale, collard greens, mustard greens, spinach

Animal sources:
Milk, yogurt, cheese, ice cream, sardines, salmon

Iron

- RDA: 15 mg
- Formation of hemoglobin, which RBCs use to carry oxygen to all cells in the body

Vegetarian sources:
Dried beans, nuts, spinach, whole grains, strawberries

Animal sources:
Beef, liver, chicken, tuna, shrimp

Zinc

- RDA: 12 mg
- Protein synthesis, DNA replication
- Many enzyme reactions

Vegetarian sources:
Legumes, seeds, nuts

Animal sources:
Meat, poultry, oysters, eggs, milk products

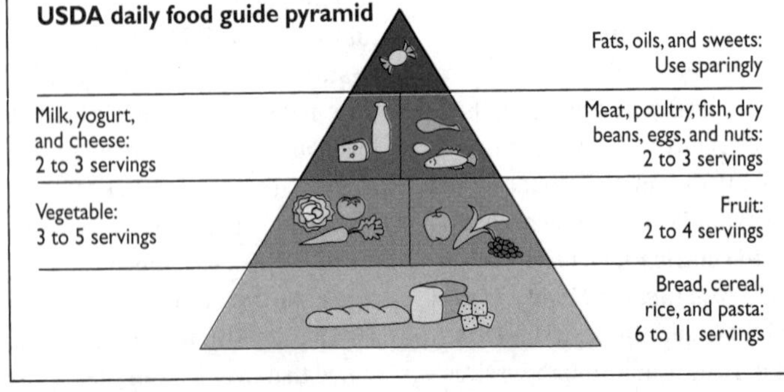

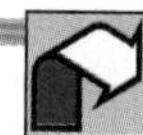

PREVENTION POINTER

Dietary guidelines for Americans

Aim for fitness

- Healthy weight
- Sensible portion sizes
- Physical activity each day

Build a healthy base

- Start with choosing foods from the Food Guide Pyramid.
  - Different foods contain different nutrients. No single food can supply all the nutrients in the amounts you need. Note that the daily recommendations differ depending on age, gender, and level of activity.
  - Increase your calcium intake. Be sure to consume at least 1,000 mg of elemental calcium daily either from food sources high in calcium or from supplements. This amount is required to continue building bone mass that peaks by age 35 and to maintain bone mass through the premenopausal years. It's important to check labels because calcium amounts vary according to their forms. For example, calcium phosphate contains 40% elemental calcium, while calcium gluconate contains 90% elemental calcium.
- Choose a variety of grains daily, especially whole grains.
  - Foods made from grain help form the foundation of a nutritious diet and may help protect against many chronic diseases. Whole grains are also high in fiber and promote normal bowel function. Many whole-grain products are also enriched with folic acid, a B vitamin that reduces the risk of neural tube defects in the fetus when consumed before and during early pregnancy.
- Choose a variety of fruits and vegetables daily.
  - Fruits and vegetables provide essential vitamins, minerals, and fiber and are naturally low in fat and calories.
- Keep food safe to eat.
  - Safe means that the food poses little risk of food-borne illness. Pregnant women as well as young children, older persons, and those with chronic diseases or immune deficiency are at highest risk for food-borne illnesses.

Choose sensibly

- Choose a diet that's low in saturated fat and cholesterol and moderate in total fat.
  - Some fat is needed in the diet to help provide energy, to assist in the absorption of the fat-soluble vitamins (A, D, E, and K), and to provide a necessary ingredient for the production of certain hormones (such as estrogen and testosterone). It's important to choose fat-sensible foods. Some fats, especially saturated fats and trans fats, increase the risk of coronary heart disease by raising serum cholesterol. In contrast, unsaturated fats (found mainly in vegetable oils, most nuts, olives, and avocados) don't increase cholesterol level. Aim for a total fat intake of no more than 30% of total daily calories.
- Choose beverages and foods to moderate your intake of sugars.
  - Foods that are high in sugars but low in essential nutrients primarily contribute calories to the diet. Foods containing sugars and starches can promote tooth decay.
- Choose and prepare foods with less salt.

(continued)

Dietary guidelines for Americans *(continued)*

– Sodium plays an essential role in regulating the body's fluid and electrolyte balance and blood pressure. Many studies in diverse populations have shown that a high sodium intake is associated with higher blood pressure. Most adults consume way too much salt. The body needs only a small amount of salt to meet sodium needs—less than ¼ tsp daily. Choosing primarily fresh foods and then adding only small amounts of salt during food preparation is one way to limit daily salt intake.

- If you drink alcoholic beverages, do so in moderation.

  – Alcoholic beverages supply calories but few nutrients. Alcohol intake is associated with high blood pressure, stroke, violence, suicide, increased risk of motor vehicle crashes, and certain types of cancer. Even one drink per day can slightly raise the risk of breast cancer. Alcohol consumption during pregnancy raises the risk of birth defects, especially fetal alcohol syndrome—the leading cause of congenital mental handicaps. Excessive intake can lead to altered judgment, dependency, cirrhosis of the liver, pancreatitis, and cellular damage to the brain and heart. Moderation is defined as no more than one drink per day for women and no more than two drinks per day for men. This limit is based on differences between the sexes in both weight and metabolism

mately 4,000 pregnancies affected by neural-tube defects each year could be prevented by adequate intake of folic acid throughout the periconceptional period. In addition, small increases of other vitamins and minerals are required during pregnancy. Vitamin and mineral supplementation generally meets these additional needs.

SPECIAL NEEDS

Vegetarianism can be a healthy nutritional option. In fact, in its dietary recommendations for cancer prevention, the American Cancer Society states that one should "eat a variety of health foods, with an emphasis on plant sources." Even so, a vegetarian diet must be well-balanced, including eating a variety of foods, such as grains, fruits and vegetables, beans, nuts and seeds, and a small amount of fat with or without dairy products. Vegans, who eat no dairy or eggs, should pay special attention to their calcium, vitamin B_{12}, and vitamin D intake by eating fortified foods or taking vitamin and mineral supplements. Of course, exposure to direct sunlight is a major source of vitamin D, so dietary intake isn't important if sun exposure is adequate. Vegetarian and vegan diets can also meet the nutrient and calorie needs of pregnant and lactating women with careful dietary planning and appropriate vitamin and mineral supplementation.

SPECIAL NEEDS

It's important to remember that eating patterns are influenced by culture, religious proscriptions, personal preferences, and financial barriers to obtaining desired food. These issues must be considered when giving recommendations for food choices and food preparation.

Stress reduction

The proven link between stress and the development and course of illness guides many treatment methods for such diseases as hypertension and depression and has even proved useful in modulating local inflammatory processes. In the past, our innate stress-alarm system encouraged us to fight or run away when faced with danger, the "fight-or-flight" response. In today's world, when commonly faced with more ambiguous stresses, this fight-or-flight response is not only inappropriate but usually not possible.

Some causes of stress include financial insecurity, job loss, discrimination, and the threat of war. Stressors specific to women include pregnancy and childbirth, balancing career and children, and sexual discrimination and abuse within society, in the workplace, and at home.

Stress can influence any system in the body and aggravate any chronic disease. Women who have such physical complaints as tiredness, frequent headaches, insomnia, and neck, back, and shoulder pain commonly have underlying psychological distress. Unfortunately, women and their health care providers rarely recognize these symptoms as stress. Consequently, a timely diagnosis isn't made and appropriate interventions aren't initiated.

Many women who experience stress-related health problems have low self-esteem and have been socialized to derive their self-esteem from caring for others. It's essential that a woman considers her own needs and how best to fulfill them and to set aside some time each day for herself.

The effects of stress can be minimized in various ways, including exercise, a healthy diet, meditation, massage, changes in sleep routine, and improved time management. It's also important to identify the causes of negative or excessive stress and change as many of those negative influences as possible. Some women may require referral for stress management or counseling from a trained professional.

Illness prevention

Preventing illness in the adult female involves dealing with chronic health problems that are especially prevalent in women, including obesity and heart disease. In addition, cessation of self-destructive behaviors, such as smoking and alcohol and drug abuse, becomes even more imperative as the adult female ages.

Chronic health problems

Obesity and heart disease rank among the most common health problems affecting young to middle-age women in the United States. While being closely related to each other (obesity is a significant risk factor in developing heart disease), these conditions are also related to many other acute and chronic conditions that are particularly harmful to a woman's health and well-being.

Obesity

Among women in the United States, obesity is more common than normal body weight. The prevalence of obesity among adults in the United States increased by 1% each year during the 1990s. In addition, women of racial and ethnic minorities as well as women of lower socioeconomic status are disproportionately affected by obesity.

Overweight or obese status is determined by calculating body mass index (BMI), the weight in kilograms divided by the height in meters squared (kg/m^2). This index approximates the amount of fat stored in the body. Using this definition, a BMI of less than 18 is considered underweight, a BMI of 18.5 to 24.9 is considered normal, 25 to 29.9 is overweight, and greater than 30 is obese. Based on these definitions, more than 60% of American adults are overweight or obese. (See *Are your patients at a healthy weight?*)

Moreover, obesity is associated with a significant increase in morbidity and mortality. A woman who is overweight or obese is at a substantially increased risk for morbidity from a number of conditions, including hypertension, dyslipidemia, type 2 diabetes mellitus, coronary artery disease, stroke, gallbladder disease, osteoarthritis, sleep apnea, and respiratory problems as well as endometrial, breast, and colon cancers. The link between obesity and endometrial and breast cancer is suspected to be the increased amount of estrogen produced by adipose tissue. Obesity results in more adipose tissue, which, consequently, produces more estrogen that increases the risk of these cancers. The CDC estimates that obesity and related lifestyle issues cause 300,000 deaths per year. Research has shown that the mortality risk in obese women increases in proportion to the degree of obesity, highlighting the need for early and effective intervention.

Other factors, such as gender, race, economic status, and genetics, may play a role in causing obesity. Even so, obesity is essentially a disease of energy imbalance, where "energy in" exceeds "energy out." The World Health Organization recently concluded that the fundamental causes of the obesity epidemic worldwide are reductions in spontaneous and work-related physical activity and overconsumption of high-fat, energy-dense foods. Attention to these environmental factors forms the cornerstone of obesity treatment.

Provider's role

Health care providers should target those individuals at risk for developing obesity and employ measures to correct the problem. Weight loss can be achieved through dietary intervention, physical exercise, and behavior modification. The search for an optimal diet is almost a national pastime. Considerable evidence exists that diets low in saturated fats and high in fruits, vegetables, and high fiber–con-

Are your patients at a healthy weight?

Body mass index (BMI) measures weight in relation to height. The BMI ranges shown here are for adults. Although they aren't exact ranges of healthy and unhealthy weights, they show that health risk increases at higher levels of overweight and obesity. Even within the healthy BMI range, weight gains can carry health risks for adults.

Directions: Find your patient's weight on the bottom of the graph. Go straight up from that point until you come to the line that matches her height. Then look to find her weight group.

■ Healthy weight
BMI from 18.5 up to 25 refers to a healthy weight.

■ Overweight
BMI from 25 up to 30 refers to overweight.

■ Obese
BMI 30 or higher refers to obesity. Obese persons are also overweight.

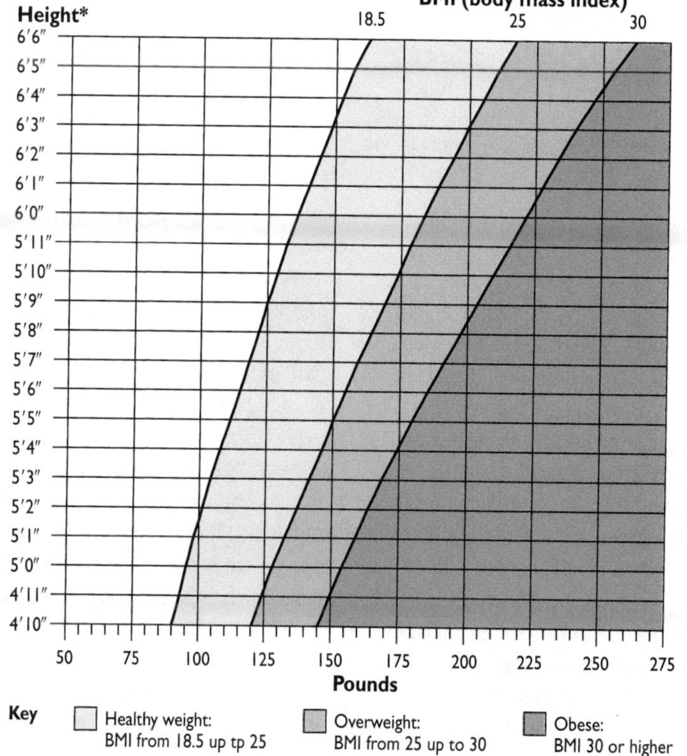

*Without shoes. Without clothes.

Source: Report of the Dietary Guidelines Advisory Committee on the Dietary Guidelines for Americans, 2000.

taining carbohydrates are safe and effective for weight loss, weight maintenance, and overall health. This type of diet is associated with satiety and reduced risk of chronic disease. Explain to the patient that the key message in diet planning is that a diet isn't something to follow for 8 days, 8 weeks, or 8 months. Rather, it should form the basis of everyday food choices throughout life. Many studies demonstrate that obese adults can lose about 1 lb (0.5 kg) per week and achieve a 5% to 15% weight loss by consuming 500 to 1,000 calories fewer per day than the caloric intake required for the maintenance of their current weight. For women, if calories are reduced to 1,200 per day, a wide variety of nutrients can be incorporated into the diet while still allowing for weight loss.

Health care providers need to stress to patients that while high-protein diets seem to be the latest weight-loss trend, most medical literature doesn't support their superiority over a high-carbohydrate, low-fat diet. The American Dietetics Association and the American Heart Association recommend a diet of 30% fat (with no more than 10% saturated fat), 15% to 20% protein, and 55% to 60% carbohydrates. The effectiveness of commercial weight-loss programs is also questionable. In fact, the only program that has demonstrated a long-term benefit is Weight Watchers. This program demonstrated that — 5 years after the initial weight loss period — 18.8% of the participants studied maintained a loss of at least 10% of their body weight, 42.6% maintained a loss of at least 5% of their body weight, and 70.3% were still below their initial weight. Other commercial programs, such as Jenny Craig, TOPS Club Inc., Overeaters Anonymous, Inc., and Nutrisystem, haven't published any official data or outcome statistics regarding the efficacy of their recommendations.

Again, it's important for health care providers to point out to patients that physical activity is an integral part of any weight-loss program. Physical activity burns fat and calories and increases muscle tone and metabolism. (See *Physical activity and calories.*)

In addition to dietary intervention and physical exercise, health care providers should incorporate all weight-loss programs with behavior modification in the form of one-on-one sessions with a therapist or group therapy. The best programs help the patient identify the cause of her weight gain in order to gain control over situations that cause her to overeat. Provide behavior modification techniques such as self-monitoring, which involves keeping a food diary — recording where eating occurred, what the portion size was, and how many calories were consumed. Exercise and any physical activity should also be recorded in the diary. Another behavior modification technique to teach a patient is called stimulus control, which aims to help the patient to avoid buying tempting foods, to plan ahead by shopping with a list and buying only what's on the

PREVENTION POINTER

Physical Activity and Calories

Activity	Calories burned per hour*
Bicycling, 5 mph	174
Walking, 2 mph	198
Swimming, 20 yds/min	288
Golf (twosome, carrying clubs)	324
Walking, 4½ mph	440
Tennis, singles	450
Swimming, 45 yds/min	522
Racquetball	588
Bicycling, 13 mph	612
Jogging, 6 mph	654
Running, 10 mph	1,280

*These figures are for a person who weighs 150 lb (68 kg).

mph = miles per hour yds = yards min = minute

list and, when eating out, to decide in advance not to order certain foods, such as the fattening dessert after the meal. Finally, relapse prevention is a technique that involves social support — vital to any weight-loss program — and the "buddy system," which involves a family member, friend, or a weight-loss counselor who can give support to the patient when needed to avoid a relapse.

When adequate weight loss isn't achieved by lifestyle changes, the health care provider may initiate drug therapy as an option. Current guidelines recommend that pharmacologic agents are appropriate for treating obesity in people with a BMI greater than 30. If serious risk factors (such as elevated cholesterol) or such disorders as hypertension, coronary heart disease, and type 2 diabetes are present, weight-loss drugs may be initiated at a BMI of 27 to 29.9. Two drugs (orlistat, an inhibitor for fat absorption, and sibutramine, which enhances satiety) are approved for long-term use in treating obesity. These drugs typically produce a weight loss of approximately 10%. Even this modest loss can lead to improvements in diabetes and cardiovascular risk factors. However, both drugs may have adverse effects, and it's important to counsel patients on these adverse effects. For example, orlistat causes GI problems, including flatus, oily spotting, abdominal pain, fecal urgency, fecal incontinence, and a slight reduction in the levels of fat-soluble vitamins. These effects are connected to the amount of fat ingested; reduced fat in the diet results in fewer adverse effects. Adverse effects of sibutramine include dry mouth, insomnia, headache, constipation, and restlessness. These effects are mild and usually resolve within a few weeks. However, a small number of patients taking sibutramine experience a significant elevation in blood pressure; therefore, it's necessary to routinely monitor blood pressure in anyone taking this drug. Encourage patients taking these drugs to participate in behavior modification; the effectiveness of these drugs is significantly improved when coupled with these techniques.

Lastly, health care providers can turn to surgical interventions, such as gastric bypass surgery, for patients with a BMI greater than 40 for whom other methods of treatment have failed, particularly if serious obesity-related complications are present.

Heart disease

Heart disease is, by far, the principal cause of death in men and women. However, the onset, distribution, and presentation of the disease may differ in women and men. Although heart disease develops approximately 10 to 15 years later in women than in men, the annual number of deaths caused by heart disease is greater in women. The delay in the development of heart disease among women is commonly attributed to the protection derived from endogenous estrogen (estrogen produced in the body).

The major risk factors for heart disease are the same for women and men and include elevated serum lipids (such as cholesterol, low-density lipoprotein [LDL], and triglycerides), hypertension, diabetes, obesity, sedentary lifestyle, and smoking. (See *Normal cholesterol levels.*) Prevalence of these risk factors increases with age and may further increase with menopause. Even so, many of these factors are present years before menopause. For example, about 50% of women are hypertensive by age 45, and obesity is a common, growing problem in young women. About 25% of adult women, regardless of age, report no regular sustained physical activity, and abnormal serum lipids are commonly detected years before menopause. Women's LDL cholesterol levels tend to rise with menopause, and high-density lipoprotein (HDL) cholesterol levels are thought to play an important role in the development of heart disease in women.

Provider's role

As a health care provider, identifying a woman's risk of heart disease early in life and intervening at the initial stages of the disease process is the op-

Normal cholesterol levels

Cholesterol levels are measured in milligrams (mg) of cholesterol per deciliter (dl) of blood.

HDL cholesterol levels

A low HDL level (less than 40 mg/dl) is strongly associated with increased heart disease risk for women. A level of 60 mg/dl is considered protective against heart disease.

Triglycerides

Levels that are borderline high (150 to 199 mg/dl) or high (200 mg/dl) may require treatment.

Level	Desirability
Total cholesterol	
Less than 200 mg/dl	Desirable
200 to 239 mg/dl	Borderline high
240 mg/dl and above	High
LDL cholesterol	
Less than 100 mg/dl	Optimal
100 to 129 mg/dl	Near optimal/above optimal
130 to 159 mg/dl	Borderline high
160 to 189 mg/dl	High
190 mg/dl and above	Very high

timal way to reduce her risk. The American Heart Association and the American College of Cardiology have published the Guide to Preventive Cardiology for Women. This guide has identified pregnancy and the preconception period as the "optimal time to review a woman's risk factor status and health behaviors to reduce future cardiovascular disease." For instance, during pregnancy, a woman may be more motivated to adopt healthy lifestyle habits such as stopping smoking. Therefore, this may be the right time for a health care provider to examine a woman's risk factors and behaviors to further prevent future disease.

Studies have shown that women are less likely than men to be evaluated for cardiovascular risk factors. Women are also less likely to receive adequate counseling and treatment about risk factor control after modifiable risk factors have been identified — even in women with established heart disease. In some cases, adverse trends in risk factors are more concerning in women. For example, smoking rates are declining more slowly in women than in men.

Health care providers should teach patients about how to reduce their risk of heart disease by following simple guidelines for modifying risk factors. (See *AHA and risk reduction.*)

Recent studies have provided increasing evidence that diet plays a crucial role in heart disease prevention. Studies on fish oil supplements (omega-3 fatty acids) have demonstrated that these supplements have an independent effect on heart disease risk. Unfortunately, the majority of data available to date has examined only the cardiac benefits of omega-3 fatty acids in men. Researchers from the Harvard School of Public Health have recently analyzed the dietary patterns of the 84,688 participants enrolled in the Nurses' Health Study. They found that the more frequent the intake of fish, the greater the reduction in heart disease risk (21% reduction for those consuming fish 1 to 3 times per month, climbing to a 34% reduction for those with intake of more than 5 times per week).

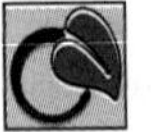

ALTERNATIVE THERAPIES

Current research indicates that soy intake lowers the risk of heart disease and atherosclerosis in women by lowering arterial blood pressure. The positive effects are attributed to phytoestrogens, a plant-based, estrogen-like compound found in soy. Over the past decade, antioxidants (vitamin E, vitamin C, and beta-carotene) have been found to possibly protect against heart disease. However, a more recent study published in the *Journal of the American Heart Association* has shown that antioxidant vitamins E and C and beta-carotene, alone or in combination, don't protect against heart disease and actually blunt the response to cholesterol-lowering drugs.

In addition to diet and physical exercise, health care providers can initiate drug therapy to lower a patient's cholesterol or treat hypertension. Research suggests that, in those with diabetes or a prior cardiovascular event such as a myocardial infarction, lipid-lowering therapy (statins) may be beneficial, regardless of the presence or absence of elevated cholesterol.

Self-destructive behaviors

Self-destructive behaviors, such as cigarette smoking and alcohol and drug abuse, are commonly initiated in adolescence. Continuation of these behaviors steadily increases the risks of morbidity and mortality in the adult female. Stopping these behaviors must be emphasized for successful treatment of associated disorders.

Cigarette smoking

In the United States, smoking is responsible for 400,000 deaths each year, or one in every five deaths. Currently, approximately 22% of adult women smoke — 13% of which are Hispanic, 21% are Black, and 24% are White. Young adults, ages 18 to 44, have the highest smoking rates. As of 1998, 28% of young adults were smokers. The deadliest risks from

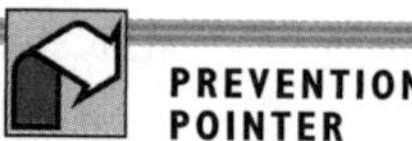

PREVENTION POINTER

AHA AND RISK REDUCTION

The American Heart Association (AHA) suggests that women who haven't had any cardiac procedures or events follow these guidelines:

Cigarette smoking—Stop smoking and avoid passive smoke inhalation.

Physical activity—Include 30 minutes (or more) per day of moderate intensity physical activity.

Nutrition—AHA Step I diet for healthy women: ≤ 30% fat (8 to 10 g saturated) intake; <300 mg/day cholesterol intake; limit sodium intake to 6 g/day or less; 25 to 30 g/day total dietary fiber intake; five or more servings of fruit and vegetables per day.

Weight management—Achieve and maintain desirable weight; target body mass index (BMI): 18.5 to 24.9 kg/m^2; waist circumference in women with BMI 25 to 34.9 kg/m^2: < 88 cm (35 in).

Blood pressure management—Maintain blood pressure <140/90 mm Hg (optimal: <120/80 mm Hg); persons with blood pressures greater than 120 mg Hg systolic or 80 mm Hg diastolic now are considered prehypertensive, thus necessitating lifestyle modifications to reduce blood pressure. In pregnant women, minimize short-term risk for elevated blood pressure with effective therapy that's safe for both mother and fetus.

Lipids/lipoprotein management—Lower-risk women (without cardiovascular disease): low-density lipoprotein (LDL): <160 mg/dl (optimal <130 mg/dl); higher-risk women (two or more risk factors): LDL: >130 mg/dl (<100 mg/dl in women with cardiovascular disease), high-density lipoprotein (HDL): ≥40 mg/dl, and triglycerides <150 mg/dl.

Diabetes management—Maintain blood glucose: before meals 90 to 120 mg/dl and at bedtime 100 to 140 mg/dl; maintain HbA_{1c} (an indicator of glucose control) < 7%; maintain LDL <130 mg/dl (<100 mg/dl with cardiovascular disease); maintain triglycerides <150 mg/dl; control blood pressure.

smoking are cancer of the lungs, throat, and mouth. Research also indicates that smoking is associated with increased risk for cervical cancer. Interestingly, cervical cancer rates are lower in ex-smokers when compared to current smokers, suggesting that the risk is reversible after smoking cessation. Smoking is also a major risk factor for heart and cerebrovascular disease. Middle-age women who smoke are three times more likely to die of coronary artery disease and five times more likely to die of a stroke than nonsmoking women. Smoking is also associated with pregnancy-related complications. It's a major cause of intrauterine growth retardation in the developed world, accounting for an estimated 30% of cases. An increase in spontaneous abortions, stillbirths, and neonatal deaths as well as other pregnancy complications, such as placenta previa and abruptio placentae, are linked to smoking.

Smokers who use hormonal contraceptives are also at increased risk for myocardial infarction, subarachnoid hemorrhage, and stroke. Hormonal contraceptive use alone increases this risk, which is further increased with age, especially after age 35. Thus, the risk is substantially greater in those women who take hormonal contraceptives, are age 35 and older, and smoke cigarettes. In addition, women who smoke are at increased risk for postmenopausal osteoporosis and fractures and also have more prominent skin wrinkling than nonsmokers, regardless of their history of sun exposure.

Provider's role

The health care provider should encourage all patients to refrain from tobacco use. Smoking cessation at any time is always beneficial — even after age 65 or after the development of a smoking-related disease. Even so, more than 90% of smokers know that smoking is harmful to their health yet continue to smoke. Smoking cessation is difficult for several reasons, most significantly the psychoactive, addictive action of nicotine contained in cigarettes. In addition, smoking is a habit, a behavior that has become an integral part of a daily routine. Smokers also use cigarettes to cope with stress; therefore, quitting smoking is equated with the loss of a valuable coping tool.

As health care providers, it's essential to help a patient stop smoking by identifying the activities that trigger her desire, teaching her to anticipate and handle urges to smoke that will occur, and offering alternative coping strategies for handling stress. For many, finding a substitute for smoking is the key to quitting. For example, if a woman smokes for stimulation or a lift, encourage her to take a brisk walk or perform moderate exercise as a healthy substitute; if she smokes for relaxation or to relieve tension, encourage her to begin an exercise program, start a new hobby, or perform deep-breathing exercises.

Two effective methods of smoking cessation — pharmacotherapy and behavioral counseling — work best when used together. The major therapies approved by the U.S. Food and Drug Administration (FDA) for use in achieving cessation include nicotine replacement therapy (such as a patch, gum, inhaler, or nasal spray) and antidepressants such as bupropion (Wellbutrin). Health care providers should use effective counseling methods to teach problem-solving techniques, provide social support, and help build confidence in the smoker's ability to quit. These skills can be taught in group sessions, individual counseling, or even over the telephone. It's also important for health care providers to address barriers to smoking cessation, which may include fear of failure, nicotine withdrawal, concern regarding weight gain, lack of social support for quitting, and presence of comorbid disorders, such as depression and substance abuse.

Alcohol and drug abuse

Alcohol and drug use and dependence are highly prevalent in the general population. Data from the National Comorbidity Survey indicate that

18% of noninstitutionalized women ages 15 to 54 will have been diagnosed with substance abuse or dependence during their lifetime and that 6.6% will have been diagnosed within the past 12 months.

In the United States, alcohol is abused more than any other substance, with approximately 4 million individuals being alcohol dependent. According to the 1998 National Household Survey on Drug Abuse, approximately 2.7 million women abuse alcohol, which is about one-third of all those who have alcohol abuse or dependence disorders. Alcohol abuse in women is associated with adverse pregnancy outcomes, high-risk sexual behavior, accidents and injuries, depression, domestic violence, child abuse, family problems, and employment issues. Other health problems associated with alcohol abuse include higher rates of liver disease, heart disease, cancer, and osteoporosis.

A higher proportion of body fat in women than in men as well as differences in total body water content and relative amounts of gastric alcohol dehydrogenase (a stomach enzyme that breaks down alcohol before it reaches the bloodstream) create differences in the way women and men metabolize alcohol. Thus, a woman who drinks the same amount as a man will have a higher level of alcohol in her blood. These differences may explain the earlier appearance and increased severity of complications from drinking seen in women compared to men. Interestingly, the majority of alcohol-related adverse events occur in women who aren't alcohol dependent, although these women generally drink too much and too often.

Alcohol and pregnancy

There's no known safe level of alcohol use during pregnancy. Maternal alcohol consumption is a leading preventable cause of birth defects and childhood disabilities in the United States. Women who drink two or more drinks per day during their pregnancy are at increased risk for spontaneous abortions, low–birth weight infants, preterm labor, and perinatal mortality. Infants born to mothers who drink during pregnancy are at increased risk for fetal alcohol syndrome characterized by severe physical, behavioral, and cognitive abnormalities. Infants of alcoholic mothers may also be at increased risk for cardiac, skeletal, renal, ocular, and auditory defects.

Provider's role

When assessing patients for alcohol abuse, it's important to first identify specific risk factors, including a family history of alcoholism, history of physical or sexual abuse, other substance use, and a young age at first intoxication. A history of eating disorders, depression or anxiety disorders, divorce, and a partner with heavy alcohol or drug use also raises the concern that there may be an alcohol problem.

A number of studies have shown that a "moderate" amount of alcohol helps protect against heart disease.

Most experts say that moderation means no more than one drink per day for women and two drinks for men. The National Institute of Alcohol Abuse and Alcoholism defines "at-risk drinking" for women to be more than 7 drinks per week or more than 3 drinks per occasion.

To treat problem drinking, health care providers can employ a number of successful treatment models. To begin, a brief 5- to 10-minute counseling session has been found to reduce alcohol use in women by 20% to 30%. Other effective interventions include guided self-change programs, cognitive therapy, behavioral therapy, and the 12-step program. The intervention may be offered as outpatient, inpatient, or residential treatment. Additionally, family therapy is commonly helpful in assisting the family to learn more about the disease of alcohol dependence, deal with their anger and anxiety, and participate in the recovery process.

Reproductive issues

Women have been attempting to control their fertility since the beginning of recorded history. The adult woman's health and well-being are directly affected by issues of reproduction. It's important to understand that what a woman experiences in her reproductive health can greatly impact her overall health. Unplanned pregnancies, sexually transmitted disease (STDs), and infertility continue to plague our society in spite of education, awareness, and technological advances. Women play a vital role in the prevention and promotion of their reproductive health. This section will cover contraception, infertility, and STDs.

Contraception

Today, women have more contraceptive choices than ever before, yet American women have more unplanned pregnancies (more than 50% of pregnancies are unplanned) and more abortions (1.3 million per year) than women in most industrialized countries. The willingness and ability to use a method of contraception are influenced not only by the efficacy of that particular method but also by possible adverse effects and concerns regarding medical risks, cost, availability, life circumstances, and culture. In addition to abstinence and coitus interruptus, there are four types of contraception: hormonal methods, intrauterine devices, barrier methods, and sterilization.

Hormonal contraception

Hormonal contraceptive methods available in the United States include oral contraceptives, Depo-Provera, Lunelle, the NuvaRing, and the Ortho Evra contraceptive patch. Hormonal methods contain either a combination of estrogen and a form of progesterone, or progesterone alone. These hormones act primarily to prevent ovulation and to thicken the cervical mucus so that the sperm can't reach and fertilize the egg.

Oral contraceptives

Two types of oral contraceptive pills exist — one that contains both estrogen and a progestin and a progestin-only pill, also called the "mini pill." For women who don't miss any pills, oral contraceptives are 99.9% effective against pregnancy in the first year; however, the typical range is 95% to 97% effective against pregnancy in the first year. The "mini pill" has about the same efficacy (95% to 97%) and about 99.5% for those who take it correctly. In addition to its benefits as an effective reversible contraceptive, this method generally results in lighter, more regular periods.

Hormonal contraceptives also have many advantages beyond contraception, such as decreased risk of ovarian and endometrial cancer, pelvic inflammatory disease, benign breast disease, ectopic pregnancy, dysmenorrhea, iron deficiency anemia, and acne. Growing evidence also suggests that oral contraceptives may help prevent osteoporosis by slowing or preventing loss of bone mineral density in the premenopausal years.

Women may experience minor adverse effects from oral contraceptives, including nausea, breast tenderness, and irregular spotting after pill initiation. These effects generally subside after 3 months of use. A more serious complication associated with combined pill use is the risk of venous thromboembolism (VTE). This risk is associated with the dose of estrogen included in the combined form; increased estrogen equals increased risk. Even so, the risk of VTE from taking oral contraceptives is only half of the VTE risk associated with pregnancy. However, women taking the pill who have underlying blood coagulation disorders, such as factor V Leiden mutation and protein C and S deficiency, are at significantly higher risk for VTE. In addition, women with a personal history of thromboembolic disease or with a known coagulation disorder shouldn't take pills that contain estrogen. The progestin-only pill is a good choice for women who have contraindications to or experience adverse effects from estrogen.

Low-dose pills (such as 0.45 mg estrogen or less) don't increase the risk of myocardial infarction or stroke in healthy, nonsmoking women, regardless of age. However, preexisting hypertension is a significant additive risk factor for stroke in pill users. Despite studies that have shown that current users of pills are slightly more likely to be diagnosed with breast cancer, the consensus is that pills don't cause breast cancer. Some postulate that the increased risk may be attributable to a detection bias (more breast examinations and more mammography in pill users, who must undergo regular examinations to obtain a prescription). Others theorize that oral contraceptives promote preexisting cancer cells. The Collaboration Group conducted the largest collaborative study of the risk of breast cancer and concluded that women with a strong family history of breast cancer don't increase their risk of breast cancer by taking birth control pills. This was also the conclusion of the Nurses

Health Study and the Cancer and Steroid Hormone study.

Depo-Provera

Depo-Provera is a long-acting, injectable, progestin-only method of contraception. It's administered by I.M. injection of 150 mg every 3 months (11 to 13 weeks). The initial dose should be given during the first 5 days of menses, and pregnancy should be excluded. In women who receive their injection on time, the pregnancy rate is less than 1%.

Depo-Provera is a good choice of contraception for women who have trouble remembering to take daily hormonal contraceptives. A progestin-only method is also particularly valuable for use in women with estrogen-related contraindications, such as a history of thromboembolic disorders, hypertension, coronary artery disease, or cerebrovascular disease, and those over age 35 who smoke. Progestin-only methods can also be used immediately postpartum with no significant impact on the quality or quantity of milk production, unlike hormonal methods containing estrogen that, if used before the establishment of lactation, can diminish the quality and quantity of breast milk.

The major drawback of Depo-Provera is menstrual cycle irregularity. Approximately 30% of women develop irregular bleeding, specifically during the first 3 months of use, and 70% of women become amenorrheic after 2 years. Increased appetite, weight gain, acne, and depression are other adverse effects. Prolonged use may also result in decreased bone density. It's important to note that return to baseline fertility is excellent after using Depo-Provera; however, an average delay of 9 to 10 months occurs between the last shot and conception.

Lunelle

Lunelle is a fairly new, long-acting method of contraception administered I.M. It contains estrogen and progestin and is given every 28 to 30 days. As with Depo-Provera, it's a very effective method of contraception, with a pregnancy rate of 0.02%. Most women have regular monthly bleeding, although many have some irregular spotting during the first 3 months of use. Returning for injections on a regular schedule will result in the most regular menses. Approximately 6% of women discontinue Lunelle due to weight gain, although the weight gain is typically less than that experienced with Depo-Provera use.

NuvaRing

The NuvaRing is another method that's good for women who want to avoid daily dosing requirements. It's a contraceptive ring placed in the vagina and left in place for 3 weeks, then removed for 1 week. Menses occur during the week the ring is removed from the vagina. Each month, a new ring is used and shouldn't be removed for intercourse. Hormones, similar to those in birth control pills (estrogen and progestin), are gradually released out of the ring and are absorbed through the vagina into the circulation.

Most women continue to have regular menstrual cycles while using the ring. However, device-related problems, such as vaginal discomfort during intercourse, vaginal discharge, and vaginitis, were reported by 2% to 5% of women and expulsion of the ring occurred in 2%. Other hormone-related adverse effects included headache, nausea, weight increase, and breast pain. The efficacy of the NuvaRing is similar to oral contraceptives.

Ortho Evra patch

The Ortho Evra contraceptive patch contains hormones similar to birth control pills. Each patch is worn for 1 week and must be changed on the same day of the week, three times per month, with the 4th week patch-free. Menses occur during the patch-free week. The patch can be placed on the arm, abdomen, or buttocks but shouldn't be placed on the breast. The effectiveness of the patch in typical users is more than 99%. Women using the patch can continue to participate in such normal activities as bathing, exercising, and swimming without worrying that the patch will come off.

The incidence of partial or complete patch detachment is less than 3%. Research indicates improved compliance with patch users when compared to oral contraceptive users. Most women have regular menstrual periods, although some patch users may experience irregular spotting. A small percentage of women (2.6%) discontinued using the patch because of application site reactions. Women weighing more than 198 lb (89.9 kg) aren't good candidates for the patch because of decreased efficacy.

Intrauterine contraception

Intrauterine contraception is accomplished through two kinds of intrauterine devices (IUDs) available in the United States: the T380A intrauterine copper contraceptive (ParaGard) and the progestin-releasing IUD (Mirena). The ParaGard is effective for 10 years and the Mirena for 5 years. The effectiveness of both IUDs is superior to that of hormonal contraception, with a pregnancy rate of less than 1%. Both IUDs primarily prevent fertilization by interfering with sperm motility, although a secondary effect of inhibition of implantation can't be completely excluded. The major benefits of the IUD are its high effectiveness, long-term ease of use, and lack of systemic adverse effects. The Mirena has the additional benefits of decreasing both heavy bleeding and cramping that may be associated with the menstrual period.

The major risk associated with IUD use is pelvic inflammatory disease. This risk is most prominent in the first 3 weeks after IUD insertion and in women who are at risk for STDs. Women using an IUD should immediately report any unusual lower abdominal pain, vaginal bleeding, or vaginal discharge. Other problems that may occur, primarily with the ParaGard, include an increase in cramping and menstrual bleeding. These problems may diminish with short-term use of a nonsteroidal anti-inflammatory drug such as ibuprofen. The IUD is best suited to women who have had a child and are in a stable and mutually monogamous relationship. The device can be removed at any time. Its effects are rapidly reversible, so another method of contraception must be initiated immediately if pregnancy isn't intended.

Barrier methods

Barrier methods have historically been the most widely used contraceptive technique. When used during intercourse, these methods prevent sperm from reaching the egg. Barrier methods include the male and female condom, the diaphragm, and the cervical cap. It's recommended that both the diaphragm and the cervical cap be used in combination with spermicides. Spermicides shouldn't be used alone because they provide limited protection against pregnancy. The World Health Organization recommends that women at high risk for HIV infection shouldn't use spermicides that contain nonoxynol 9. According to the CDC, frequent use of spermicides containing nonoxynol 9 has been associated with genital lesions, which may in turn be associated with an increased risk for HIV transmission. When either the male or the female condom is used as the primary contraceptive method, information and a prescription for emergency contraception should also be provided.

Male condom

The male condom is 85% to 95% effective in preventing pregnancy and is the only method that effectively protects against the transmission of STDs, including HIV and herpes. The major disadvantage of the condom is that it must be applied immediately before intercourse when the penis is erect, which inhibits full compliance. Other concerns associated with the condom are that it blunts sensation and that it may break. Allergic reactions to latex may also occur. Use of polyurethane condoms, although associated with increased breakage and slippage, avoids such reactions.

Female condom

The female condom is a disposable, single-use pouch made of polyurethane, which lines the vagina. An internal ring in the closed end of the pouch covers the cervix and an external ring remains outside the vagina, partially covering the perineum. Although studies are lacking, this condom is also believed to reduce the risk of STD transmission.

Diaphragm

The diaphragm is a dome of latex or polyurethane inserted in the vagina to cover the cervix and is generally used in combination with a spermicide. It comes in different types and sizes and must be professionally fitted. It should be placed in the vagina no longer than 6 hours before coitus and left in place for at least 6 hours after the last act of sexual intercourse, although it can remain in place for up to

24 hours. Failure rates for diaphragm users vary from as low as 2% per year of use to as high as 23%. This method is rarely associated with even minor adverse effects, although some women may experience vaginal irritation due to sensitivity to latex or the spermicide. Urinary tract infections are two to three times more common among diaphragm users than among women using hormonal contraceptives. An advantage of the diaphragm is that it reduces the risk of certain STDs, including gonorrhea, chlamydia, cervical dysplasia, and pelvic inflammatory disease. No data are available regarding the effect of diaphragm use on the transmission of HIV/AIDS.

Cervical cap

The Prentif Cavity-Rim Cervical Cap is a thimble-shaped, latex device with a small groove in its inner surface that creates suction to keep the cap on the cervix. Studies have demonstrated the cervical cap to be about as effective as the diaphragm, although, efficacy is significantly reduced in parous women. The most common cause of failure is dislodgment of the cap from the cervix during sexual intercourse. It's somewhat more difficult to fit than the diaphragm (it comes in four sizes) and more difficult to insert (it must be placed precisely over the cervix). A small amount of spermicide is placed inside the cap before insertion, and the cap can be left in place for up to 48 hours. An odor may develop if the cap is left in place too long. The cap must be left in place for at least 8 hours after sexual intercourse to ensure that no motile sperm are left in the vagina. No documentation that cervical caps protect against STDs exists.

Provider's role

Health care providers should perform a thorough assessment of patients' sexual history and current use of contraceptives. Based on these findings, they should counsel female patients on all available contraceptive options, along with their benefits and disadvantages as well as teach about preventing STDs.

Sterilization

Sterilization is the predominant method of contraception throughout the world and is used by more than one-third of American couples. Female sterilization, also called *tubal ligation*, permanently blocks or removes a portion of the fallopian tubes, thereby preventing fertilization. It's generally performed by laparoscopy under general anesthesia in an outpatient surgery setting or immediately postpartum within 48 hours of delivery. Laparoscopic sterilization can be achieved with tubal occlusion by bipolar cautery, silastic bands, clips, or removal of a portion of the tube.

The effectiveness of sterilization depends on the method used, the skill of the surgeon, and the patient's age. The typical failure rate during the first year is less than 1%. Up to 50% of failures are caused by technical errors in the methods used. The methods that had the highest failure rates were bipolar cautery and the clip. In addition, women younger than age 35 were 1.7 times more likely to become pregnant than women over age 35. An additional benefit of tubal sterilization is a decrease in the risk of ovarian cancer. Evidence from the Nurses' Health Study indicated that tubal sterilization was associated with a 67% reduced risk of ovarian cancer.

If failure does occur, an increased risk that the pregnancy will be ectopic exists. In addition, complications from the surgical procedure include infection, hemorrhage, and vessel or organ injury and death. The procedure has an extremely small mortality (1 to 2 per 100,000 procedures), which is most commonly a complication of general anesthesia.

Male sterilization (vasectomy) is safer, easier, and less expensive, and has a lower failure rate than female sterilization. This method involves severing the vas deferens, the tube through which sperm travels from the testes to the penis. The most popular method is the "no scalpel" technique. This approach is fast and less invasive than other methods, and is also associated with fewer complications. It involves an ultrasound device with three parts: a water balloon that covers the skin through which chilled water runs to keep the skin from burning; a clamp that holds the vas deferens in place; and an ultrasound machine that focuses sound waves on the vas deferens. At the point of focus, the ultrasound energy creates intense heat, which heats up the tissue of the vas deferens so that it closes. Then healing of the tissue creates scar tissue that further blocks the vas deferens.

Failure rate of the vasectomy in the first year is less than 1%. To improve efficacy, a couple should continue to use some other form of birth control until at least two sperm counts show no sperm in the semen — which usually requires 20 or more ejaculations. Hematomas, bruising, and wound infections are the most common adverse effects associated with this procedure.

Fears about vasectomy increasing the risk of prostate cancer, the most common cancer among men, have convinced some men not to undergo the procedure. Based on a number of studies conducted over the past decade, a link between vasectomy and prostate cancer is unlikely.

Tubal sterilization and vasectomy are permanent methods of contraception and should be utilized only in individuals committed to never again producing children. Reversal of both procedures is costly, and failure rates are high.

Infertility

Infertility is generally defined as the inability to conceive after 1 year of sexual intercourse without using contraception. Infertility may be due to specific male or female factors or, in many cases, may be multifactorial. Approximately 10% to 20% of couples in the United States are infertile. Age is an important associated factor. Many couples are delaying childbearing to pursue their education and careers. Approximately one-third of women who defer pregnancy until their middle to late 30s will have an infertility problem. In younger adults, infertility has other causes. Sometimes the cause is simple, such as not having intercourse at the optimal time. More commonly, causes include tubal blockage, anovulation, such pelvic factors as adhesions or endometriosis in women, and a low sperm count or low sperm motility in men.

Provider's role

Health care providers can perform several diagnostic tests to help evaluate infertility. One test that a patient can perform is keeping a basal body temperature chart to determine both the presence of and the time of ovulation. Other diagnostic tests include a postcoital test to assess the cervical mucus and the presence of motile sperm; semen analysis to assess the volume, viscosity, and pH of the semen and analyze the sperm for number, motility, and morphology (structure and form); and hysterosalpingogram, an X-ray that evaluates the contours of the uterine cavity and assesses the patency of the fallopian tubes. Laparoscopy is also used to confirm diagnosis of pelvic adhesions or endometriosis. Use of laser technology may effectively treat the problem at the same time. Hysteroscopy is used to diagnose and treat intrauterine lesions (such as endometrial polyps or adhesions) that may reduce fertility. This procedure uses a uterine endoscope to visualize the uterine cavity directly. Additional tests that evaluate the pituitary or thyroid gland should also be included in assessing women who have menstrual irregularity.

Numerous treatments are available for infertility, and many of the causes are correctable. About 50% of the couples who seek help are eventually able to have a child. However, treatments are typically expensive and may involve emotional and ethical issues. It's important to discuss with your patient and her partner any treatments before pursuing a particular course of action. Referral to a fertility specialist may be necessary. Also, support groups such as RESOLVE, a national fertility education and support network, can offer guidance. Treatment options include drug therapy for anovulation, surgery to treat pelvic adhesions or endometriosis as well as to correct intrauterine factors (such as removal of submucous fibroids), and assisted reproductive technologies. Assisted reproductive technologies are used when other treatment options have been exhausted. The options include artificial insemination, in vitro fertilization (transfer of an embryo into the uterus), gamete intrafallopian transfer (transfer of mature ova/sperm into the fallopian tubes), and zygote intrafallopian transfer (transfer of a zygote into the fallopian tubes). This technology may include the use of donor gametes.

Sexually transmitted diseases

Each year, more than 15 million cases of STDs occur in the United States. Of those, teenagers and young adults (under age 25) have the highest number of new STD cases each year. Although STDs commonly occur in younger individuals, they know no age. If left untreated, STDs put a woman at risk for such conditions as ectopic pregnancy, infertility, adverse pregnancy outcomes, and chronic pelvic pain.

In addition to these conditions, the emotional impact of contracting an STD can affect a woman's self-image and well-being. It's important to emphasize to women that sexual health promotion involves preventative measures, such as reducing one's risk of STDs by using male condoms, getting appropriate screening, and avoiding sexual contact with at-risk partners.

Risk factors for STDs include a history of multiple sexual partners, a previous STD, a sexual partner with other partners in the preceding 3 months, use of illicit drugs, and use of nonbarrier contraceptives. Individuals who have one or more of these risk factors should also receive appropriate screening such as HIV testing.

Provider's role

Health care providers must make every effort to prevent the acquisition and spread of STDs. As part of routine care, the provider should ask the adult female patient about her sexual behavior and counsel her regarding sexual practices and STDs. The most reliable preventive measure, apart from abstinence, is long-term monogamy with an STD-free, monogamous partner. Other preventive measures include the correct use of condoms; knowing who one's partner is; being observant (not having sexual contact with anyone who has genital or anal sores, a visible rash, a discharge, or any other sign of a sexually transmitted infection); being informed (recognizing the symptoms of STDs and seeking medical treatment immediately); being responsible (if exposed to a sexually transmitted infection, not having sex again until after visiting a health care provider, and if infected, informing one's partners and advising them to seek medical attention); getting vaccinated against hepatitis B; and informing other sexual partners about an STD, if present.

This section explores the most common STDs reported in the United States.

Chlamydia

Chlamydia is the most common bacterial STD in the United States, causing about 4 million infections each year. In women, untreated chlamydia can cause serious complications, including pelvic inflammatory disease (a condition that can lead to infertility), ectopic pregnancy, and possible infection of the eyes, if they come in contact with genital secretions of an infected person. Unfortunately, most women infected with chlamydia have few or no symptoms, and without testing and treatment, the infection can continue for months or even years. Symptoms, when they occur, can include abnormal discharge or bleeding from the vagina, dysuria, or pain in the lower abdomen. The good news is that chlamydia is easy to detect with appropriate testing and treatment with antibiotics. Deoxyribonucleic acid (DNA) amplification techniques are the test of choice in screening women (and men), because of their high sensitivity and specificity. Azithromycin (Zithromax), a long-acting antibiotic, is the treatment of choice. Its one-time dosing schedule makes it convenient for patients and decreases the problem of noncompliance.

Gonorrhea

Gonorrhea is also caused by a bacterial infection and, like chlamydia, frequently causes no symptoms in women. An estimated 600,000 cases occur annually in the United States. The STD is spread by direct contact with infected mucous membranes in the genitals, mouth, and throat. Women with symptomatic infection may report vaginal discharge, dysuria, abnormal uterine bleeding, or labial pain or swelling. A sore throat may be the presenting symptom if the infection is contracted through oral sex; rectal pain or discharge, if contracted through anal sex. Gonorrhea can also cause pelvic inflammatory disease (which can result in infertility), ectopic pregnancy, and chronic pelvic pain. The recommended diagnostic test is by DNA amplification techniques. Many antibiotics are effective for treatment, including cefixime (Suprax), ceftriaxone (Rocephin), and ciprofloxacin (Ciloxan). However, there has been an increase in quinolone-resistant gonorrhea to ciprofloxacin in parts of Asia, the Pacific, and the West Coast of the United States. Therefore, it's important to obtain a recent travel history, including sexual partner history, to ensure appropriate antibiotic therapy. Patients infected with gonorrhea often are infected with chlamydia. Thus, it's recommended that patients treated for gonococcal infection also be treated routinely with an effective regimen against chlamydia.

Human papillomavirus

Human papillomavirus (HPV) is probably the most common viral STD among young, sexually active individuals. About 5.5 million Americans become infected with HPV each year. More than 30 types of HPV can infect the genital tract, and most infections are asymptomatic. Visible warts are usually caused by HPV types 6 and 11, while other HPV types (such as types 16, 18, 31, 33, and 35) have been strongly associated with abnormal Papanicolaou (Pap) tests and cervical neoplasia in women. One study suggested that nearly 40% of college-age women have HPV lesions on their cervix. The primary goal of treating visible genital warts is the removal of symptomatic warts. In most patients, treatment can result in a wart-free period. Research indicates that treatment of genital warts reduces, but doesn't eradicate, infectivity. A number of different treatments can remove visible warts, including such provider-administered treatments as cryotherapy, trichloroacetic acid or bichloracetic acid, podophyllin, and surgery. Patient-applied treatments include podofilox and imiquimod. Detection of precancerous changes in the cervix can be found with a Pap test, and treatments to prevent the development of cancer include DNA testing and colposcopy.

Herpes simplex virus

Genital herpes is a recurrent, lifelong viral infection. At least 50 million individuals in the United States have genital herpes simplex virus (HSV) infection. The two types of HSV that cause genital infection are HSV-1 and HSV-2, with most cases of recurrent genital herpes caused by HSV-2. Many people who become infected are asymptomatic — the typical painful blisters and sores are absent. The infection is highly contagious, and transmission can occur with or without the presence of visible sores. In fact, persons unaware that they have the infection or who are asymptomatic when transmission occurs transmit most genital herpes infections. Pregnant women must be especially careful because herpes can be transmitted during childbirth, resulting in severe health problems for the neonate. The diagnosis of genital HSV infections is usually missed if based only on clinical signs and symptoms. Diagnostic tests, such as viral culture and serologic tests, are necessary to assist in making the correct diagnosis.

At present, no cure for HSV infection exists. The major goal of treatment is to decrease its symptoms, time for healing, and viral shedding. Antiviral therapy, when initiated at the onset of symptoms, offers clinical benefits to most patients and is the mainstay of managing primary and recurrent HSV. Effective treatment of recurrent herpes requires initiation of therapy within 1 day of lesion onset, or when prodromal symptoms (such as tingling, itching, or pain that precedes some outbreaks) occur. If a patient has more than six recurrences per year, daily suppressive antiviral therapy should be considered. Quality of life commonly improves with this type of therapy when compared to episodic treatment. Patients should be advised to abstain from sexual activity with uninfected partners when lesions or prodromal symptoms are present.

Trichomoniasis

Trichomoniasis is an infection caused by a one-celled organism, called a protozoan. About 5 million cases occur each year in the United States. In women, trichomoniasis can cause vaginal itching, redness, and a frothy, yellow-green discharge. The infection may also cause pain or discomfort during sexual intercourse or urination. Trichomoniasis may increase the risk of infection with HIV. It's usually cured with an antibiotics such as metronidazole.

Syphilis

Syphilis is one of the oldest STDs, with records going back as far as the time of Columbus's voyage. An estimated 70,000 new cases of this bacterial infection occur annually in the United States, and 1 in every 7,000 to 10,000 neonates born in the United States has congenital syphilis. The primary manifestation of syphilis is a painless chancre or ulcer that occurs at the site where the bacteria enters the body — the genital region, mouth, rectum, vagina, or cervix. When the chancre or ulcer appears on the cervix or rectum, it commonly goes unnoticed and therefore undiagnosed. Without treatment, the chancre resolves spontaneously within 5 weeks. Most women present with symptoms during the secondary phase of the infection. Signs of secondary syphilis appear 2 to 8 weeks after the appearance of the chancre. This phase is characterized by nonspecific flulike symptoms and a non-itching rash. Lymphadenopathy may be present during both the primary and secondary phases. Without treatment, the signs and symptoms of secondary syphilis resolve within 2 to 10 weeks and the infection becomes latent. Tertiary, or late-stage syphilis, can develop many years after the initial infection, with symptoms that can mimic many other diseases (such as cardiovascular disease or neurologic disease). Diagnosis is accomplished with either dark-field microscopic examination of exudate from the chancre or serologic tests for secondary, latent, and tertiary syphilis.

Long-acting penicillin is the treatment of choice for syphilis, although other antibiotics may be used in the nonpregnant, penicillin-allergic patient. The dosage and the length of treatment depend on the stage and clinical manifestations of the disease. Penicillin is the only therapy with documented efficacy for syphilis during pregnancy. Pregnant women with syphilis who report penicillin allergy should undergo skin testing to verify a penicillin allergy. If the skin test is positive, desensitization to penicillin is recommended, and the patient should then be treated with the appropriate penicillin dosage. There's an increased incidence of HIV infection in people with syphilis; therefore, everyone with syphilis should be counseled on HIV infection, and HIV testing should be recommended. Patients should be reexamined both clinically and serologically for test of cure at 6 months and 12 months following treatment. If signs and symptoms persist or recur or if the serologic titers increase, the treatment has failed or reinfection has occurred. These patients should be retreated and reevaluated for HIV.

Recommended screening

Medical experts agree that good health depends on improved access to and increased use of clinical preventive services — including immunizations, screening tests for early detection of disease, and education about healthful habits and injury prevention. It's estimated that only 1% to 3% of the annual health care bill in the United States today is used toward preventive services. This lack of awareness could be attributable to contradictory screening recommendations, causing confusion among patients, health care providers, and public health officials.

The U.S. Preventive Services Task Force (USPSTF), a multidisciplinary expert panel appointed by the government, reviewed available evidence about preventing illness and then made recommendations regarding content of screening based on age-groups and risks of specific diseases or conditions. The overall conclusions of the USPSTF are that (1) interventions that address patients' personal health practices are vitally important; (2) the clinician and the patient should share decision making; (3) the clinician should be selective in ordering tests and providing preventive services; and (4) preventive services need not be delivered exclusively during preventive visits. This section presents current screening recommendations for cancers of the breast, cervix, endometrium, and skin; diabetes; and elevated cholesterol. As a health care provider, make sure that your adult female patients are receiving the appropriate screening for their age and level of risk factors involved. This section also discusses screening a female patient for depression and domestic abuse.

Cancer

Cancer — the uncontrolled growth of abnormal cells in the body — is the second-leading cause of death in women in the United States. As cancer cells grow, they divide rapidly, tend to be aggressive, and usually occur in the breast, skin, lungs, or reproductive systems. Breast and lung cancer are the leading cancer killers of women. (See *Top 10 cancer sites in the adult female.*)

Breast cancer

In 2003, updated breast cancer screening guidelines were issued by the American Cancer Society (ACS). The new guidelines stress education, especially in high-risk women about mammography and other screening methods in older women, and clarification on the role of the breast self-examination (BSE). Once considered by the ACS as the most reliable method of detecting beast cancer, the BSE lacks evidence. Mammography remains the most proven form of screening and has consistently reduced deaths from breast cancer. In addition, clinical breast examination (CBE) should remain part of a woman's periodic health examination. Genetic testing for breast cancer is another option for women considered to be at high risk for breast cancer, although it's generally undertaken only if the information gleaned from the testing would lead to additional steps not otherwise taken.

The CBE is widely recommended as a tool to differentiate normal breast tissue from a discrete breast mass and as a complement to regular mammography screening. It also provides wo-

Top 10 cancer sites in the adult female

Breast	Ovary
Colon and rectum	Pancreas
Leukemia and lymphomas	Thyroid
Lung	Urinary
Melanoma of the skin	Uterus

men and their health care providers an opportunity to discuss any changes in their breasts, risk factors, and early detection testing. CBE should be performed about every 3 years for women in their 20s and 30s and annually for women ages 40 and older.

Mammography screening has shown considerable evidence that it reduces mortality in women ages 50 to 74. Data regarding mammography in women under age 50, however, is controversial. Fifty isn't a magic number, but it does correspond to the approximate time of menopause. Premenopausal women have an increased density of breast tissue, which may influence the accuracy of mammography. The USPSTF, after review of the research, found evidence that mammography screening every 12 to 33 months significantly reduces mortality from breast cancer. The evidence is strongest for women ages 50 to 69, although most studies also indicate a mortality benefit for women ages 40 and 49. As a result of this review, the USPSTF recommends that women age 40 and older consider having screening mammography every 1 to 2 years. For low-risk women younger than age 40, screening mammography isn't recommended. For high-risk women (women with a strong family history) under age 40, screening mammography should be started between ages 30 and 35 or 10 years before the age at which a mother or sister was diagnosed.

Provider's role

In the past few years, preventive options have emerged that may decrease the risk of breast cancer specifically in women who are considered to be at high risk. Any woman whose risk assessment indicates an increased risk of breast cancer should be given information about the benefits and risks of breast cancer prevention therapies. Options that health care providers should discuss with all of their adult female patients include lifestyle change (such as diet, physical activity, and alcohol consumption) and chemoprevention (such as tamoxifen).

Cervical cancer

An estimated 13,000 cases of invasive cervical carcinoma were diagnosed in 2002, with more than 4,000 deaths occurring. As Pap screening has become more prevalent, an increase in the diagnosis of preinvasive cervical lesions and a decrease in the diagnosis of invasive carcinoma have occurred. Cervical cancer risk is closely linked to sexual behavior and to infection with certain types of HPV, a sexually transmitted disease. Women who have had many partners or have a partner who has had many partners, who initiated sex at an early age, who participate in unprotected sex, or who smoke tobacco are at increased risk for cervical cancer.

The Pap test is a simple procedure that involves collecting a small sample of cells from the exterior cervix and the endocervical canal and then smearing the sample onto a glass slide or placing it in a special solution for laboratory analysis. The traditional Pap test is associated with at least a 20% false-negative (negative with cancer actually present) result. Studies have shown that the use of liquid-based technologies, such as ThinPrep and AutoCyte Prep, improves detection rates.

A continuing controversy in cervical cancer screening is the frequency of testing. The ACS and the American College of Obstetricians and Gynecologists recommend initiation of screening 3 years after first vaginal intercourse. Virginal women should be counseled regarding risks and benefits of screening; however, cervical cancer is extremely rare in this group of women. If no recent history of an abnormal Pap exists, the screening recommendation is as follows: (1) if using liquid-based cytology, screen every 2 years until age 30, then every 2 to 3 years; or (2) if using conventional Pap tests, screen yearly until age 30, then every 2 to 3 years. The rationale for these recommendations is that the highest rates of high-grade squamous intraepithelial lesion (HSIL) occur in younger women, while HSIL is less common in women age 30 and older. The ACS also recommends that a Pap test be performed every 6 months for 1 year, then yearly if the woman is HIV positive or is immunocompromised by organ transplant, chemotherapy, or chronic steroid use, because the progression rates from HSIL to cancer is more rapid in immunocompromised women. In women age 70 and older with an intact cervix, three normal Pap tests, and no abnormal smears within 10 years before age 70, there's no need for further testing. Also, in women with a total hysterectomy for a benign condition (such as fibroid tumors of the uterus), there's no need for further testing. The current USPSTF recommendations state that cervical cytology screening should be performed every 3 years for sexually active women.

Because HPV has a strong link to cervical cancer in women, recently the FDA approved a new screening test. This test is performed at the same time as the regular Pap test and is used for women whose Pap results indicated atypical squamous cells of unknown origin (or ASC-US), an abnormality that can't be readily explained. The goal of this additional test is to help distinguish women at increased risk from those at extremely low risk of developing cervical cancer.

Provider's role

All adult female patients should be screened for cervical cancer. An important fact to remember is that the greatest risk of dying from this type of cancer is caused by the failure to be screened. Also, for women who are at risk for sexually transmitted infections, teach them that the best way to prevent cervical cancer is to always use a condom during sexual intercourse.

Endometrial cancer

In the United States, endometrial cancer is the most common malignant disease of the female genital tract. An estimated 39,300 cases were diagnosed in 2002, with 6,600 deaths occurring. The incidence rates are higher among White women when compared to Black women, although Black women have nearly twice the mortality rate. Abnormal uterine bleeding or spotting is an early symptom of endometrial cancer, while pelvic pain and mass and weight loss are symptoms that usually occur in later stages of the disease. High cumulative exposure to estrogen is the major risk factor for the development of endometrial cancer. Estrogen-related exposures include estrogen replacement therapy (without progestins), tamoxifen (a drug used for reducing the risk of breast cancer), early menarche, late menopause, nulliparity, and a history of failure to ovulate — all of which have been shown to increase the risk of endometrial cancer. Other risk factors include infertility, diabetes, gallbladder disease, hypertension, and obesity.

Provider's role

There's no recommended routine screening test for endometrial cancer. Most women are diagnosed because they have symptoms. Perform testing for endometrial cancer with an endometrial biopsy in the following women: women who experience postmenopausal bleeding; posmenopausal women with endometrial cells evident on the Pap test; women who chronically fail to ovulate and who present with heavy, irregular bleeding; and perimenopausal women with intermenstrual bleeding. It isn't necessary to perform an endometrial biopsy before initiating hormone replacement therapy or estrogen replacement therapy unless the woman is experiencing these signs and symptoms. With women on tamoxifen, routine screening isn't recommended for those who are asymptomatic.

Skin cancer

Skin cancer is the most common of all cancers. The ACS estimates that more than 1 million cases of highly curable basal cell or squamous cell cancer oc-

ABCDs of melanoma

A simple **ABCD** rule outlines the warning signals of melanoma:
A is for asymmetry: One-half of a mole or birthmark doesn't match the other.
B is for border: The edges are irregular, ragged, notched, or blurred.
C is for color: The pigmentation isn't uniform but may have varying degrees of brown or black, or sometimes red
D is for diameter greater than ¼": Any sudden or progressive increase in size should be of concern.

The most important warning sign for skin cancer is a spot on the skin that's changing in size, shape, or color. Other warning signs include a sore that doesn't heal, a new growth, the spread of pigment to surrounding skin, redness or new swelling beyond the border of a mole, change in sensation (itchiness, tenderness, or pain), and change in the surface of a mole (scaliness, oozing, bleeding, or the appearance of a bump or nodule).

cur annually. The most serious form of skin cancer, melanoma, was estimated to occur in about 53,600 individuals in 2002, with an estimated 9,600 deaths occurring. Melanoma occurs 10 times more often in Whites than in Blacks. Risk factors for skin cancer include excessive exposure to ultraviolet radiation; fair complexion; occupational exposure to coal tar, pitch, creosote, arsenic compounds, or radium; family history; and multiple or atypical moles.

Provider's role

Health care providers should instruct their patients to perform monthly skin self-examination as recommended by the ACS. Teach a patient that the best time to do this simple examination is after a bath or shower. Tell her to use a full-length mirror and a hand mirror to check her skin from head to toe. (See *ABCDs of melanoma.*) Perform a clinical examination every 3 years for patients between ages 20 and 40 and annually for those age 40 and older.

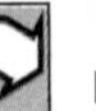

PREVENTION POINTER

Prevention of melanoma is key. Advise patients to limit or avoid exposure to the sun during the midday hours (10 a.m. to 4 p.m.). Caution patients, when they are outdoors, to cover as much skin as possible and use a sunscreen with a sun protection factor (SPF) of 15 or higher.

Diabetes

Each year, about 625,000 Americans are diagnosed with type 2 diabetes. Diabetes occurs in more than 50% of women. If undetected and untreated, it can lead to blindness, heart disease, kidney disease, nerve and blood vessel damage, and pregnancy-related problems. The American Diabetes Association recommends screening of adults for type 2 diabetes at 3-year intervals beginning at age 45. Screening at an earlier age and screening more frequently should be considered in patients with a BMI ≥ 25; who have a parent or sibling with type 2 diabetes; patients who are Black, Hispanic, or Native American (these ethnic groups are at increased risk for type 2 diabetes); patients who gave birth to a neonate weighing more than 9 lb (4.1 kg) or who developed gestational diabetes; patients who have high blood pressure; and patients who have an HDL ("good") cholesterol level of 35 or below and a blood triglyceride level of 250 or higher.

Provider's role

In addition to cancer screening, health care providers must monitor the diets of their adult female patients based on age and risk factors, such as family history or high BMI. A fasting plasma glucose test is the recommended screening test. A result of 126 mg/dl, repeated at least once, is a diagnosis for diabetes. The former ADA guidelines set the cutoff at 140 mg/dl. Yet current research now shows that serious adverse effects linked to diabetes begin with glucose levels in the mid-120s.

Cholesterol

Several studies have established that lowering cholesterol levels can reduce the incidence of coronary artery disease. Women's LDL cholesterol levels tend to rise with menopause, and HDL cholesterol levels are thought to play an important role in the development of heart disease in women.

Screening tests for cholesterol generally include total cholesterol, LDL cholesterol, and HDL cholesterol. LDLs carry cholesterol throughout the body, dropping it off where it can be used for cell metabolism. Cholesterol carried by LDL that isn't used, metabolized by the liver, or excreted may accumulate in the arterial walls and form plaques. Over time, plaques decrease the blood flow, a condition known as *atherosclerosis*, which increases the risk of blood clots. Conversely, HDLs circulate throughout the bloodstream, picking up cholesterol and bringing it back to the liver for reprocessing or excretion.

Provider's role

Health care providers should monitor the adult female patient for the risk of high cholesterol. Based on the USPSTF guidelines, it's strongly recommended that routine cholesterol screening (total cholesterol and HDL cholesterol) be performed every 5 years in women age 45 and older. Women ages 20 to 45 with risk factors for coronary heart disease (see "Heart disease" earlier in this chapter) should also be screened. To lower the risk of heart disease, the desirable level for total cholesterol should be less than 200 mg/dl and the level of HDL cholesterol should be greater than 40 mg/dl. If an LDL cholesterol level is also included, a level lower than 100 mg/dl is optimal. With cholesterol levels outside the normal range, cholesterol-lowering measures should be instituted.

Depression

Occurring twice as frequently in women as in men, depression is a common and serious psychiatric disorder. Major depression is one of the 15 leading causes of disability in industrialized countries and has been shown to increase the risk of morbidity and mortality in individuals with coronary heart disease. It's estimated that 15% of those diagnosed with severe depression will die by suicide. Mental illness of any type, including depression, still carries a powerful stigma and, as a result, usually goes underreported, underrecognized, and undertreated. It's safe to say that nearly everyone has experienced a transient, self-limited depressed mood, especially when related to an adverse life event. However, when no apparent reason for depression exists, these individuals are commonly thought of as self-indulgent, lazy, selfish, or ungrateful. Research has shown that women, when stressed, tend to brood about problems and internalize them (whereas men turn to external sources of distraction such as sports). It's suggested that this brooding and rumination tend to make depression worse in women.

Depression, whether triggered by life circumstances, by abrupt hormonal changes, or by no discernible cause, is associated with characteristic changes in the brain. These changes can be treated and reversed with psychotherapeutic and psychopharmacologic therapies. Difficulties in a relationship are commonly cited as a precipitant to a major depressive episode. Other factors that may bring about depression in women include single parenting, infertility, poverty, physical and sexual abuse, job discrimination, and chronic illness. Medications, such as certain cardiovascular drugs (thiazide diuretics) or anti-infective agents (sulfonamides) may also be associated with depression. (See *Diagnosing depression.*)

Provider's role

Generally, health care providers should treat mild to moderate depression in an adult female patient with psychotherapy or antidepressant medication, while a more severe depression is best treated with a combination of psychotherapy and medication. Psychotherapies that have been shown to be effective with depression include cognitive therapy, behavioral therapy, and interpersonal psychotherapy. Studies have shown that all prescription antidepressants available have statistically equal effectiveness in treating depression, although the selective serotonin reuptake inhibitors, such as fluoxetine (Prozac) and paroxetine (Paxil), cause fewer adverse effects than the older tricyclic antidepressants (TCAs) such as amitriptyline (Elavil). Antidepressant medication should be continued for at least 9 to 12 months. Some evidence exists that supports their use for 1 to 2 years. Consider long-term antidepressant medication in patients with three or more previous episodes of major depression.

Diagnosing depression

Depression is diagnosed when the patient experiences five of the following symptoms every day and lasting most of the day for at least 2 weeks:

- sad or irritable mood, weeping
- changes in appetite and weight (typically, both are reduced)
- changes in sleep (typically, early-morning awakening without feeling rested)
- loss of energy
- difficulty concentrating
- psychomotor slowing or agitation
- feelings of helplessness and hopelessness
- feelings of worthlessness and guilt
- thoughts of death or suicide.

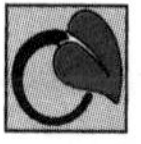

ALTERNATIVE THERAPIES

An alternative treatment option to traditional therapy for depression is the herb St. John's wort. There has been a significant amount of evidence indicating that it's effective in treating mild to moderate depression, equal to the effectiveness of TCAs but with fewer adverse effects. However, recent clinical trial results found that St. John's wort was no more effective than a placebo. Adverse effects associated with St. John's wort are generally mild and include GI symptoms and fatigue. This herb shouldn't be taken with other antidepressant medications.

Domestic violence

Domestic violence, or intimate-partner violence, is the leading cause of injury to women in the United States. Affecting 1 to 4 million women each year, it's responsible for approximately 30% of female murders. Despite the prevalence of domestic violence and the potential for fatality, this health hazard is commonly overlooked. Domestic violence not only involves physical abuse but is also intertwined with psychological and sexual abuse. (See *Understanding types of abuse*, page 106.) The aim of the violence is to assert control and power. Neither the batterer nor the victim fits a distinct personality or socioeconomic profile; rather, battering is considered a set of learned, controlling behaviors and attitudes. Most batterers are verbally abusive between violent episodes; this abuse alone can indicate domestic violence. Although all women are at risk for domestic abuse, a history of alcohol or substance abuse and mental illness in either partner has been correlated with increased risk of domestic violence. A major risk factor is pregnancy. For many women, the abuse starts during pregnancy; for women with a prior history of partner abuse, the violence commonly escalates during this time.

UNDERSTANDING TYPES OF ABUSE

- **Physical:** includes slapping, pushing, hitting, kicking, biting, or punching
- **Emotional:** involves name-calling, insulting, and degradation, especially in public
- **Sexual:** can be in the form of rape or forcible sexual contact
- **Threats:** occur with statements such as "If you don't . . . I'll kill you."
- **Intimidation:** involves gestures, looks, destroying property, and causing fear
- **Isolation:** can be in the form of keeping the victim from seeing or talking to others, especially family members; not allowing her to go out by herself; and forcing her to account for her whereabouts every single minute
- **Economic:** putting restraints on the victim by giving her a money allowance or not allowing her to work

Provider's role

Health care providers should look for obvious signs of abuse, including multiple injuries that are centrally located, bruises at different stages of healing, and evidence of sexual assault. Injured genitalia, breasts, or abdomens are especially common in abused pregnant women. Many times, however, the signs and symptoms of abuse aren't so obvious. Look for vague or chronic symptoms, such as headaches, abdominal or pelvic pain, fatigue, and shortness of breath, which are present in many abused women. Also, screen the female patient for eating disorders, depression, and anxiety, which are common in abused women. (See *Screening females for domestic violence.*)

Women who hesitate to admit to experiencing domestic violence may feel shame, guilt, and fear. When abuse is detected, it shouldn't be ignored. The health care provider needs to acknowledge the problem and take it seriously. Assess the level of danger that the woman might be facing. Encourage the abused woman to develop a safety plan, and have information about local shelters and hotlines available. The safety plan may include teaching her children to dial 911 during an emergency, keeping extra items (such as clothes and car keys) with a friend or family member, hiding money in an accessible place, and opening a personal bank account.

A woman who discloses abuse may not necessarily be ready to leave the relationship. Financial concerns, religious beliefs, children, and both love and fear of the partner may make it difficult for her to leave. The greatest risk of severe injury or death typically exists when the woman expresses her intentions to leave the abuser and after she leaves the situation.

It's crucial for health care providers to document evidence of domestic violence. Describe and document symptoms and wounds and the

Screening females for domestic violence

Routine screening for domestic violence should be a part of all patient–health care provider visits. Three simple questions during an annual examination can elicit important information about abuse. Ask the female patient: How is your home situation? Do you feel safe? Has your partner ever hurt you in any way?

Answers to these questions may reveal domestic abuse, which should be acknowledged and taken seriously. The female patient may feel guilt, shame, and fear. It's your role to document the abuse and offer help in the form of referrals for assistance or resources for her to contact.

circumstances of an assault in vivid terms based on the woman's own words. Identify the perpetrator by name and relationship to the victim in the documentation. Also, document conversations about abuse as well as referrals for assistance or recommended resources.

If violence against an elderly person (age 60 or older), a child younger than age 18, or a disabled person has occurred, or if you uncover a sexual assault, the incident must be reported to state authorities. California, Utah, and Colorado require the mandatory reporting of all cases of intimate-partner abuse.

Assessing and caring for the adult female

A complete assessment includes a health history, physical examination, and appropriate laboratory tests. The time of the assessment is also an excellent opportunity for teaching and counseling.

The components of a complete health history include obtaining demographic and biographical information; the reason for the visit; the past medical and surgical history, including obstetric and contraceptive history; family history; psychosocial history; and a review of systems that includes a thorough past and present history of each. The history should also include a nutritional assessment, fitness assessment, occupational assessment, and stress assessment. (See *Prevention assessment in the adult female*, page 108.)

The second component of an in-depth assessment involves the physical examination. The tools of assessment — inspection, palpation, percussion, and auscultation — are used to evaluate each body system. Before the examination, explain all procedures and ensure privacy. The examination should be gentle, systematic, and sensitive to the patient's needs in such ways as helping to move her from a lying position to a sitting position. The minimum examination should in-

Prevention assessment in the adult female

Nutrition assessment: Have the patient describe a 24-hour diet recall of food and drink intake, which helps to determine the balance and adequacy of nutrients. It helps to correlate diet patterns with other history, physical examination, and diagnostic test findings — for example, high fat intake may be correlated with obesity and elevated cholesterol levels.

Fitness assessment: Assess whether the patient's intensity and duration of physical activity is sufficient to meet therapeutic cardiovascular levels. Healthy women should participate in an aerobic activity for a minimum of 30 minutes every day.

Occupational assessment: Ask the patient about the type and duration of her work, environmental risks (such as exposure to toxins, chemicals, or excessive heat or cold), and work-related stress, all of which have an overall effect on her health and wellness. For example, exposure to asbestos can lead to chronic lung disease. Determining environmental exposures is especially important for pregnant women.

Stress assessment: Assess the patient's stress level. Signs of excessive stress, such as mood swings, disposition changes, and physical signs and symptoms, often are correlated with other assessment findings, such as sleep, appearance, nutrition, use of medications, and substance abuse.

clude assessment of blood pressure, height and weight, lymph nodes, thyroid, heart, lungs, breasts, abdomen, extremities, and the pelvic examination. For women over age 40, a rectal examination should also be included. Timing of the examination is also critical — for example, changes in the size, nodularity, and tenderness of the breasts occur related to hormonal changes in the menstrual cycle. Therefore, breast examination may need to be repeated after the end of the woman's menstrual cycle.

The third component of assessment is performing routine screening tests, including the Pap test, a gonorrhea and chlamydia screening, mammography, hematocrit and hemoglobin, fasting plasma glucose, cholesterol and lipids, stool hemoccult, urinalysis, endometrial sampling, and thyroid testing. The decision to perform each of these tests depends on the patient's age, lifestyle, and presence of risk factors.

The annual examination is also an excellent time to update immunizations, if needed. A tetanus-diphtheria booster is recommended every 10 years. Relatively few cases of tetanus occur in the United States; however, the disease, which is commonly fatal, can develop after even a minor wound or scratch in adults who aren't immunized. Hepatitis B vaccination also should be considered in any adult at high risk, including health care workers who are exposed to blood or blood products, injection drug users, people with a history of sexual contact with multiple partners, and people with STDs.

Communicating with the adult female

As her health care provider, remember that the adult female patient commonly serves as her family's caregiver, providing care for her children, grandchildren, or even elderly parents. Knowing that a woman may be in charge of making the health care decisions for more people than just herself makes establishing the line of communication even more important during her visit. Traditionally, women have more physician visits per year than do men. This stems from their reproductive needs, their tendency to seek help for problems, and their higher risk of depression. Consequently, health care providers see adult females more often and need to learn to communicate effectively with them and help them to become more comfortable with talking openly. Women may seek more information about their own and their family's health and medications. They may intend to ask more questions, but given the competing priorities on their time, they may hesitate to get the answers they need if they can't be obtained quickly. Keep this in mind to ensure that the female patient receives the proper answers and direction necessary for her health and well-being and that of her family.

In a 1998 study by researchers at the Mayo Clinic, 57% of patients were females while 74% of physicians were male. The study found that the communication between a male physician and his patient during a routine office visit runs more smoothly if that patient is also male. It also found that "failures [of physicians] to identify the patient's main reason for the visit occurred more frequently in female patients." Another study found that female physicians tended to have longer visits with their patients and were more "patient-centered" than male physicians. Because women are such a central focus as primary caretakers, health care providers — male and female alike, nurses and physicians — must learn to communicate effectively with their female patients.

Selected references

ACS News Center. (2003, March). "FDA Approves New Cervical Cancer Screening Test: Test for HPV Now Combined with Pap Smear" [Online]. Available: *www.cancer.org* [accessed May 27, 2003].

Aflalo-Calderon, B. (2002). "HRT, Women, and Heart Disease: What We Need to Know About Prevention," *Heartbytes* [Online]. Available: *www.medscape.com/viewarticle/440744.* [accessed October 15, 2002].

American Cancer Society. Cancer Facts and Figures 2003 [Brochure]. Atlanta: American Cancer Society 2003.

American Cancer Society. (n.d.). "Detecting Skin Cancer" [Online]. Available: *www.cancer.org* [accessed May 27, 2003].

American Cancer Society. (n.d.). "How Is Endometrial Cancer Diagnosed?" [Online]. Available: *www.cancer.org* [accessed May 27, 2003].

American Cancer Society. (n.d.). "What Are the Risk Factors for Cervical Cancer?"

[Online]. Available: *www.cancer.org*. [accessed May 27, 2003].

American Cancer Society. (n.d.). "What Are the Risk Factors for Endometrial Cancer?" [Online]. Available: *www.cancer.org* [accessed May 27, 2003].

American Heart Association. (2002). "Physical Activity in Your Daily Life; Tips for Exercise Success; Physical Activity and Cardiovascular Health Fact Sheet; Body Composition Tests; Physical Activity Calorie Use Chart" [Online]. Available: *www.americanheart.org/presenter.jhtml?identifier=2155* [accessed May 16, 2003].

Asher, J., et al. "Detection and Treatment of Domestic Violence," *Contemporary OB/GYN* 9:61-71, September 2001.

Bessesen, D., and Kushner, R. *Evaluation and Management of Obesity*. Philadelphia: Hanley & Belfus, Inc., 2002.

Breslin, E.T., and Lucas, V.A. (eds). *Women's Health Nursing Toward Evidence-Based Practice*. St. Louis: W.B. Saunders Co., Elsevier Science, 2003.

Brown, G.B., et al. "Antioxidant Vitamins and Lipid Therapy: End of a Long Romance?" [Online]. *Arteriosclerosis, Thrombosis, and Vascular Biology: Journal of American Heart Association* 22(10):1535-46, October 2002.

Byers, T., et al. "American Cancer Society Guidelines on Nutrition and Physical Activity for Cancer Prevention: Reducing the Risk of Cancer with Healthy Food Choices and Physical Activity," *CA A Cancer Journal for Clinicians* 52(2):62-119, March/April 2002.

Cahill, CA. "Women and Stress," *Annual Review of Nursing Research* 19:229-48, 2001.

Carlson, K.J., et al. (eds.). *Primary Care of Women*, 2nd ed. St. Louis: Mosby Year–Book, Inc., 2002.

Chobanian, A.V., et al. "The Seventh Report of the Joint National Committee on Prevention, Detection, Evaluation, and Treatment of High Blood Pressure," *JAMA* 289(19): 2560-72, May 2003.

Collins, A. (2000-2003). "Vegetarian Diet Nutrition: Dietary Guidelines, Vegetarian & Vegan Nutrition Advice" [Online]. Available:*www.annecollins.com/vegetarian-diet-nutrition.html* [accessed May 18, 2003].

Committee Opinion No. 267. "Exercise During Pregnancy and the Postpartum Period," *Clinical Obstetrics and Gynecology* 46(2):496-99, June 2003.

Cunningham, F.G., et al. (eds.). *Williams Obstetrics*, 21st ed. New York: McGraw-Hill Book Co., 2001.

DeCherney, A.H., and Nathan, L. *Current Obstetric & Gynecologic Diagnosis & Treatment*, 9th ed. New York: Lange Medical Books, 2003.

Fleming, M. *Identification of At-Risk Drinking and Intervention with Women of Childbearing Age: A Guide for Primary-Care Providers*. Bethesda, Md.: National Institute on Alcohol Abuse and Alcoholism Publication Distribution Center, 1999.

Fugh-Berman, A., and Cott, J.M. "Dietary Supplements and Natural Products as Psychotherapeutic Agents" [Online]. *Psychosomatic Media* 61(5):712, September-October 1999.

Gerard, M. "Domestic Violence: How to Screen and Intervene," *RN* 63(12):53-56, December 2000.

Hu, Frank B. "Overweight and Obesity in Women: Health Risks and Consequences," *Journal of Women's Health* 12(2):163-72, 2003. [Online]. Available: *www.medscape.com/viewarticle/452831* [accessed May 22, 2003].

Klauer, J., and Aronne, L.J. "Managing Overweight and Obesity in Women," *Clinical Obstetrics and Gynecology* 45(4):1080-88, December 2002. [Online]

O'Meara, A.T. "Present Standards for Cervical Cancer Screening [Gynecologic Cancer]," *Current Opinion in Oncology* 14(5):505-11, 2002.

Speroff, L., and Darney, P.D. *A Clinical Guide for Contraception*, 3rd ed. Philadelphia: Lippincott Williams & Wilkins, 2001.

Stotland, N.L., and Stotland, N.E. "Focus on Primary Care: Depression in Women," *Obstetrical & Gynecological Survey* 54(8):529-25, August 1999. [Online]

Swartzberg, J.E., and Margen, S. *The UC Berkeley Wellness Self-Care Handbook: The Everyday Guide to Prevention and Home Remedies.* New York: Rebus Inc., 1998

United States National Academy of Sciences, National Research Council. "Vegetarianism: Nutritional Guidelines," 1997. Available: *www.nutrition.cornell.edu/foodguide/guidelin.html* [accessed May 18, 2003].

Wenger, N.K., et al. (2003). "The Importance of Identifying and Reducing Cardiovascular Risk Factors in Women" [Online]. *Medscape from WebMD.* Available: *www.medscape.com/viewprogram/2223_pnt* [accessed May 20, 2003].

CHAPTER 4

Health promotion and illness prevention in the older adult female

Overview

Midlife, generally considered to be the years from ages 45 to 64, is an important phase in a woman's life. During this time, the "perimenopausal-menopausal transition" takes place, marking a major passage for women when their childbearing years come to an end. In the United States today, an unprecedented number of women are reaching midlife. For this group, an ever-increasing life expectancy has underscored the importance of promoting health and preventing disease. However, at the same time, health care professionals who work with this growing segment of the population have the unique opportunity to focus on the special needs of these aging women while making a significant impact on the public's health.

The middle years typically represent some of the most challenging and rewarding of a woman's life. For many, by this time childbearing and child rearing have been largely completed, and they're "free" to pursue other interests, such as career, travel, hobbies, or education. As women move beyond their responsibilities as parents, they commonly approach this period of life with a renewed energy and eagerness as they embrace the opportunity to develop new interests and focus on their personal growth and interpersonal relationships.

Midlife is also a time in which many women experience major life situations that demand considerable energy and resources. Aging parents, struggles with loneliness, and self-concept issues impacted by a media-driven society that's obsessed with "staying young" are just a few issues that women face. However, current trends suggest a resurgence of focus on women in midlife. Today, more than ever, the health care arena is embracing this developmental time in a woman's life, offering more educational programs and strategies she'll need to care for herself and her family.

During midlife, women commonly seek health care advice in dealing with myriad physical changes and hormonally linked symptoms they're experiencing. Although usually equipped with many strengths, including a wealth of life experiences, the motivation for learning, and an interest in gaining health promotion strategies to improve their well-being, women face the daunting challenge of sifting through information accessible through the Internet and other media sources. They may become overwhelmed or confused by the extensive health care options — as well as opinions — available and seek guidance concerning such issues as hormone replacement therapy, complementary and alternative therapies, and stress management.

Overview of the older adult female

Commonly termed the "mature years," this time in a woman's life offers opportunities for happiness and self-actualization along with challenges for achieving and maintaining optimal health through wellness-focused activities and lifestyle choices. The Administration on Aging reports that the most rapidly growing age-group in the United States consists of persons age 65 and older, three out of five of which are women. Subsequently, the fastest growing subgroup comprises individuals over age 85. To put this into perspective, in 1995 there were 3.6 million persons in America age 85 and older. By the year 2040, an estimated more than 12 million people will be age 85 and older, and by 2050, an estimated two-thirds of all Americans age 85 and older will be women.

It has been documented that the older adult female focuses more on how she feels rather than her state of physical health, the extent of her medical problems, or her ability to carry out activities of daily living. In 1995, researchers met with a group of elderly women whose ages ranged from 70 to 91 and asked them this question: "What does being healthy mean to you?" Their findings revealed the following: "Health involves the appreciation of life, experiencing joy, and happiness. To be free from sickness doesn't guarantee health. Likewise, health can be experienced despite chronic illness and disability, because being healthy is a philosophy or way of living."

For older adult females, health care focuses on maximizing independence, vigor, and life satisfaction. Strategies for health promotion among this age-group are essential to prevent complications and decrease the risks that adversely affect quality of life. Older adult females must receive proper education for health promotion and illness prevention that's tailored to address the physical, sensory, mobility, sexual, and psychosocial changes that accompany the aging process. The goal for females age 65 and older is to maintain independence and physical activity, which frequently boosts self-esteem, decreases depression and anxiety, and enhances overall well-being and quality of life.

Health promotion

In the past, little attention was given to promoting health among adult female patients. However, with the increasing number of women reaching midlife and living well into the 9th and 10th decades of life, renewed interest has occurred in the development of programs designed for this growing population.

As women age, their risk of developing certain disorders increases. Health promotion in the form of diet, exercise, nutrition, and stress management, along with screening and early detection, are crucial to a woman's health. The most important determinant of a woman's health is the woman herself; by making smart decisions in partnership with her health care provider, she can change her well-being and the overall quality of her life.

It's also important to point out that, according to the Administration on Aging, although health prevention, screening, and early detection are the cornerstones to women's health, high out-of-pocket costs and a lack of information about their potential benefits prevent two-thirds of older women from taking advantage of the many preventive health services available.

Morbidity and mortality

During midlife, women may experience their first chronic illness. Many of the health conditions that commonly occur first during these years foreshadow future problems that may be associated with significant morbidity and mortality as women age. Heart disease — the leading cause of death in women — is responsible for more deaths than breast, ovarian, and uterine cancers combined. According to the Society for Women's Health Research, as a woman approaches menopause, her risk of heart disease parallels a man's risk.

For middle-age to older women, the leading causes of death continue to be heart disease, cerebrovascular disease, malignant neoplasms, chronic obstructive lung disease, liver disease, influenza and pneumonia, accidents, diabetes, suicide, and homicide. The National Center for Health Statistics reports that during the middle and later years, more than 10% of women experience various chronic conditions, including arthritis, hypertension, chronic sinusitis, skeletal deformity or orthopedic impairment, and heart disease. Women suffer more disability as they grow older than do men, and their major reasons for hospitalization are heart disease, malignant neoplasms, cholelithiasis, benign neoplasms, psychoses, and diabetes.

During the middle and older years, females face three major risk factors for significant morbidity and mortality: smoking, sedentary lifestyle, and inadequate nutrition. Avoiding or ceasing risky behaviors linked to health problems is the key to prevention for women of all ages. Traditionally, women are the primary caregivers and health care decision makers for their families, so by engaging in preventive activities, not only do they reap the benefits themselves, but so do their families. Stopping smoking, modifying the diet, maintaining ideal body weight, and getting regular exercise will have the greatest effects on reducing the incidence of death and disease in women.

Smoking

It has been well documented that smoking is associated with a number of health conditions, including lung cancer, coronary artery disease, cerebrovascular disease, peripheral vascular disease, cervical cancer, hypertension, osteoporosis, various respiratory diseases, and accidents and injuries stemming from fires caused by an unattended lighted cigarette.

According to the Report of the Surgeon General published by the Centers for Disease Control and Prevention, from ages 45 to 74, a woman's annual risk for death more than doubles among continuing smokers compared to persons who have never smoked. In this age-group, postmenopausal women who currently smoke also have lower bone density than women who don't smoke. Over time, smoking decreases a woman's level of estrogen, putting her at risk for osteoporosis and thereby increasing the incidence of hip fractures.

Exercise and fitness

Exercise contributes to good health in a variety of ways. Consistent physical activity can lower the risk of a number of conditions that are influenced by obesity and a sedentary lifestyle. Exercise helps prevent or delay age-related illnesses, such as cardiovascular disease, and is therapeutic in managing such chronic conditions as hypertension, arthritis, diabetes, respiratory disorders, and osteoporosis. In addition to helping women maintain a desirable weight, exercise helps promote stress reduction and an overall sense of well-being. Physical activity — even assisting with household chores — not only enhances body functioning but also promotes a sense of self-worth by providing an outlet for productivity. It also improves body image, boosts self-esteem, and elevates overall mood. Lack of exercise can produce such psychological effects as decreased mental stimulation, increased feelings of hopelessness, depression,

Hazards of inactivity for the older adult female

Increasing the activity level of older women may be challenging because of medical conditions, including muscle pain, joint pain, fatigue, and other symptoms associated with various health problems common in later life. However, the hazards of a sedentary lifestyle are particularly harmful, especially for older women.

Physiologic effects	Complications
Decreased blood flow	▪ Postural hypotension, hypertension, hyperlipidemia
Decreased chest expansion and ventilation	▪ Hypostatic pneumonia, respiratory infections
Reduced muscle strength, tone, and endurance	▪ Arthritis, joint stiffness, weakness, fatigue
Demineralization of bones	▪ Fractures and falls (increased risk)
Slow GI motility	▪ Constipation, poor appetite
Slow metabolism	▪ Weight gain, obesity
Poor skin turgor	▪ Pressure ulcers

increased dependency, isolation, reduced opportunities for socialization, and low self-esteem. (See *Hazards of inactivity in the older adult female.*)

Various exercises are beneficial for middle-age to older women. Aerobic activities, which increase the amount of oxygen delivered to the muscles, provide cardiovascular improvement. Anaerobic exercise, such as weight training, improves individual muscle mass without placing stress on the cardiovascular system and increases caloric expenditure. Because of the concern about cardiovascular and bone health, weight-bearing aerobic activities, such as walking, are ideal. Through regular exercise, women can improve their sense of well-being while strengthening and toning muscles, building endurance, and improving balance, all of which lessen their likelihood of injuries and falls.

As women age, their limitations on activity level increase. In 2001, women age 45 and older were twice as likely to report activity limitations as females ages 18 to 45, and they had the highest rate of activity limitations. Some older women may hesitate to initiate or adhere to an exercise program because they fear injury. Others may worry about exacerbating a current medical condition, disability,

Exercise guidelines for older females

Before initiating an exercise program for the older female adult, first, perform a physical examination to detect any conditions that could adversely affect or be affected by the exercise program (such as heart disease or stroke). Then, consult a physician about the appropriateness of the exercise program. Finally, discuss the following guidelines with the patient to prevent injuries or falls and to maximize the benefits of her exercise program:

- Assess the patient's current activity level, range of motion, muscle strength and tone, and response to physical activity; modify the exercise program based on these factors.
- Develop an exercise program that matches her interests, hobbies, abilities, and limitations; make it one that she can realistically master.
- Plan a wide range of activities, such as brisk walking, dancing, swimming, aerobic exercises, or bicycling; focus on exercises with good speed and rhythm.
- To prevent trauma, avoid recommending exercises (such as running and jumping) that require resistance, produce stress on an immobilized joint, or cause strain or stress on the joints; older females are prone to fractures.
- Pace the exercise program throughout the day, if she tires easily.
- Encourage her to wear proper-fitting, shock-absorbing shoes with traction soles to prevent blisters, joint pain, and falls.
- Have her perform warm-up exercises and gentle stretching for at least 10 minutes immediately before exercising.
- Begin her exercise program gradually, and increase the activity level according to her tolerance.
- Tell her to allow herself plenty of time for exercise because it may take longer for her to perform it.
- Ensure that she allows for a cooling-down period; it may take longer for her to cool down.
- Caution her to stop and immediately contact her physician if she has any shortness of breath, dizziness, fainting, chest pains, or palpitations.

or sensory impairment. The four most common conditions reported by these women as causing activity limitation are arthritis, back and neck problems, heart problems, and hypertension.

Provider's role

Health care providers should address a woman's personal beliefs and concerns about exercise. Strategies to help promote exercise in this age-group include encouraging a woman to find a companion when engaging in physical activities, finding out whether she has proper transportation to participate in an exercise program, building on her prior activity habits, and tapping into her existing skills.

When creating an exercise program with older women, health care providers should choose a program that best matches the individual's needs, interests, and ability. (See *Exercise guidelines for older females.*) Although physical activity and exercise are beneficial, they can also be harmful if not individualized for the older female's age, health, and physical limitations. Many factors — such as underlying diseases, fragility, altered balance, poor vision, and use of certain medications — can contribute to injuries and falls. Discuss exercise guidelines and household safety tips to prevent injuries and falls and to maximize the exercise program.

SPECIAL NEEDS

Compared with the general population, older women with disabilities and chronic illnesses are less likely to exercise. Address these disabilities and illnesses before developing an individualized physical activity program. Diminished bone mineral density caused by the long-term use of steroids for such conditions as lupus erythematosus or arthritis; decreased bone mass caused by osteoporosis; joint instability and pain from scoliosis or arthritis; and elasticity and decreased blood supply caused by menopausal skin changes all may put older women at risk for fractures, joint pain, and skin breakdown. Physical activities such as those performed in a swimming pool may be more desirable than such exercises as walking or weight training.

Nutrition

Nutrition plays a vital role in the health of women of all ages. It's one area of a woman's life that, for the most part, can be readily modified to reduce risks of certain chronic diseases. Nutritional assessment and counseling remains a cornerstone of effective health promotion. *Healthy People 2010*, the national health initiative, identified the following two broad goals for Americans: to increase the quality and years of healthy life and to eliminate health disparities.

Nutrition is particularly significant to women across their life span. Promoting health and preventing chronic disease are associated with a person's diet and body weight, which can help prevent some of the 10 leading causes of death for middle-age and older females — including heart disease, cancer, stroke, diabetes mellitus, kidney disease, chronic liver disease, and cirrhosis. Osteoporosis, another disability particularly significant to women, is associated with a lifelong dietary deficiency of calcium. Diets high in animal fats and low in fruits and vegetables have been associated with colon cancer, in addition to a sedentary lifestyle and obesity. An increased body mass index and excessive weight gain are associated with diabetes mellitus, which is a risk factor for coronary artery disease. Also, obesity is linked directly to acute coronary syndrome in women.

Despite the information available about proper nutrition, eating habits haven't necessarily improved. An individual's food preferences are the result of a complex process that develops over a lifetime. The food habits of Americans are as diverse as the country's ethnic and cultural groups. Each ethnic group in the United States has its own culturally based foods and food habits.

Many cultural factors influence diet. Dietary habits are shaped by global events, such as food production and distribution systems, as well as by personal lifestyle factors, such as income, occupation, nutritional knowledge, health, religious beliefs, education, rural or urban residence, and ethnic identity.

SPECIAL NEEDS

When working with women of diverse ethnic backgrounds, health care providers should have an understanding of specific food preferences and common methods of preparation. For example, many Mexican people living in this country eat a diet similar to the traditional diet of their homeland. Customary foods include eggs, beans, or meat and tortillas or pan dulce for breakfast. Lunch, typically a large meal, may consist of beans, tortillas, and meat, or a soup or stew; dinner may be a lighter meal of tortillas, beans or meat, and rice or potatoes. Fruits, such as bananas, oranges, mangoes, guava, pineapple, strawberries, and melon, are generally preferred as a snack or dessert. Because the adult female typically prepares meals for herself and her family, she may not be aware of the alternatives to health food preparation. Recent immigrants may not know how to prepare canned or frozen foods and may choose instead to grill and fry foods rather than bake or broil them.

Provider's role

When planning nutrition for middle-age to older adults, health care providers should consider that physiologic and psychological characteristics (age, gender, perceived body image, and state of health) strongly influence personal food habits. As women age, their food preferences and their ability to consume and digest foods change. Metabolism slows down, and caloric needs decrease. Older women may discover that their tolerance for fatty or highly spiced foods has diminished. Some may also find purchasing, selecting, preparing, or eating healthy foods difficult.

Health care providers should also consider an older woman's state of health, living situation, and economic situation, all of which influence her nutritional intake. For example, chronic diseases (such as diabetes) require restriction of certain foods. An individual who's sick may not be hungry or may find preparing or eating nourishing food difficult. Older women also may have difficulty chewing because of tooth loss, poor-fitting dentures, or simply the loss of taste buds, which makes eating unpalatable. Women living alone may decide that food preparation for only one requires too much energy and isn't worth the effort. Some women living on Social Security may have poor nutritional intake because they may not be able to afford healthy foods.

As women age, the nutrients needed to maintain optimal nutritional status remain high, but caloric needs decrease because of diminished activity levels and lowered metabolic rates. An older female's diet should be dense in nutrients to provide the essential components of foods with fewer calories. As is true with younger women, older women benefit from a diet consisting of fruits and vegetables, low-fat meats, fortified dairy products, and enriched and fortified high-fiber

Special Nutrient Needs for Older Females

Calcium
Recommended daily allowance (RDA): 1,200 mg
Sources: nonfat dairy products (milk, yogurt, cheese), leafy, green vegetables (spinach, collard greens, broccoli)

Vitamin D
RDA: 400 International Units (IU) for adult females ages 51 to 70; 600 IU for those over age 70.
Sources: sunlight; vitamin D–fortified nonfat or low-fat milk

Vitamin B_{12}
RDA: 2.4 mcg
Sources: vitamin B_{12}–fortified foods (breakfast cereals), fermented miso, milk, yogurt, fish, vitamin B_{12} supplements

breads and cereals. Because fats, sweets, and alcohol are high in calories but low in essential nutrients, their consumption should be limited. On average, the older woman needs about 1,600 calories per day. The older female also has special needs for calcium, vitamin D, and vitamin B_{12} to keep bones strong. (See *Special nutrient needs for older females.*)

For help in selecting proper nutritional choices for female patients, the Food Guide Pyramid provides a graphic illustration of the adequate daily number of servings from various food groups. It emphasizes balance, moderation, and variety in foods that meet the recommended daily allowances and Dietary Reference Intakes. The pyramid can be modified to meet women's ethnic preferences by using foods customary to their culture.

Researchers at Tufts University developed a new Food Guide Pyramid for Older Adults, which they believe more accurately reflects the nutritional needs of healthy adults age 50 and older, with a particular focus on those age 70 and older. That pyramid limits saturated fats across all populations to protect against heart disease. For women age 50 and older, the newly modified food guide pyramid adds eight servings of water to the base of the pyramid (to reduce the risk of dehydration caused by a decreased sense of thirst, common in older adults), increases dairy servings to three (rather than two) per day, and recommends calcium, vitamin D, and vitamin B_{12} supplements. (See *Food Guide Pyramid for Older Adults.*) The new recommended daily allowances for vitamin B_{12} specify that fortified foods or supplements provide most of this vitamin for persons age 50 and older.

Researchers have recently reported that a high intake of refined carbohydrates, such as white bread and white rice, can create significant problems with the body's glucose and insulin levels. Replacing refined carbohydrates with monounsaturated or polyunsaturated "healthy" fats is believed to lower the risk of heart disease. Nutritionists have since proposed a new food pyramid that encourages the consumption of healthy

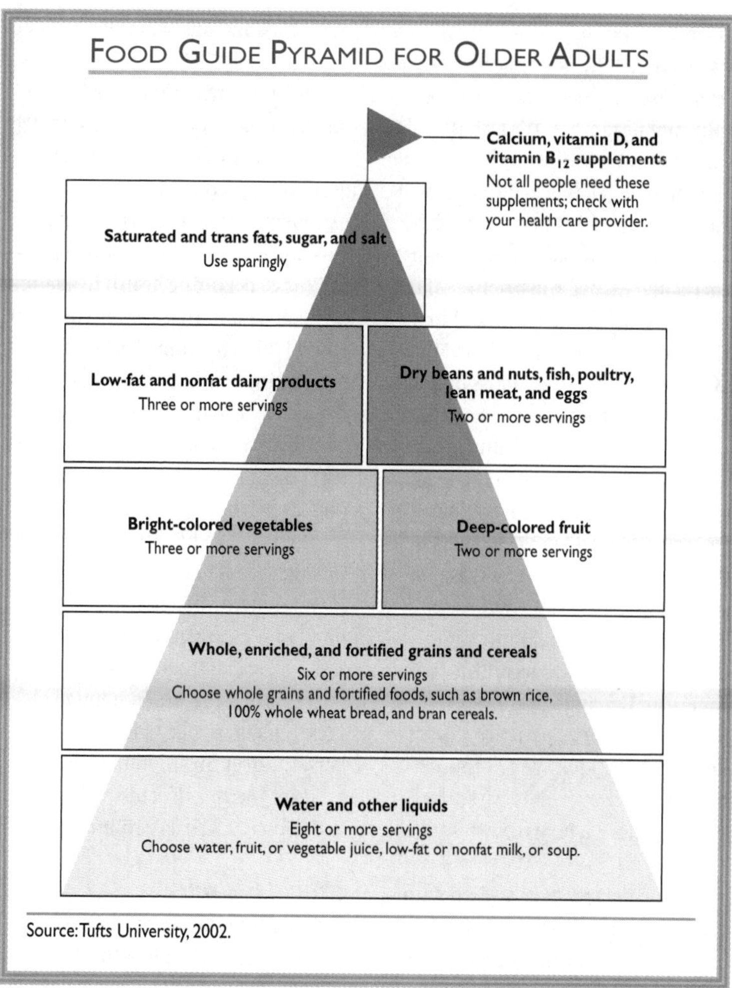

Source: Tufts University, 2002.

fats and whole-grain foods while avoiding refined carbohydrates, butter, and red meat. The U.S. Department of Agriculture's Center for Nutrition Policy and Promotion is currently reassessing the Food Guide Pyramid, which will be published in 2005.

Stress reduction

Stress is a complex, dynamic process that combines periods of "ups and downs" with periods of recovery. Usually, it causes no permanent adverse effects; however, chronic stress — stress without any recovery period — can cause problems. Chronic stress is associated with diminished life satisfaction, the development of mental disorders, and the appearance of such stress-related illnesses as cardiovascular disease, GI disorders, low back pain, and headaches. It's also linked to a reduced functioning of the immune system, which has been implicated in the development of cancer. Stress of even short duration is believed to produce a heightened constriction of the cardiac vessels, which can lead to high blood pressure, decreased blood flow to the heart muscle, and loss of normal heart rhythm.

Many social factors influence a woman's experience of stress, which, in turn, influences her overall health and sense of well-being. Social isolation has been shown to increase the risk of heart disease as well as the likelihood of survival following a heart attack. In fact, according to the American Psychological Association, individuals who experience a heart attack and live alone are 1.5 times more likely to have a second heart attack than are those who live with someone else.

While the stress associated with young adulthood generally diminishes with advancing age, other sources of stress become more prevalent as one ages. Some middle-age women may experience "empty nest syndrome" when grown children leave the home; others may be "sandwiched" between caring for an older relative while raising children or grandchildren. Caregiving takes a tremendous toll on the adult female. In addition, middle-age women are remaining in the workforce longer, making the role of caregiver a difficult one to balance and one that causes undue stresses.

Older women are particularly vulnerable to stressful life events, which tend to occur in the later years. The death of a spouse or a close family member (particularly one's own parents and even a child), personal injury or illness, declining health in a family member, and retirement are common among this age-group. Difficulty in performing routine activities of daily living may occur because of diminished sensory acuity, decreased dexterity and strength, loss of flexibility, or increased fatigue. Older women may begin to neglect positive health behaviors that would otherwise enhance their strength and resilience, such as proper nutrition, physical activity, rest, and social interaction. As the stressors of daily life compound, depression may strike, which can adversely affect the immune system and increase the risk of acute and chronic infections as well as chronic disease.

Provider's role

Health care providers must pay special attention when helping middle-age to older women reduce their stress levels. Accumulated stress associated with the hassles of daily living and major life events commonly translates into an increased morbidity and mortality during old age, especially when an individual already has poor coping methods. Stress produces systemic effects on the cardiovascular, GI, neurologic, endocrine, and immune systems. Because of their increased vulnerability to disease, it's important to help older women use existing coping mechanisms effectively or to teach them new coping strategies.

Employ techniques that will increase the woman's resistance to stress through psychological or physical conditioning. Physical stress resistance involves participating in regular, ongoing physical activity. Psychological stress resistance is multifaceted and, depending on the individual, may involve strategies to enhance her self-esteem, improve her assertiveness, or help her set realistic goals or explore other coping resources.

Many older women must cope with changes related to chronic disease in addition to the myriad changes that accompany the normal aging process, including changes in employment status and a shift from independence to dependence. The woman's personality, attitude, life experiences, and willingness to adapt to change will help her to cope with changes brought on by advancing age. To help her deal with stress, teach her to identify its sources, recognize how it affects her, avoid its harmful effects, and deal with it when it occurs. Help her to understand that some events are out of her control but that strategies exist to deal with the stresses that can be controlled. These include managing her time and commitments, establishing a strong system of social support and effective coping strategies, and leading a healthy lifestyle.

Sexuality

In the past, it was assumed that both women and men experienced a decrease in sexual feelings and enjoyment as they grew older. Stereotypical images of older adults portrayed them as sexless and as either uninterested in sex or incapable of sexual intercourse. Although various factors affect older women's ability to remain sexually active, they're physically able to maintain a sexually active lifestyle and many can and do enjoy the pleasures of sexual intercourse and intimacy. (See *Factors affecting sexuality in older women*, page 124.) With more men seeking treatment for erectile dysfunction, an inevitable condition of aging, women have also come to recognize that the effects of menopause and aging shouldn't hamper sexual happiness. For most women, sexuality can be as enjoyable and fulfilling during the years following menopause.

Sexual responsiveness reaches a peak for women in their late 30s and can remain on a high plateau into their 60s. Some women report an increased sexual desire after menopause because the fear of unwanted pregnancy commonly frees them to be more sexually expressive and responsive.

Provider's role

During menopause, many women do experience changes in libido (sex drive), reduction in vaginal lubrication, discomfort during sexual intercourse, and changes in orgasmic response. As health care providers, offer solutions, such as the use of vaginal lubricants (K-Y, Astroglide) or creams (Replens) that are specifically formulated for menopausal vaginal discomfort and

Factors affecting sexuality in older women

Sexual functioning is influenced by many biologic and psychosocial factors.

Biologic factors
- Partner's loss of desire or potency
- Menopause (decreased hormone production, affecting sexual responsiveness)
- Decreased vaginal lubrication and thinning of vaginal walls
- Drug use (antihypertensive, chemotherapeutic agents, central nervous system, and hormonal medications)
- Depression (decreased desire)
- Poor physical health

Psychosocial factors
- Death of a partner
- Stress (physical or emotional)
- Sexual abuse
- Substance abuse
- Alcoholism
- Low self-esteem
- Ageism
- Physical characteristics (feeling unattractive because of skin wrinkling or sagging, graying or loss of hair, weight gain, tooth loss)

allow many older women to continue to enjoy sexual intercourse. Suggest to the female patient that lengthening foreplay may promote enhanced vaginal lubrication as well. For women who experience a significant decrease in sex drive along with vaginal symptoms, offering estrogen replacement therapy (ERT), often in the form of a vaginal cream, may help. Low-dose vaginal estrogen cream (conjugated estrogen [Premarin] or estradiol [Estrace]) has been shown to significantly improve symptoms associated with vaginal dryness and also reduce the incidence of urinary tract infections. Advise the female patient not to use progestins while on ERT. Explain to her that the estrogen cream is inserted into the vagina daily for 3 weeks, followed by twice-weekly administration. In addition to vaginal creams, a tablet that contains a low dose of estradiol (Vagifem) is also available, which is inserted in the vagina twice per week.

Another method to offer female patients is the vaginal ring (Estring), a newly introduced silastic device that delivers estrogen (estradiol) locally to the vagina. The vaginal ring is inserted for 3 months and is changed by either the woman or her health care provider.

Hormone therapy is also effective in treating some of the sexual problems women experience with menopause. It can relieve vaginal atrophy and hot flashes and also decrease pain and burning during intercourse, thereby improving her sexual experience. Recent studies have shown that lower doses of estrogen may be used to alleviate menopausal symptoms successfully. One study found that conjugated equine estrogens plus medroxyprogesterone acetate were as effective in reducing vasomotor symptoms and vaginal atrophy as the commonly prescribed doses of 0.625 mg conjugated equine estrogens. Interestingly, these hormonal therapies not only treat sexual problems associated with menopause but are effective for contraception, which may be needed because many women remain fertile during and even beyond menopause. (See *Contraceptive choices for older women*, pages 126 and 127.)

Encourage the use of natural remedies, changes in diet, and lifestyle modifications to improve the symptoms associated with vaginal dryness. Sexual activity increases blood flow to the vagina, increases elasticity and lubrication of the vaginal tissues, and maintains muscle tone. It has been demonstrated that perimenopausal women who experience orgasm, by any means, 3 or more times per month are less likely to experience vaginal atrophy than those who have intercourse fewer than 10 times per year.

ALTERNATIVE THERAPIES

The plant-based, estrogen-like compound found in soy (known as *phytoestrogens*) is believed to enhance sexual functioning. Supplements of vitamins C and E can also produce an estrogenic effect to help women relieve the symptoms of menopause that can inhibit sexuality. However, women who have hypertension shouldn't take vitamin E.

Menopause

Menopause marks the last 10 to 15 years of reproductive aging in a woman. In 2001, the Stages of Reproductive Aging Workshop (STRAW), a forum sponsored by the North American Menopause Society (NAMS), developed a staging system that divides these years into seven stages: five precede and two follow the final menstrual period. While the menopausal model developed by this group can be applied to all women, STRAW emphasized that not all healthy women necessarily follow this pattern — some may move back and forth between stages, while others may skip a stage completely.

The physiologic and hormonal changes that occur during the middle years of a woman's life are called *perimenopause*, or *climacteric*. They involve the time before total cessation of menstrual periods, known as *menopause*. Although the length of the perimenopausal period varies, most women experience physical and hormonal changes for 5 to 10 years before menses cease completely. When a woman hasn't had a menstrual period for 1 year, she's considered to have reached menopause. Postmenopause refers to the time following the final menstrual period, regardless of whether the menopause was spontaneous or induced.

Although various hormonal changes signal ovarian decline, the menopausal process still isn't fully understood. The perimenopausal period varies among women and is somewhat influenced by genetics. In addition, such factors as disease, cigarette smoking, and surgical intervention can influence the timing of menopause and may even produce premature menopause. For most women, the transition usually begins during the

(Text continues on page 128.)

Contraceptive choices for older women

Method	Advantages
Less effective*	
Abstinence (periodic)	▪ Doesn't mask menopause
Condoms (male or female)	▪ Only method that protects against human immunodeficiency virus (HIV) and sexually transmitted diseases (STDs) ▪ Don't mask menopause
Diaphragms, caps	▪ Don't mask menopause
Spermicides	▪ Don't mask menopause
Effective*	
Combined oral contraceptive pills (COCs)	▪ Strongly protect against ovarian and endometrial cancer ▪ Prevent bone loss ▪ Normalize menstrual bleeding ▪ Control menopausal symptoms
Progestin-only pills (POPs)	▪ Can be safely used when estrogen is contraindicated
Emergency contraceptive pills (ECPs): COCs or POPs	▪ No medical contraindications for use by women at risk for cardiovascular disease
More effective*	
Combined injectable contraceptives (CICs)	▪ Estrogens in CICs possibly less potent than those in COCs, which may produce fewer adverse effects
DMPA: progestin-only injectable	▪ Can be safely used when estrogen is contraindicated ▪ Protects against uterine fibroids ▪ May protect against endometrial cancer
Subdermal implants	▪ Can be safely used when estrogen is contraindicated. Effective for 5 to 7 years.
Intrauterine device (IUD): Copper T 380A	▪ Effective for at least 12 years ▪ Doesn't mask menopause ▪ May protect against endometrial cancer
Levonorgestrel intrauterine system (LNg-IUS)	▪ Effective for at least 7 years ▪ Reduces menstrual bleeding ▪ Complements hormone replacement therapy
Sterilization (male or female)	▪ May protect against ovarian cancer ▪ Doesn't mask menopause

* Effectiveness is defined here as: "less effective" for most users (becoming "effective" when used consistently and correctly), "effective" for most users (becoming "more effective" when used consistently and correctly), and "more effective" for all users. Definition of effectiveness adapted from "Contraceptive efficacy," In Hatcher, R.A., Trussell, J., Stewart, F., et al., eds. *Contraceptive Technology,* Seventeenth Revised Edition. New York: Ardent Media, 1998.

Disadvantages
▪ Determining fertile days difficult if menses are irregular ▪ No protection against HIV and STDs
▪ Must be used correctly with each act of intercourse
▪ Devices possibly difficult to fit in older women ▪ Protection against HIV and STDs unknown
▪ No protection against HIV and STDs
▪ Not appropriate for women at risk for cardiovascular disease ▪ Mask menopause ▪ No protection against HIV and STDs
▪ Requires stricter compliance than for COCs ▪ No protection against HIV and STDs
▪ Not meant for repeated use ▪ No protection against HIV and STDs
▪ Not appropriate for women at risk for cardiovascular disease ▪ No protection against HIV and STDs
▪ May make bleeding patterns unpredictable ▪ No protection against HIV and STDs
▪ May make bleeding patterns unpredictable ▪ No protection against HIV and STDs
▪ May add to menstrual bleeding problems ▪ Insertion may be more difficult in older women ▪ No protection against HIV and STDs
▪ Insertion may be more difficult in older women ▪ No protection against HIV and STDs
▪ Irreversible ▪ No protection against HIV and STDs

Adapted with permission from Family Health International. Retrieved December 5, 2003 from *www.fhi.org/pic/olderwomanopt.gif.*

early to middle 40s. In American women, menstrual periods generally cease around age 50. By age 52, approximately 80% of women are no longer menstruating.

The entire menopausal transition period represents a profound change physiologically and emotionally. Hormone levels shift, readjust, and reach new balances, and the tissues and organs whose function has been influenced by the various hormones also change structurally and functionally. A woman also experiences mental and emotional changes that affect her self-image as she makes this passage into a new phase of life.

Hormonal changes

During the perimenopausal period, ranging anywhere from ages 40 to 60, hormone levels are commonly erratic, with highs and lows occurring without the usual synchronicity. The normal hormonal pattern of ovulation — when estrogen levels are elevated and progesterone levels are low — marks the decline of ovarian function when the ovaries lose their ability to manufacture large amounts of sex hormones. The physiologic feedback loop between the ovaries, the hypothalamus, and the pituitary glands loses its synchronicity. Progesterone levels undergo the most dramatic drop during menopause because the production of progesterone depends on ovulation and the development of the corpus luteum.

Although small amounts of estrogen continue to be produced by the ovaries for up to 10 years following the end of menses, a woman's body uses other means for estrogen production. Androgens produced by the adrenal glands are converted by the woman's fat cells into estrogens. Androgens are female forms of "male-type" hormones that are created by the ovaries and the adrenal glands. They're responsible for the maintenance of muscle strength and the sex drive (libido). As estrogen and progesterone levels fall during menopause, the effects of the androgens commonly become more pronounced. For example, androgens can cause the increase in facial hair that's commonly noticed during midlife. Other hormonal changes may produce a decrease in muscle mass with a relative increase in the amount of fat tissue as well as symptoms of low libido.

Menopausal signs and symptoms

Many common signs and symptoms are associated with menopause. For most women in midlife, alterations in the menstrual cycle herald the beginning of the menopausal transition. During this time, women may experience vasomotor symptoms (such as hot flashes) and other physical changes that occur in the skin, hair, breasts, and vagina.

The menstrual cycle

It's rare for a woman to simply stop bleeding. More commonly, menstrual periods become progressively less regular. They may occur closer together or become farther apart, and the volume of blood flow may be heavier or become lighter. Midcycle spotting may also occur. This change in bleeding pattern is largely caused by a lack of ovulation, which interrupts the production of progesterone and thereby causes the uterine lining to be sloughed off irregularly. Also, without ovulation, a longer than usual release of estrogen may occur, which may overstimulate the growth of the endometrium, causing bleeding to be heavier or more prolonged. The uterine lining may also grow with irregular or thickened areas and may not slough off completely or evenly, causing the woman's menstrual periods to stop and start again.

Although irregular periods are a normal part of the perimenopausal process, any heavy bleeding should be investigated. Nonmalignant uterine fibroid tumors, a frequent cause of increased bleeding, are common in perimenopausal women, as is cervical or uterine cancer. If heavy bleeding is an ongoing problem and cancer has been ruled out, low-dose oral contraceptives, progesterone alone, or another form of hormone replacement therapy may be initiated. If fibroid tumors are the cause of heavy bleeding, surgery may be necessary. Remind women that although fertility declines during the perimenopausal period, conception can occur until menopause is complete; thus, contraception choices should be discussed.

Vasomotor symptoms

One of the hallmark signs of menopause is the occurrence of vasomotor symptoms commonly known as "hot flashes" or "flushes." Hot flashes are the most common symptom reported by 50% to 75% of women in menopause. For some, hot flashes are a problem for only 1 or 2 years. However, 10% to 15% of women characterize their hot flashes as debilitating. In many non-Westernized cultures, hot flashes either don't occur or are so minimal they're barely noticed. In the United States, women seek medical attention for hot flashes more often than for any other symptom of menopause.

The experience of a hot flash is distinct. It may begin with a feeling of pressure in the head, followed by a warm feeling rising from the chest to the neck and face. The heat for some may be a highly intense, hot, burning sensation followed by sweating that can be profuse. The frequency of hot flashes can vary from 1 or 2 per week to 1 or 2 per hour, averaging 4 minutes per "flash." They may be accompanied by palpitations, weakness, fatigue, faintness, or dizziness.

Although causing discomfort, hot flashes in and of themselves are completely harmless. They may, however, cause a profound disruption in sleep, which exacerbates other menopausal symptoms, including mood swings, fatigue, and memory loss.

Other body changes

A variety of body changes occur during menopause. (See *Body changes during menopause*, page 130.) The diminishing levels of estrogen affect many tissues in a woman's body. Her skin and mucous membranes of various

Body changes during menopause

Hair growth
- Thinning of scalp hair
- Darkening or thickening of other body hair such as facial hair

Skin
- Loss of firmness, tension, and fluid
- Decrease in melanocytes, which give skin pigment
- Increasing sensitivity to sun exposure
- Increasing drying and roughness

Bone
- Becoming progressively more porous and brittle
- Increasing risk of osteoporosis
- Becoming more subject to fractures, especially the shoulder, upper arm, and hip

Breasts
- Glandular tissue replaced with fat
- Loss of fullness, causing flattening and drooping

Reproductive system
- Few remaining follicles (egg cells) in ovaries
- Decreasing size of reproductive organs
- Thinning, less-lubricated vaginal mucosa
- Increasing susceptibility to infection because of vaginal pH changes
- Disappearing endometriosis

Urinary system
- Thinning of tissues in bladder and uterus
- Increasing risk of urinary tract infections

parts of the body become dry, rough, and wrinkled as the fatty layer beneath her skin shrinks, causing decreased elasticity and moisture. The skin also produces less melanin and can burn more easily. Also, the increasing predominance of androgens often causes a darker, thicker, more wiry type of hair to appear on the pubis, underarms, chest, lower abdomen, and back. Some women report the appearance of facial hair during this time. The hair on the head may become dry, and pubic and axillary hair may grow thin.

During menopause, a woman's breasts go through changes that cause them to shrink, lose fullness, flatten, and drop, with the nipples becoming smaller and flatter. Vaginal changes may accompany perimenopause, or they may not occur until 5 to 10 years following menopause. The mucous membranes, previously supported by estrogen stimulation, become thin and more fragile. The vagina loses its rough texture and dark pink coloration; it becomes smooth and pale and eventually shortens and narrows, causing vaginal itching or soreness. As the production of cervical mucus diminishes, the vagina lubricates more slowly, causing painful intercourse. An alteration occurs in the normal vaginal flora, which increases the likelihood of urinary tract infections.

Other body changes during menopause cause symptoms of joint pain, the onset of or worsening of migraine headaches, dry mouth, bloating, indigestion, and gas. During this time, changes in sleep patterns are extremely common, with insomnia occurring either alone or as a result of hot flashes. Mood swings, forgetfulness, lack of concentration, and depression may be present — all of which commonly have multiple causes. Estrogen affects the brain neurotransmitter serotonin, which influences mood. Improved cognitive function has been associated with estrogen use. Many menopausal women experience weight gain caused by a sedentary lifestyle and poor dietary habits.

Cultural differences in and perceptions of menopause

In 1900, the average age of menopause for American women was 46 and the average life expectancy was 51, although many women lived much longer. Today, menopause marks not the end of life but rather a transition into another phase with a potential life span of an additional 30 to 50 years. Because most women will spend one-third of their lifetime after menopause, it's important that researchers discover how the natural process of aging interacts with the hormonal changes of menopause, as well as how diet and lifestyle influence the aging process and the menopausal transition. Interestingly, other cultures experience lower incidences of osteoporosis and heart disease, and women in those cultures commonly transition through menopause with fewer uncomfortable symptoms than American women. Through the study of other cultures, much can be learned about the differences in and perceptions of menopause.

How culture influences women's perceptions of midlife isn't well understood. It's known that a woman's lifestyle and social interaction are an important influence on her physical and emotional health. What's more, in some cultures, as a woman grows older, her social status becomes elevated and she's valued as a life expert.

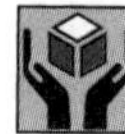

SPECIAL NEEDS

Certain cultures view women in a different light. For example, Mexican American women, who commonly live into their late 70s, are considered "old" after menopause. Yet, with advancing age, they become greatly respected sources of wisdom to their families and in their communities. Likewise, in Korean culture, elderly and widowed women are highly respected and generally live with their adult children and grandchildren. Conversely, in other cultures, a woman's social status decreases with advancing years and she may be considered a devalued and unworthy contributor to society. For example, while elderly Russian women aren't given more respect than their younger counterparts, they're an important source of financial support and of child care. Elderly Colombian women are respected but aren't necessarily seen as sources of wisdom in the community.

Cross-cultural studies have shown that the menopausal experience is highly influenced by the attitudes of the culture and the community in which women live. In the United States, attitudes toward menopause and aging are beginning to change. For many traditional cultures throughout the world, menopause represents a time for women to assume leadership roles in the community based on their increased wisdom. American women can learn to embrace the perspectives of other cultures and begin to view menopause as an opportunity to enhance self-perceptions and create a positive image for other older women.

Menopause is a natural, inevitable process, and women have control over how they pass through this period of life. By developing a lifestyle that helps to ease uncomfortable symptoms and by minimizing the risks of chronic disease by stopping smoking, maintaining an appropriate weight through exercise and diet, limiting alcohol intake, and reducing stress, women can enjoy maximal health during and beyond menopause.

Illness prevention

Preventing illness in the middle-age to older adult female involves addressing the many changes — both physical and emotional — involved in the aging process.

Chronic health problems

Middle-age to older adult females face a number of chronic health problems, including osteoporosis, depression, heart disease, obesity, anorexia, osteoarthritis, urinary incontinence, and eventually the problems of sensory and cognitive impairment (which may include Alzheimer's disease). Facing these conditions can be challenging; however, if prepared with appropriate information about the benefits of a healthy lifestyle — including regular physical exercise, smoking cessation, and better nutrition — these women have a better chance of preventing or postponing these chronic health problems.

Osteoporosis

Osteoporosis is a chronic disease that causes bone to become weak and thin or porous; *osteopenia* is a condition of a diminished amount of bone tissue. These conditions increase women's susceptibility to debilitating bone fractures. While osteoporosis is neither caused by nor brought on by menopause, it does occur most commonly with advancing age. Women can lose up to 20% of their bone mass in the 5 to 7 years after menopause. Osteoporosis is a preventable disease, one that may occur before, during, or after menopause. The development of thin or porous bone is a process that occurs over time when the body loses bone faster than it can produce it. This process should be viewed across the lifetime of a female, particularly from a preventive standpoint.

Reported statistics in the United States show that approximately 44 million adults have osteopenia or osteoporosis. Of this group, an estimated 10 million (8 million women and 2 million men) have osteoporosis and 34 million have osteopenia, a condition that places them at a greater risk for developing osteoporosis. These conditions vary among ethnic groups; Asian Americans and Whites are more commonly affected than are Blacks.

Among non-Hispanic Black women age 50 and older, 5% have osteoporosis and 35% have osteopenia. Among Hispanic women age 50 and older, 10% have osteoporosis and 49% have osteopenia. Among non-Hispanic White women and Asian American women age 50 and older, 20% have osteoporosis and 52% have osteopenia.

Osteoporosis represents a major health threat for women. In the United States, the incidence of osteoporosis-related fractures has increased over the past 20 years. Most fractures occur at the femoral neck, vertebrae, and distal radius. Hip fractures pose the greatest risk. It's estimated that approximately 12% to 20% of cases will result in death within 1 year following a hip fracture and that more than half won't return to independent living.

Osteoporosis occurs when the normal balance of bone formation and bone resorption is disrupted. In women and young adults, bone growth and calcium deposition is a continuous process, and bone mass generally reaches a peak around age 30. As women age, bone loss gradually occurs because of an imbalance in bone tissue and metabolism. Estrogen deficiency and calcium and vitamin D deficiency worsen the situation as women age. During the first 5 or 6 years following menopause, women lose bone six times more rapidly than men. By age 65, one-third of women have experienced a vertebral fracture; by age 81, one-third have suffered a hip fracture. At age 80, it's estimated that women have lost approximately 47% of the trabecular bone (which is the porous type of bone found in the vertebrae, hip, and all articulating joints).

In addition to the aging process, osteoporosis may also result from endocrine diseases (such as diabetes, hypogonadism, overactive thyroid, and hyperparathyroidism), rheumatoid arthritis, and chronic lung disease. Also, certain prescription drugs — including corticosteroids, anticoagulants, and some diuretics as well as some over-the-counter aluminum-containing antacids — can contribute to bone loss. It's also been reported that excessive caffeine intake increases calcium excretion and that excessive alcohol use interferes with calcium absorption and depresses bone formation. (See *Risk factors for osteoporosis,* page 134.)

Provider's role

According to recommendations established by the U.S. Preventive Services Task Force and the National Osteoporosis Foundation, health care providers should routinely screen all women older than age 65 for osteoporosis. (See *Osteoporosis prevention and treatment,* page 135.) Women with risk factors should be screened beginning at age 60. In the United States, women typically reach menopause around age 51, and most bone loss occurs during the first 5 to 7 years after cessation of menses. Thus, it may be prudent to begin screening at an earlier age. Insurance carriers commonly will support bone

Risk factors for osteoporosis

Women have a higher risk of osteoporosis than men. In addition to gender, other risk factors include:

- advancing age
- postmenopausal status
- inactive lifestyle
- small bone structure
- low calcium intake
- smoking
- excessive alcohol consumption
- medications (glucocorticoids, for arthritis and asthma; antiseizure medications; sleeping pills; some hormones used to treat endometriosis; and some cancer drugs)
- excessive thyroid hormones
- race (White and Asian women have higher risks)
- endocrine disorders.

mineral density (BMD) measurements in postmenopausal women who aren't using hormone replacement therapy and who have other risk factors for bone loss.

Health care providers should assess all adult female patients for the risk of osteopenia and osteoporosis. In recent years, peripheral densitometry scans of the forearm, heel, and finger have become widely used because they're inexpensive and readily available in many offices and outpatient clinics. However, the "gold standard" for the measurement of BMD and the diagnosis of osteopenia and osteoporosis is the sophisticated test known as central dual X-ray absorptiometry. This test assesses the BMD in the spine, hip, and waist. It's also used to monitor treatment progress. Be sure to reassess adult female patients' BMD every 3 to 5 years. For certain women, such as those who are undergoing treatment for osteoporosis and those who are immobilized, BMD should be measured more often — for example, every 6 to 24 months.

In addition to assessing patients' BMD, teach them about the advantages of weight-bearing physical exercise, which has been directly related to overall bone mass, and the benefits of certain vitamins for preventing osteoporosis.

PREVENTION POINTER

Women who regularly engage in exercise programs that include weight bearing and muscle strengthening can help prevent postmenopausal bone loss and reduce their risk of falling. It's believed that the bone-building effect of exercise results mainly from the repetitive physical stress applied to the bones. With weight-bearing exercise, pressure is placed on the bones either by the weight of the body or by the force of muscular contractions. Effective exercises, which are generally safe and contribute to cardiovascular health and bone mass, include walking, stair climbing, gardening, weight lifting, and low-impact aerobics. Regular exercise should be performed for at least 30 minutes three or four times a week. Patients should also be encouraged to adopt good eating

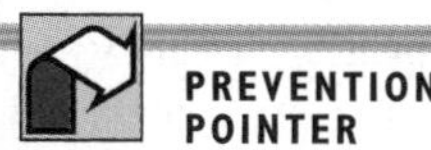

PREVENTION POINTER

OSTEOPOROSIS PREVENTION AND TREATMENT

Treatment and overall prevention of osteoporosis may involve the use of estrogen replacement therapy (ERT), calcitonin, or bisphosphonates.

ERT has long been considered the most important strategy for preventing osteoporosis in postmenopausal women who have low or normal bone mineral density. However, estrogen's influence on bone is short-lived, thus necessitating long-term treatment in order to preserve the benefits of bone mineral density. Treatment typically consists of a daily dose (0.625 mg) of conjugated equine estrogens or its equivalent; however, recent studies have suggested that lower doses (for example, 0.45 or 0.3 mg) also protect bone. In addition, using oral contraceptives during the premenopausal and perimenopausal stages can increase bone mineral density after menopause.

Calcitonin, a synthetic version of a hormone secreted from the cells of the thyroid gland, inhibits the action of osteoclasts and decreases bone resorption. Because it hasn't proven effective in early postmenopausal women, calcitonin must be considered more of a treatment than a preventive agent.

Bisphosphonates are synthetic forms of a class of compounds found in the body that bind to the crystals in the bone matrix and inhibit bone resorption. Risedronate (Actonel) and alendronate (Fosamax) are two bisphosphonates that have been approved to prevent and treat postmenopausal osteoporosis. Women who can't or who choose not to take ERT are good candidates for this therapy. Bisphosphonates inhibit normal physiologic bone resorption as well as abnormal bone resorption, thereby halting bone loss, increasing bone mineral density, and reducing the risk of spinal and nonspinal fractures. These medications have proven to be the only therapy to date to reduce fractures that occur outside of the spine.

habits, to limit alcohol intake, and to avoid smoking.

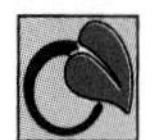

ALTERNATIVE THERAPIES

Diets composed primarily of plant-based, unprocessed whole foods contribute to the prevention of osteoporosis. Examples of these foods include legumes, fresh fruits and vegetables, whole grains, nuts, and seeds. They provide a rich supply of nutrients in the right proportions to enhance absorption and use. Many vitamins (such as B_6, K, C, and D) and minerals (including calcium, manganese, magnesium, boron, and zinc) play an important role in maintaining bone mass and preventing osteoporosis.

Calcium

Aging is accompanied by a decrease in synthesis of vitamin D by the skin. This problem is exacerbated by the common tendency of older people to decrease their exposure to the sun. Sun exposure of as little as 10 to 15 minutes per day can positively impact bone health by improving calcium absorption and use. Dietary sources of vitamin D include fish, eggs, liver, corn flake cereal, and dairy products. The National Academy of Sciences (NAS) has provided the following recommendations for vitamin D supplementation:

- age 50 and younger: 200 IU/day
- ages 51 to 70: 400 IU/day
- age 70 and older: 600 IU/day
- intake not to exceed 2,000 IU/day.

Recommendations for daily calcium intake were developed by the National Institute of Health Development Panel on Optimal Calcium Intake in 1994. The recommendations were then revised by the NAS in 1997, in response to concerns that most Americans weren't getting enough calcium to prevent osteoporosis during the later years. Specific calcium recommendations for women are:

- ages 25 to 50: 1,000 mg/day
- postmenopausal using exogenous estrogen: 1,000 mg/day
- postmenopausal not using exogenous estrogen: 1,500 mg/day
- age 65 and older: 1,500 mg/day.

The NAS also issued a precaution that the maximum daily intake should be 2,500 mg/day. Risks of exceeding this limit include the potential for the accumulation of calcium deposits in soft tissues, such as the kidneys and arteries, and impaired absorption of other vital minerals, such as iron, zinc, and manganese.

When considering dietary sources of calcium, most women are aware that dairy products are rich in calcium. However, it's important to point out that the animal protein in these products can interfere with the body's ability to absorb the calcium. Explain to them that other substances that inhibit calcium absorption are found in wheat bran, raw spinach, salt, caffeine, alcohol and tobacco, and fructose (found in many soft drinks). Good nutritional sources of calcium include sardines, soy, canned salmon, tofu, collard greens, broccoli, sesame seeds, tahini, and molasses. Reishi, an edible fungus known to herbalists as the "mushroom of immortality," has been used to strengthen bones and tendons. Soy milk, rice, and orange juice, along with many other products, are now available with extra calcium added.

Instruct your patients about the many calcium supplements currently available. Calcium citrate preparations provide 21% elemental calcium. This supplement may be taken with or without meals. Calcium carbonate provides approximately 40% elemental calcium and should be taken with meals. While calcium citrate tends to be better tolerated, it's a more expensive form of calcium supplement. Calcium carbonate is adequately absorbed by most people unless they have a problem with insufficient stomach acid. Dolomite or bone meal–based products should be avoided because they may contain lead and other toxic heavy metals. Antacids aren't the best sources of calcium because they can cause other problems (such as kidney stones) and they may aggravate other medical conditions as well. Some antacids also contain aluminum, which can cause the body to lose calcium. If problems with constipation occur, a combined calcium-magnesium supplement should be taken. It's recommended that, for best absorption, supplements should be taken in divided doses of no more than 500 mg of calcium with each meal.

Depression

Assessment of the middle-age to older adult female for depression is vital because this condition constitutes a major health problem in this age-group. During their lifetime, women are likely to experience depression twice as often as men. In many cases, depression accompanies other serious mental disorders, such as borderline personality disorder, eating and substance abuse, and anxiety disorders. Depression may be related to biochemical alterations, or it may stem from various social and economic issues unique to women.

Older women are more likely to experience depression related to loss associated with the death of a spouse or close family member, personal injury or illness, change in health status of a family member, or retirement. Age-related difficulties of daily living may result from diminished sensory acuity, decreased dexterity and strength, reduced flexibility, lack of energy and stamina, declining physical strength and health, retirement, and a reduced income. Elderly women may neglect to engage in health behaviors, including proper nutrition and rest, adequate exercise, and social interaction, all of which enhance physical and mental functioning and an overall sense of well-being. Be alert for clues of physical complaints that sometimes stem from depression and loneliness, which put older women at greater risk for misdiagnosis and inappropriate treatment.

In addition, older women must learn to adopt and adapt to a new social setting and lifestyle. Because of the decreased physical abilities that accompany aging as well as the common issues of social isolation and economic difficulties, it's highly recommended that older women be routinely screened for depression.

ALTERNATIVE THERAPIES

Herbs have been used throughout history to control physical difficulties, soothe emotional problems, facilitate the body's adaptation response to illness, and promote overall mental well-being. Women may benefit from the use of herbs by decreasing depression and restoring psychological harmony and balance. Since ancient times, foods and herbs have been used to support healing of the body, mind, and spirit, yet how they bring about emotional changes remains unknown. (See *The benefits of herbs,* page 138.)

Heart disease

Heart disease remains the number one killer of older American women. This disease includes coronary heart disease, stroke, heart failure, hypertension, and other diseases of the heart and vascular system. According to the American Heart Association, during the past 20 years, improved prevention and treatment has reduced the annual number of cardiovascular deaths

The benefits of herbs

A number of herbs have been shown to reduce symptoms of depression in women.

- Black cohosh — Native to North America, this plant has been used in the United States since the late 1700s for a variety of problems, including pain, colds, hives, sleep disturbances, and menstrual irregularities. It may be given as an ethanol extract, which is believed to reduce the symptoms of many menopause-related problems, including sweating, hot flashes, irritability, insomnia, and depression.
- St. John's wort — Whether taken internally or applied externally, this plant is best known for its use in promoting the healing of bruises and sprains, enhancing concentration, and treating nervous and psychiatric disorders. It's believed that older women who feel lonely and sad may benefit from drinking tea made with St. John's wort. This herb is recommended for mild to moderate depression. Other herbal remedies that are believed to reduce depression are feverfew, ginkgo biloba, lemon balm, sage, and Siberian ginseng.
- Aromatherapy — This process involves the use of essential oils from aromatic plants to enhance the health of a person's body, mind, and spirit. It may be effective in reducing women's depression. Lavender essential oil, considered one of the safest and most widely used oils in aromatherapy, is believed to stimulate the appetite and help relieve depression. The essential oil of rose is used to combat emotional shock, bereavement, grief, and depression.

in men but not in women. Despite heightened public awareness of heart disease in women, the majority of women in the United States continue to underestimate their risk of dying as a result of heart disease. Risk factors include increasing age, early menopause, positive family history, elevated serum cholesterol levels, diabetes, hypertension, obesity, and such lifestyle patterns as a high-fat diet, stress, and a sedentary activity level. Many of these risk factors may be modified through changes in a woman's lifestyle.

Provider's role

Health care providers should identify a woman's risk of heart disease to prevent further complications. Studies have shown that women are less likely than men to be evaluated for heart disease risk factors. Health care providers should teach patients about how to reduce their risk of heart disease by following simple guidelines for modifying risk factors.

Western diets appear to play a large role in the development of heart disease. Modifying food intake, along with reducing, stopping smoking, and engaging in regular physical exercise, is believed to significantly benefit cardiovascular functioning. (See *Tips for modifying your patient's food intake.*)

Obesity

Maintaining an ideal body weight constitutes a major strategy in disease prevention among women of all ages.

Tips for modifying your patient's food intake

Along with reducing stress, exercising regularly, and stopping smoking, women can reduce their risk of heart disease by modifying their diet following these guidelines:

- Eat foods high in fiber.
- Eat foods high in omega fatty acids (such as salmon and tuna).
- Include garlic and soy in the diet.
- Limit fat intake.
- Limit alcohol and caffeine.
- Avoid white-flour products.

Throughout the course of their lives, many women struggle with weight issues at one time or another. Obesity, defined as a body weight that's 20% over the ideal, has become a significant health issue for an increasing number of Americans. As the number of overweight and obese individuals has climbed, the occurrence of many common health conditions has increased as well. Recent studies show that 50% of adults in the United States are overweight or obese; this number reflects a 25% increase over the past 30 years.

Excess weight has been seen in conjunction with rising rates of cardiovascular disease, type 2 diabetes mellitus, hypertension, stroke, hyperlipidemia, osteoarthritis, and certain cancers. Obesity is also a factor in other disorders, including breathing difficulties, varicose veins, and gout. Individuals who are extremely obese have shorter life expectancies.

Provider's role

Health care providers should teach overweight patients that short-term approaches to weight loss are rarely successful. Instead, management of obesity requires a lifelong commitment to changes in lifestyle, behaviors, habits, and attitudes toward food and eating.

Heredity does play an important role in the predisposition to excessive weight gain, but other issues may also have an influence. These issues include a tendency to set unrealistic standards and expectations; emotional problems, such as anxiety, boredom, and feelings of powerlessness; family problems; difficulties with friends and colleagues; and approach to food selection, preparation, and consumption. All of these can influence a woman's body weight. Counsel patients toward successful weight loss with interventions that involve changing eating patterns, participating in regular physical activity, and reducing overall stress level.

Low body weight

Among elderly women, low body weight may be of concern. Aging appears to alter requirements for calories, protein, and other nutrients, which may change lean body mass, a person's level of physical activity, and intestinal absorption. Older adults may skip meals and exclude entire categories of food from their diets because of diminished appetites, inaccessibility of grocery stores, lack of energy or desire to cook, reluctance to dine alone, and problems with chewing or swallowing. Many older adults experience tooth or mouth problems that make eating fruits and vegetables difficult and unpleasant. Fiber, beneficial in maintaining proper bowel function, also reduces risk of colon cancer, decreases serum cholesterol, and improves glucose metabolism. For most older adults, the actual daily fiber intake is less than half of the recommended 20 to 35 g.

Provider's role

Because physical activity is necessary to maintain muscle mass, encourage the older adult female to remain physically active in her later years. To do so, make sure that the woman's nutritional intake is sufficient to support her regular physical activity. The diets of older women may contain inadequate amounts of protein and calories because of an inability to chew meat or the expense of protein-rich foods. Assist your patients in selecting low-cost foods that are tasty and easy to prepare and that meet the recommended nutritional requirements. They may need help interpreting food labels to enhance their product choices. Older women may also seek guidance concerning methods of food preparation that preserve flavor yet create foods that are easier to chew and swallow. Maintaining appropriate body weight is integral to the quality of health for women of all ages and is especially important in the later years.

Osteoarthritis

As women age, a number of changes take place in the musculoskeletal system. A decrease in muscle mass and tone and diminished elasticity of tendons and ligaments commonly cause a limited range of motion and prolong the time it takes to move and perform routine tasks. Women may also develop osteoarthritis, a degenerative joint disease than affects more than 20 million Americans. A common rheumatic disorder, osteoarthritis is the major cause of disability and reduced activity in persons age 50 and older. Radiographic findings show evidence of osteoarthritis in up to 85% of people age 65 and older. Contributing factors of osteoarthritis include heredity, trauma, obesity, overuse of joints, and aging.

Joints commonly affected in osteoarthritis include the large, weight-bearing and often-used joints, such as the hips and knees, the spine, and the joints of the fingers, thumb, and big toe. Osteoarthritis is a progressive disease, and women generally report symptoms of pain and stiffness associated with activity, along with bony enlargement of the affected joints. Joint pain is usually more pronounced following physical activity but diminishes after rest. If the vertebral column is involved, women typically complain of a radiating pain with muscle spasms in the extremity innervated by the affected area. Diagnosis is made by X-ray or other imaging procedures.

Provider's role

Although no cure for osteoarthritis exists, treatment centers on education and pain control, which is accomplished by medication, other pain relief methods, or surgery. Health care providers can prescribe nonsteroidal anti-inflammatory drugs, which have analgesic and anti-inflammatory effects, to reduce the woman's pain. Because joint pain diminishes with rest, women generally find they're most comfortable during the morning hours. Encourage women to exercise to avoid muscle atrophy related to nonuse and to maintain range of motion and muscle strength. Women should participate in physical activity early in the day. Suggest the application of heat or cold to the affected areas for to provide pain relief. Weight loss to decrease joint stress is also recommended for obese or overweight individuals. Many women engage in complementary therapies, such as imagery, music therapy, acupressure, and acupuncture, to reduce pain and stress. Others find symptomatic relief from homeopathic therapies, such as glucosamine and chondroitin; however, further research is needed to determine the efficacy of these therapies in the treatment of osteoarthritis. If your patient hasn't successfully managed her pain, surgery in the form of a total joint replacement may be necessary.

ALTERNATIVE THERAPIES

Acupuncture — an ancient Chinese healing therapy that involves the insertion of very fine needles — manipulates the body through minor adjustments, which results in an improved internal functioning. Traditional Asian medicine identifies 14 meridians of the body, and acupuncture aims to restore the balance of vital energy in the body along the meridians by stimulating specific junctures through the needles (which cause no bleeding or pain). Other similar Chinese healing therapies that may reduce the pain and discomfort associated with osteoarthritis include massage therapy, acupressure, and pinching or scratching techniques.

ALTERNATIVE THERAPIES

Herbs have also been successfully used to reduce symptoms of osteoarthritis. Powdered ginger, used in China for over 2,500 years, has been reported to improve joint mobility and decrease swelling and morning stiffness associated with osteoarthritis. Fresh ginger has been associated with improvement in symptoms of rheumatoid arthritis. In aromatherapy, rosemary essential oil is used for osteoarthritis and rheumatoid arthritis and as a tonic for the nerves, heart, and circulation. Other herbs used for various conditions include cayenne (or *capsicum*), the chili pepper, for myalgia, frostbite, rheumatism, backache, and muscle spasms. Topical application of capsaicin cream has been shown to reduce joint pain in persons with rheumatoid arthritis and osteoarthritis.

Urinary incontinence

In the 6th decade and later years, a number of age-related changes take place in a woman's genitourinary system. The kidneys decrease in size, function, and urinary output. Blood flow to the kidneys is reduced because of a decreased cardiac output and increased peripheral resistance. Because kidney filtration rate and tubular function are diminished, a decrease in the renal clearance of all medications occurs. Bladder size and tone are also reduced, and elderly women are more likely to experience urinary tract infections.

In general, urinary incontinence is more common among women than men because of weakened perineal muscles. During the middle-age years, many women experience stress urinary incontinence, the loss of a small amount of urine from the bladder opening. It's most likely to occur when jogging, sneezing, coughing, or laughing. During menopause, the declining estrogen supply to the estrogen-dependent tissues of the genitourinary tract results in a decrease in muscle tone and control of the bladder and urethra. Stress urinary incontinence is more likely to occur in women who have given birth vaginally. For most women, Kegel exercises, which strengthen the perineal muscles, can improve this condition.

As women age, their ability to empty the bladder becomes more difficult to control because of weakening of the bladder and perineal muscles as well as a change in brain sensation regarding the need to void. For this reason, older women may have difficulty controlling urination and may experience urinary incontinence. Older women are also more likely to suffer from urinary incontinence because they have short urethras that aren't supported by strong perineal muscles. This also puts them at greater risk for urinary tract infections.

Sexual activity improves tone and blood flow to this area. The use of a device such as a pessary, or surgical intervention, may be needed if incontinence is severe or caused by prolapse of the uterus or bladder. Urinary frequency may also occur. Relief of symptoms may be achieved with prescribed systemic estrogen therapy, low-dose vaginal conjugated estrogens, a vaginal estradiol tablet, or the vaginal ring.

Nocturia

Nocturia — the urge to urinate at night — is a common complaint that's related to kidney changes, fluid retention, and medication use. Older women commonly complain of a need to urinate within 30 minutes after lying down. This occurs because the collection of fluid held in the legs by gravity circulates through the kidneys when a recumbent position is assumed. Urine is then produced, and the woman experiences an urge to void. Because nocturia occurs with such frequency, it's important to ensure safe, easy toilet access for all older women.

Provider's role

As health care providers, it's best to manage patients' urinary incontinence individually. Remember that older women who attempt to reduce urinary leakage by limiting their fluid intake increase their risk of dehydra-

Compensating for sensory loss

Aging commonly affects an individual's senses of taste, smell, hearing, and sight. You'll need to teach your patient how to protect each of these senses and compensate for impaired function.

Taste and smell

Research shows that taste buds diminish in number and sensitivity with age. Many older adults also have difficulty distinguishing odors. Because taste and smell contribute so much to food appreciation, an elderly person may develop poor eating habits. To stimulate your patient's appetite, suggest how to arrange food attractively and encourage her to vary her diet. Suggest that she try more seasonings to bring out taste in her food. However, caution her to avoid overusing salt. If she lives alone, suggest that she try eating with friends.

Hearing

Hearing loss is a widespread problem among older adults, who sometimes fall victim to fraud when buying hearing aids without guidance from trained medical personnel. If an older adult suspects hearing loss, stress the importance of consulting an otolaryngologist or audiologist.

Sight

To help your patient preserve her sight, stress the importance of routine eye checkups to detect glaucoma and to update her eyeglass prescription. Explain how a current prescription prevents eyestrain during reading and promotes safety when driving. Encourage her to take advantage of free eye screening at a local health fair.

tion. Instead, provide them with other therapies, including bladder training programs that focus on reminding women to urinate at regular intervals, medications, and education concerning avoidance of caffeine and alcoholic beverages (which increase urinary output). Also, advise women about preferred timing of medications such as diuretics. For some, teaching perineal muscle support exercises can help. Women with unexplained difficulty controlling urination should be referred for evaluation.

Sensory impairment

With normal aging, a number of changes occur in the sensory system. (See *Compensating for sensory loss.*) Older adults experience a decrease in visual perception, a decreased elasticity of the eardrum, a diminished sense of smell and taste, and a decreased sense of touch. For most, it becomes increasingly difficult to read fine print because of eye changes that affect the focus of near and far vision.

Hearing loss is a common condition among older adults. Because high-pitched tones are usually the first sounds difficult to discriminate, it can be more effective to communicate with older adult patients by whispering, which decreases the pitch of the sounds. Older females may lose their sense of smell because of such non–age-related problems as nasal obstruction, sinus conditions, or allergies. A diminished taste perception may be associated with ill-fitting dentures, poor oral care, certain medications, tobacco, and oral disease.

Provider's role

Because red lighting is more easily detected by the cones and rods, encourage older female patients to use a red night-light to enhance their ability to see in the dark. Also, to communicate effectively, speak in a moderate volume and tone and stand directly in front of the female patient when talking with her — shouting increases the volume and pitch of the sound and proves ineffective.

Cognitive impairment

In addition to the physical changes associated with aging, older adults also experience cognitive changes. Cognition is the mental process by which a person acquires and uses knowledge. It requires many brain elements to function in harmony. Cognitive function, including concentration and memory, has been found to decrease with aging. Many factors — including genetics, lifestyle patterns, and social status — affect this decline. Pain from chronic diseases, such as arthritis, can diminish cognition as pain becomes dominant over one's body and mind. Sleep deprivation and medications that produce drowsiness may also impair cognition. According to the North American Menopause Society (NAMS), hormonal changes also produce cognitive impairment.

Areas of the brain involved in cognition include the cerebral cortex, the temporal lobes, and the limbic system. All of these areas contain estrogen receptors. Although studies done by the NAMS have supported the effects of estrogen on cognition, its exact role isn't known.

The hormones estrogen, progesterone, and androgen influence various aspects of brain function that affect neurons, glia, microglia, and neurotransmitters in many areas of the brain. Perimenopausal women commonly complain of short-term memory problems and difficulty concentrating. NAMS encourages more research to determine whether a relationship exists between estrogen loss and diminished cognitive function.

Provider's role

For most older adults, long-term memory is easier to retrieve than short-term memory. Health care providers should encourage their older female patients to use written lists, visual cues, and other memory-enhancing aids to boost their short-term memory skills. When appropriately measured with an instrument that focuses on accuracy instead of response speed, intelligence hasn't been shown to decline with age. Although cognitive abilities slow down as one grows older, they aren't lost. Thus, as health care providers, it's important to promote good health through such strategies as proper nutrition, stress reduction, social interaction, physical activity, and adequate rest to maintain older patients' optimal brain function.

Alzheimer's disease

Among the postmenopausal population, age-related dementias have become an important health problem. The incidence of dementia is expected to rise as life expectancy increases in most industrialized countries. Although dementia has multiple causes, Alzheimer's disease and vascular changes associated with decreased brain blood flow represent are two major conditions that commonly produce cognitive impairment in older adults.

The causes of Alzheimer's disease aren't well understood. The incidence of Alzheimer's disease may be reduced in women taking estrogen, although additional research in this area is needed. It has been demonstrated that certain genes make some individuals' brain cells more susceptible to damage. However, exposure to various biochemical or environmental factors may be required to set this process in motion. Some data have connected estrogen use with a reduced risk of developing Alzheimer's disease. Researchers suspect that estrogen protects the brain by acting as an antioxidant, which removes the toxic by-products of oxidation that can damage cells. Estrogen is also involved in nerve cell repair and may promote blood flow to the brain and help protect nerve cells from the damaging formation of protein plaques.

Other research has demonstrated that certain similarities exist between vascular-related dementia and Alzheimer's dementia. Individuals with vascular risk factors, such as aging, stroke, diabetes, high cholesterol, hypertension, and a high fat intake, experience a higher incidence of Alzheimer's disease. Current theory suggests that both vascular-related dementia and Alzheimer's dementia may result from a reduced cerebral blood flow.

The relationship among high cholesterol, cholesterol-lowering medications known as "statins," and Alzheimer's disease is under investigation. High cholesterol levels during midlife have been associated with a twofold risk of mild cognitive impairment during late life. A precursor to Alzheimer's disease, mild cognitive impairment is primarily characterized by memory problems; other cognitive functions remain fairly intact. A study recently completed in the United Kingdom found that persons who used statins were almost 70% less likely to experience dementia than were nonusers of these medications.

Researchers recently published their findings from their study, which involved 724 older Catholic nuns, priests, and brothers recruited from 40 churches across the United States. At the beginning of the investigation, the participants, none of whom had dementia, recorded their frequency of participation in various cognitive activities that require information processing (such as reading). Cognitive function testing was performed at the beginning and at 1-year intervals throughout the study period, which lasted approximately 4½ years. Over the course of the investigation, 111 participants developed Alzheimer's disease. After accounting for age, gender, and education, a one-point increase in cognitive activity score correlated with a 33% reduction in the risk of Alzheimer's disease, and there was a 60% reduction in specific types of memory loss. The investigators concluded that frequent cognitive stimulation is associated with a reduction in the development of Alzheimer's disease. They further concluded that a high level of cognitive activity helps prevent Alzheimer's disease, while a decrease in an individual's cognitive activity may signal its early development.

Provider's role

Because Alzheimer's disease is believed to contain a vascular component, health care providers should identify and treat vascular risk factors in women that may delay or diminish the progression of Alzheimer's disease.

It's also important to encourage women to engage in cognitively stimulating activities, which may reduce their risk of dementia.

Hormone replacement therapy

During menopause, middle-age female patients seek help for relief of menopausal symptoms with treatments such as hormone replacement therapy (HRT). As more women enter midlife, the demand for treatments of menopausal symptoms rises. The Internet and mass media advertise many traditional and alternative forms of symptom control. Women face the overwhelming challenge of sorting through this information to determine what's best for their situation. HRT and menopausal issues directly affect their health and well-being.

Provider's role

When counseling women about HRT benefits and risks, health care providers should consider a number of factors, including cardiac protection, osteoporosis prevention, short- and long-term hormone use, and other combination HRT. Educate women who are taking or considering HRT solely for the prevention of cardiovascular disease about other strategies to lower their risks of heart disease. Assess those taking HRT solely for the prevention of osteoporosis for their personal osteoporosis risk, and discuss continuing with HRT for this purpose. In these cases, bisphosphonates and calcitonin could be considered.

Short-term HRT

For female patients seeking relief of menopausal symptoms, the benefits of short-term HRT (1 to 4 years) most likely outweighs the risks. Although certain symptoms — such as hot flashes and night sweats — tend to be of limited duration for most women, other menopausal symptoms — such as vaginal dryness — generally continue throughout the postmenopausal period. Also, many women believe that estrogen helps them to feel, think, and sleep better. These women may conclude that, for them, the

Weighing the benefits and risks of HRT

Although the benefits of hormone replacement therapy (HRT) may be significant, they must be weighed against the potential risks. Older adult females considering HRT should consult with their health care provider to determine whether HRT is appropriate for them. Here's a list of some of the benefits and risks.

Benefits

- Reduces risk of osteoporosis
- Reduces risk of heart disease
- Reduces risk of urinary incontinence
- Decreases vaginal dryness and irritation
- Decreases hot flashes
- Increases feeling of well-being
- Increases energy level

Risks

- Increases risk of endometrial cancer (if using estrogen)
- Increases risk of breast cancer
- Increases risk of gallbladder disease
- May cause bloating, fluid retention, vaginal bleeding or spotting, breast tenderness, headaches, nausea, and mood changes

added benefits of fracture prevention and colon cancer reduction associated with HRT outweigh the risks. It's appropriate to discuss with patients alternatives to HRT, such as the use of vaginal lubricants, and strategies for relief from sleep disorders. (See *Weighing the benefits and risks of HRT.*)

Long-term HRT

Long-term HRT has been found to be harmful in women. A review of the studies and trials of long-term HRT found that there was an overall increase of serious adverse effects, including breast cancer, stroke, pulmonary embolism, therefore outweighing any potential benefits to disease prevention. The studies revealed that serious adverse effects occurred in 1 out of every 170 healthy women ages 50 to 59 taking HRT for 5 years, compared to the 1 in 600 women where HRT reduced the incidence of colorectal cancer and femur fractures. Additionally, in women age 60 and older, the risk of serious adverse effects was 1 in 80 compared to the 1 in 180 women where colorectal cancer and femur fractures were reduced. Therefore, the decision to continue with long-term HRT is one that must be made based on consideration of each woman's individual benefits and risks. (See *The HRT controversy,* page 148.)

HRT for vasomotor symptoms

In women who experience debilitating vasomotor symptoms, intervention with selective serotonin reuptake inhibitors (SSRIs), hormones, or other preparations may be appropriate. Clinical trials have found the following agents to be somewhat useful in relieving menopausal vasomotor symptoms:

- SSRIs (venlafaxine, paroxetine, sertraline) — have been shown to reduce

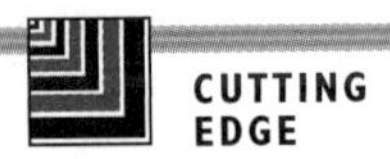

CUTTING EDGE

The HRT controversy

Hormone replacement therapy (HRT) remains a controversial issue in the treatment of menopause. It's imperative that women and their health care providers review the research findings and the current guidelines for use of HRT in making appropriate decisions concerning this therapy.

Clinical trials designed to assess the relationship between HRT and coronary artery disease events among post-menopausal women who did or did not take HRT were recently performed in the Heart and Estrogen/progestin Replacement Study (HERS), the Heart and Estrogen/progestin Replacement Study Follow-up (HERS II), and the Nurses' Health Study. Although findings from the HERS II showed that HRT didn't provide cardiac protection in women who had previously been diagnosed with heart disease, reanalysis of the data indicated that women on cholesterol-lowering statins experienced fewer problems associated with thromboembolic events.

The Women's Health Initiative (WHI) involves a primary prevention trial in healthy postmenopausal women, which has multiple arms. The purpose of this long-term clinical investigation is to evaluate the safety and effectiveness of estrogen, as well as an estrogen/progestin combination, given to healthy women. The study involves 25,000 women and was originally intended to cover a 9-year period. Participants enrolled between 1993 and 1998 with the final analysis planned for 2005. The WHI was designed to assess the major benefits and risks of HRT with regard to coronary heart disease, venous thrombotic events, breast cancer, colon cancer, and fractures. Quality-of-life issues, such as a reduction in hot flashes and vaginal dryness, weren't included in the study.

In May 2002, a 5-year follow-up of the estrogen and progestin arm of the WHI trial was halted because the predetermined boundary for invasive breast cancer was exceeded. At that time, it was concluded that the risks outweighed the benefits for the indicators that were being studied. Significantly, there was no difference in rates of mortality between the two groups (those who did receive HRT and those who did not receive HRT).

hot flashes in women with a history of breast cancer; continued research is indicated.

- Belladonna alkaloid preparation (a combination of phenobarbital, caffeine, and belladonna) — may be useful in helping women avoid sleep-related vasomotor symptoms; continued research is indicated.
- Progestin-only formulations (megestrol acetate) — may reduce hot flashes in women with a history of breast cancer; continued research is indicated.
- Topical progesterone (transdermal progesterone) — has been suggested as a useful agent in the prevention of vasomotor symptoms without producing systemic estrogenic effects; continued research is indicated.
- Clonidine (Catapres) — this antihypertensive medication acts at the cen-

tral nervous system level to reduce or eliminate hot flashes.

HRT availability

HRT is available in a variety of forms, doses, and delivery systems. Many different estrogen preparations, which include natural and synthetic agents, are used. Dosing of these medications varies from one estrogen agent each calendar day for 25 days, followed by 7 to 12 days of a progestin, to continuous estrogen dosing with intermittent progestin dosing, a regimen that tends to be more convenient for most women. Oral estrogen equivalencies include the following preparations:

- conjugated estrogens (Premarin)
- micronized estradiol (Estrace)
- esterified estrogens (Estratab, Menest)
- esterified estrogens with methyltestosterone (Estratest)
- estropipate (Ortho-Est, Ogen).

Transdermal patches, which slowly release estrogen, are applied one or two times a week to a hairless area of the skin. In general, transdermal estrogen provides the same relief of menopausal symptoms as do the oral preparations but without the adverse effects of breast tenderness or fluid retention. Transdermal estrogen is available under the brand names of Estraderm, Climara, FemPatch, Esclim, Vivelle, and Alora. Vaginal estrogen creams include Premarin, Estrace, Ogen, and Dienestrol. The Estring is a vaginal ring delivery system for estrogen.

Oral progestin equivalencies include:

- medroxyprogesterone acetate (Provera)
- medroxyprogesterone (Curretab)
- norethindrone acetate (Aygestin)
- Norethindrone (Micronor).

Combination oral estrogen-progestin preparations include Prempro and Premphase; a combined estrogen-progestin patch (CombiPatch) is also available.

Women shouldn't take ERT if they have known or suspected estrogen-dependent cancer, undiagnosed genital bleeding, active thrombophlebitis or thromboembolic disorder, active liver or gallbladder disease, or known or suspected pregnancy.

Current trends in ERT/HRT

Although ERT and HRT have proven beneficial in the treatment of postmenopausal symptoms (such as hot flashes and vaginal dryness), in response to recent research findings many women today are understandably reluctant to initiate or continue with this therapy. Adverse effects, such as breast tenderness and vaginal bleeding, are common and in many cases result in discontinuation of therapy. Other women experience problems (weight gain, mood changes) related to the progestin component of HRT prescribed for women with a uterus. Most importantly, the fear of an association between ERT/HRT and breast cancer has caused many women to be wary. Today, it's estimated that only 20% of all postmenopausal women are using HRT/ERT, and fewer than half of those who are prescribed

ERT/HRT are still taking it 1 year following initiation.

Drugs known as selective estrogen receptor modulators (SERMs) are being prescribed today for many women who choose not to use HRT. SERMs are being closely studied for their usefulness in preventing postmenopausal osteoporosis and heart disease. They act as either an estrogen agonist or an estrogen antagonist, depending on the target tissue and the particular qualities of the drug. The most familiar SERMs prescribed today are clomiphene, tamoxifen, and raloxifene — all of which are used according to their specific estrogen receptor properties. Although several SERMs are currently under investigation for use in menopause, only raloxifene (Evista) has been approved for the prevention and treatment of postmenopausal osteoporosis. The risk of thromboembolism associated with raloxifene is equal to that of supplemental estrogen. Raloxifene has also been shown to significantly reduce several risk markers associated with cardiovascular disease. Raloxifene has demonstrated value in the prevention and treatment of osteoporotic fractures. Also, breast cancer research has shown reductions with this medication in both newly diagnosed invasive breast cancer and estrogen receptor–positive breast cancer. Clinical trials are ongoing.

Alternative therapies

Many women seek out alternative therapies for their menopausal symptoms because of the associated risks involved with ERT/HRT. Because herbal supplements are generally available without a prescription, it's important to inform your patients that — because the U.S. Food and Drug Administration doesn't require oversight of herbal or botanical products — these substances haven't been subjected to rigorous testing of their safety and efficacy.

Hundreds of plants and herbs contain various forms of phytoestrogens. A few examples are legumes, flaxseed, cashews, peanuts, almonds, oats, garlic, corn, wheat, apples, sage, hops, anise, fennel, licorice, alfalfa, black cohosh, dong quai, Siberian ginseng, red clover, and soy foods. The potential adverse effects of long-term or high-dose soy isoflavone supplements are unknown. It's recommended that women who use isoflavone extracts for menopausal vasomotor symptoms (such as hot flashes) should be cautioned not to exceed 150 mg/day.

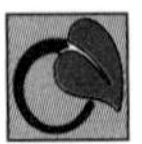

ALTERNATIVE THERAPIES

Many women use soy-based substances and herbal preparations to combat menopausal symptoms. Phytoestrogens are plant-derived compounds that are found naturally in whole plant foods and herbs; their effects on the body are similar to those of endogenous hormones. Phytoestrogens are believed to have both estrogenic and antiestrogenic benefits for women. Their use was first investigated in 1990, and a number of studies since then have examined the effects of soy protein–containing phytoestrogens on cardiovascular disease risk factors and perimenopausal symptoms; the findings are controversial. Continued research is indicated because findings from various studies have demonstrated substantial symptomatic improvement, whereas results from other studies have indicated no improvement in women's symptoms.

Provider's role

Health care providers should offer menopausal patients the option of adding whole foods to their diets because the balance of nutrients found in whole foods is better utilized by the body. There are many whole food sources of soy isoflavone, which may be more effective than extracts in preventing or reducing vasomotor symptoms of menopause. These sources include soy milk fortified with calcium and vitamin D, soynut butter, tofu, toasted soynut snacks, soy yogurt, miso (a soy paste commonly used in Japanese soups), edamame (green soybeans), and cheeses, cream cheeses and ice creams made from tofu.

Warn female patients that weight gain is likely if these substances are added to the diet rather than substituted for other food items. Stress the importance of choosing calcium-fortified soy products (such as soy milk) when possible for healthier bones. During menopause, when estrogen levels drop, these substances can act as a supplement by providing a weak estrogenic effect, thus reducing symptoms caused by lower estrogen levels. A few plants and such foods as pomegranates, dates, apples, oats, green beans, and licorice contain actual estrogens, which are similar to estrogen produced by the human body. Alert the physician to any herbs the patient is taking.

Long-term studies of black cohosh have not yet been conducted, but use of this herb to reduce menopausal vasomotor symptoms has shown some promise. A recent 6-month study involved the treatment of perimenopausal and postmenopausal women with two different doses of a black cohosh preparation. During the course of the study, the participants' menopausal symptoms decreased significantly, regardless of dose. Other studies using a specific standardized black cohosh extract have also demonstrated usefulness in reducing menopausal complaints.

The effect of black cohosh for alleviating vasomotor symptoms in women who have had breast cancer may not be consistent with its effects in healthy women. A recent clinical trial that studied the use of this herb in breast cancer survivors found that black cohosh was no more effective than a placebo in treating menopausal vasomotor symptoms. According to the American College of Obstetricians and Gynecologists, no studies have been performed to evaluate the safety of black cohosh beyond 6 months. Thus, its long-term effects are unknown, and continued research is indicated.

Some people advocate the use of the mineral boron given in a dose of 3 mg/day for menopausal vasomotor symptoms. Boron is believed to have an estrogenic effect and has also been shown to decrease calcium loss in the urine. Because boron can be toxic in

Alternative therapies to HRT

To relieve menopausal symptoms and promote health during the menopausal transition, women may choose from various complementary and alternative therapies. During menopause, Hatha yoga, acupuncture, Ayurveda, and naturopathy offer women stress relief, inner peace, calmness, relaxation, body toning, and increased energy flow.

Hatha yoga integrates physical movement with breathing and the conscious direction of energy. Yoga postures are believed to help maintain flexibility, balance moods, massage internal organs, and aid endocrine gland regulation. They also improve the suppleness of muscles and connective tissues, joint function, and bone strength. Slow, deep breathing improves tissue oxygenation and calms the mind and nervous system while enhancing balance and coordination and helping to maintain bone density.

Acupuncture, a Chinese healing art, has been successfully used to treat the menopausal symptoms of hot flashes, night sweats, insomnia, anxiety, and moodiness. Fine needles stimulate and cause the flow of energy (chi) along pathways called meridians. Acupuncture has been shown to be especially effective in regulating heavy menstrual bleeding and is believed to increase the flow of chi that supports the adrenal glands, which enhances the transition into menopause.

Ayurveda, the "Science of Life," is an ancient natural healing system from India that blends diet, herbs, bodywork, yoga, and lifestyle practices with a spiritual perspective on health and illness. It's believed that life energy, or *prana,* is enhanced through these techniques and is thus made available for healing. The life force is expressed by three biological "doshas," which represent temperament, body characteristics, digestion, and metabolism. When the doshas are unbalanced, disease follows. During menopause, special herbs are commonly used to strengthen or rejuvenate the reproductive organs, regulate the hormones, and calm the emotions.

Naturopathy is an approach to natural medicine that promotes the principles of the body-mind interconnection, focusing on diet, lifestyle, and preventive measures to promote good health. Naturopathic physicians are specially trained in clinical nutrition, botanical medicine, homeopathy, traditional Chinese medicine, acupuncture, hydrotherapy, physical modalities, and counseling. In certain states, naturopathic physicians can prescribe naturally derived and plant-based drugs such as hormones. During menopause, a diet high in phytoestrogens and soy foods is commonly recommended. Dong quai, licorice, black cohosh and ginkgo biloba are herbs that enhance hormone balance and produce relief of menopausal symptoms.

large amounts and no long-term studies have been conducted with this mineral, women should simply eat "healthy" foods that are high in boron, such as noncitrus fruits (apples, grapes, pears, cherries); leafy, green vegetables (spinach, parsley, cabbage, broccoli, beet greens); and nuts and legumes. Because of its estrogenic effect, boron shouldn't be used in women with a history of breast cancer. (See *Alternative therapies to HRT.*)

SPECIAL NEEDS

Culture directly influences how certain women experience and handle their menopausal symptoms. For example, some Black women are reluctant to use HRT and instead drink tea with lemon and water or the herb dong quai to control hot flashes. Chinese women experience fewer menopausal symptoms than do White women, which may be related to their high dietary consumption of phytoestrogens. Mexican American women view menopausal symptoms as "natural" and tend to use herbal teas instead of HRT. Arab women rely on the support of friends to help them cope with the discomfort, symptoms, and emotional issues associated with menopause. They rarely use hormones and instead seek herbal remedies, cooling drinks, humor, and disregard of symptoms during this time.

Assessing and caring for the middle-age to older adult female

Health care providers should provide regular assessment of women during the middle to older years to ensure the best possible health during this stage of life. Remember that some women may be reluctant to report certain symptoms that are embarrassing or that they believe to be associated with "old age." Such problems as incontinence, dyspareunia, or diminished libido can be difficult for them to discuss with others. More often, women may delay seeking medical care because of fear or their tendency to put the needs of their families before their own personal needs.

As women grow older, perform routine height assessments as standard practice during annual examinations. Loss of height may indicate bone loss in asymptomatic women. Identifying height loss in women in their 40s or early 50s should signal a need for further testing to determine the cause.

During the health visit, provide sufficient time for a careful review of the medical history, a discussion of any concerns, and an opportunity for counseling and education about hormone therapy, diet, vitamin and calcium supplementation, daily aspirin use, breast self-examination, mammograms, sigmoidoscopy, colonoscopy, immunization updates, the need for exercise, social interaction, and sun protection. Discuss sexuality issues and address them with sensitivity by using open-ended and reflective questions, which reassure the woman. Approach care of women during midlife and beyond with respect and reassurance, which will more than likely ensure their continued participation in seeking health care, including future visits.

Keep in mind that age-related physical changes may be associated with increased discomfort during the pelvic examination. Use a gentle, thorough approach, and consider using a small adult speculum to provide comfort in postmenopausal women. Immediately refer any postmenopausal patient with adnexal masses or vaginal bleeding to a physician for further evaluation.

Advance directives can also be introduced at any entry into the health care system. A formal statement in the medical record regarding the woman's wishes concerning life maintenance or organ donation in the event of an accident or illness is useful. Most states have laws that formalize such statements in writing. Also, a woman who wishes to delegate decision-making authority to a close friend or relative may use the Durable Power of Attorney for Health Care.

The health history for women over age 70 should include a functional assessment. When conducting the review of systems, ask the older adult patient about her daily self-care activities, such as walking, getting to the bathroom, bathing, dressing, eating, and combing her hair. Also ask her about driving, use of public transportation, availability of a telephone, methods of securing groceries and preparing meals, and medications she's taking.

Communicating with the middle-age to older adult female

Effective communication between the health care provider and the patient is an essential component of health promotion activities. Knowledge of cultural differences in communication is a key feature in the development and effective implementation of any wellness program. Verbal and nonverbal communication styles, body language, and posturing, as well as meanings and usage of words, vary across cultures, genders, and ages. When working with the older woman, consider such factors as her cultural heritage, her ability to read and write, her level of cognitive functioning, and her physical limitations, all of which may affect your level of communication with her.

Communicating with the older adult female may be difficult because of age-related hearing loss. Hearing aids can help. Make sure that the devices are being worn consistently and, if applicable, that they have working batteries. Directly facing the woman when speaking with her enhances communication; it also helps if you speak in a low-pitched, moderate-volume tone toward her best side of hearing. Avoid shouting, and minimize all background noises as best as possible.

Because many feel that hearing aids demonstrate visual evidence of aging, women may hesitate to seek evaluation for hearing loss. It's always important to ensure privacy if a referral for further evaluation is made. Reassure the adult female patient that hearing aids today are typically smaller, less obtrusive, and not as noticeable.

Caring for housebound patients

Because of illness or disability, women may be become housebound. Make sure that your housebound patients have the proper help when arranging for visits. With the expanding availability of home health care services, a schedule of regular visits can

be individualized to meet the housebound patient's needs. Providing care in the home creates a unique opportunity for assessment of the woman and her family in their own environment. As the health care provider, you are able to observe how various physical, psychosocial, and spiritual factors — as well as resources and potential hazards may influence the woman's health status. Home visitation also provides a chance to evaluate health-related issues within the context of the woman's daily life. This information can prove invaluable in the continued refinement of appropriate interventions.

Health care providers who visit housebound women commonly deal with populations of great cultural, social, and economic diversity. To deliver sensitive, appropriate care, you must develop an understanding of the cultural practices unique to various ethnic groups. If you encounter language differences, ensure that you have an interpreter available to facilitate effective communication.

It's commonly believed that the need for sleep in older adults diminishes with advancing age. Instead, the sleep pattern of older individuals usually varies from earlier times in their lives. If your patient experiences a lack of sleep, it may lead to irritability, increased fatigue, and an enhanced sensitivity to pain. Offer relief in the form of a warm bath, a back rub or foot rub, a glass of warm milk, or a glass of wine (if not contraindicated) to enhance relaxation and induce sleep. Avoid sleep medications, which can cause adverse effects.

Medication management may be difficult for older persons and their family members. Housebound patients commonly take many medications for various ailments and chronic conditions, which can interact and produce dangerous adverse effects. Also, take into account any over-the-counter medicines, along with other extracts, elixirs, herbal teas, cultural healing substances or other home remedies that the woman may commonly use. Educate the female patient and her family about her medications and their potential adverse effects to promote health maintenance and safety in the home.

Health promotion for housebound patients is a challenging yet rewarding endeavor. Such issues as environmental safety, physical activity, social support, nutrition, sleep and rest, and proper management of medications must all be addressed. Be aware that social isolation can significantly contribute to depression and other health risks, so it's essential to help the older female patient to strengthen or develop her social support system.

Selected references

Administration on Aging. *Aging into the 21st Century.* Washington, D.C.: U.S. Bureau of the Census, 2001.

American College of Obstetricians and Gynecologists (ACOG) Practice Bulletin. "*Selective Estrogen Receptor Modulators,*" Number 39, 5-15. Washington, D.C.: ACOG, October 2002.

American College of Obstetricians and Gynecologists (ACOG) Practice Bulletin.

"*Use of Botanicals for Management of Menopausal Symptoms*," Number 28, 1-10. Washington, D.C.: ACOG, June 2001.

Aroian, K.J. "Russians," in *Caring for Women Cross-Culturally*. Edited by St. Hill, P., et al. (eds). Philadelphia: F.A. Davis Co., 2003.

Berman, R.R., and Goldstein, I. "Female Sexual Dysfunction," *Urology Clinics of North America* 28(2):405-16, May 2001.

Bushnell, C. "Alzheimer's Disease and Dementia: New Insights," *The Female Patient* 28(1):46-48, 2003.

Cutson, T., and Meuleman, M. "Managing Menopause," *American Family Physician* 61(5):1391-400, 1405-1406, March 2000.

De la Torre, J. "Alzheimer Disease as a Vascular Disorder: Nosological Evidence," *Stroke* 33(9):2147-48, September 2002.

Dennerstein, L., et al. "Are Changes in Sexual Functioning During Midlife Due To Aging or Menopause?" *Fertility & Sterility* 76(3):456-60, September 2001.

Drug Facts and Comparisons. St. Louis: Wolters Kluwer, 2002.

Ferraro, K.F., and Su, Y. "Financial Strain, Social Relations, and Psychological Distress Among Older People: A Cross-cultural Analysis," *Journal of Gerontology B Psychology Science Social Science* 54(1):53-55, January 1999.

Feskanich, D. "Walking and Leisure-Time Activity and Risk of Hip Fracture in Postmenopausal Women," *JAMA* 288(18): 2300-2306, November 2002.

Fylstra, D.L. "Postmenopausal HRT and Cardiovascular Disease: The Heart of the Matter," *Patient Care for the Nurse Practitioner* (special ed.) *Perspectives on Menopause and HRT* pp 4-7, Winter 2003.

Gass, M. "Overview and Implications of the Women's Health Initiative," *The Female Patient Supplement* pp 4-8, January 2003.

Goldstein, I. "Menopause and Women's Sexual Health," *Council on Hormone Education* 1(1):1-8, 2003.

Jacobson, J.S., et al. "Randomized Trial of Black Cohosh for the Treatment of Hot Flashes Among Women with a History of Breast Cancer," *Journal of Clinical Oncology* 19(10):2739-45, May 2001.

Jick, H., et al. "Statins and the Risk of Dementia," *Lancet* 356(9242):1627-31, November 2000.

Kaunitz, A.M. "Combination Hormone Replacement Therapy and the Women's Health Initiative," *The Female Patient* 27(4):14-16 November 2002.

Lenze, E.J., et al. "Co-morbid Anxiety Disorders in Depressed Elderly Patients," *American Journal of Psychiatry* 157(5): 722-28, May 2000.

Li, S., and Holm, K. "Perimenopause and the Quality of Life," *Clinical Nursing Research* 9(1):6-23, February 2000.

Libster, M. *Delmar's Integrative Herb Guide for Nurses*. Albany, N.Y.: Delmar Learning, 2002.

Lindsay, R., et al. "Effect of Lower Doses of Conjugated Equine Estrogens with and Without Medroxyprogesterone Acetate on Bone in Early Postmenopausal Women," *JAMA* 287(20):2668-76, May 2002.

Liske, E., et al. "Physiological Investigation of a Unique Extract of Black Cohosh *(Cimifugae racemosae rhizoma)*: A 6-month Study Demonstrates No Systemic Estrogenic Effect," *Journal of Women's Health Gender-based Medicine* 11(2):163-174, March 2002.

Maricic, M. "Identifying Women at Risk for Osteoporotic Fractures," *Patient Care for the Nurse Practitioner Special Edition* pp 4-10, December 2002.

Martin, L., and Jung, P. *Taking Charge of the Change: A Holistic Approach to the Three Phases of Menopause*. Albany, N.Y.: Delmar Learning, 2002.

Menopause Core Curriculum Study Guide. Cleveland: North American Menopause Society, 2000 & 2003.

Mishell, D.R., and Mendelsohn, M.E. "Introduction: The Role of Hormone Replacement Therapy in Prevention and Treatment of Cardiovascular Disease in

Postmenopausal Women," *American Journal of Cardiology* 89(12 supp.):1E-4E, June 2002.

Mokdad, A.H., et al. "The Spread of the Obesity Epidemic in the United States, 1991-1998," *JAMA* 282(16):1519-22, October 1999.

Moore, A. "Menopausal Health Strategies: Focus on Osteoporosis," *American Journal for Nurse Practitioners* 7(2):9-21, February 2003.

Nakajima, S. "Using HRT to Prevent and Treat Osteoporosis," *Patient Care for the Nurse Practitioner* (special ed.) *Perspectives on Menopause and HRT* pp 8-10, Winter 2002.

National Osteoporosis Foundation. *The Physician's Guide to Prevention and Treatment of Osteoporosis.* Washington, D.C.: National Osteoporosis Foundation, 2000.

Neustadt, D.H. "Osteoarthritis," in *Conn's Current Therapy*. Edited by Rakel, R.E., and Bope, E.T. Philadelphia: W.B. Saunders Co., 2003.

Northrup, D.T. "Self-care: Re-examining the Myth," in *Transforming Health Promotion Practice.* Young, L.Y., & Hayes, V. Philadelphia: F.A. Davis Co., 2002

Onega, T. "How Does Menopause Alter the Primary Care of Women?" *Journal of the American Academy of Physicians Assistants* 13(4):42-44, 47-48, 51-54 passim, April 2000.

Owens, A.F., and Tepper, M.S. "Chronic Illnesses and Disabilities Affecting Women's Sexuality," *The Female Patient* 28(1):45-50, 2003.

Pietraniec-Shannon, M.A. "Nursing Care of Elderly Patients," in *Understanding Medical-Surgical Nursing*, 2nd ed. Williams, L.S., & Hopper, P.D. Philadelphia: F.A. Davis Co., 2003

Rhoads, S. "Perimenopause: A Time for Diligent Cancer Screening," *Advance for Nurse Practitioners* 10(2):65-67, February 2002.

Sawin, K.J. "Health Care Concerns for Women with Physical Disability and Chronic Illness," In *Women's Health: A Primary Care Clinical Guide*, 2nd ed. Youngkin, E.Q., & Davis, M.S. Stamford, Conn.: Appleton & Lange, 1998.

Sinclair, B.P. "Health Promotion and Prevention," in *Maternity & Women's Health Care,* 7th ed. Lowdermilk, D.L., et al. Philadelphia: Mosby Year–Book, Inc., 2000.

Speroff, L. " Management of the Perimenopausal Transition," *Contemporary OB/GYN* 45(10):10-24, 2000.

"Summaries for Patients: Screening for Osteoporosis: Recommendations from the U.S. Preventive Service Task Force," *Annals of Internal Medicine* 137(6):159, 2002.

Utian, W.H. et al. "Relief of Vasomotor Symptoms and Vaginal Atrophy with Lower Doses of Conjugated Equine Estrogens and Medroxyprogesterone Acetate," *Fertility & Sterility* 75(6):1065-79, June 2001.

Weed, S.S. *New Menopausal Years: The Wise Woman Way, Alternative Approaches for Women.* Woodstock, N.Y.: Ash Tree, 2002.

Wilson, R., and Mendes de Leon, C. "Participation in Cognitively Stimulating Activities and Risk of Incident Alzheimer Disease," *JAMA* 287(6):742-48, February 2002.

Wyman, J.F. "Treatment of Urinary Incontinence in Men and Older Women," *American Journal of Nursing* 103(3):26-35, March 2003.

PART II

Diseases and disorders

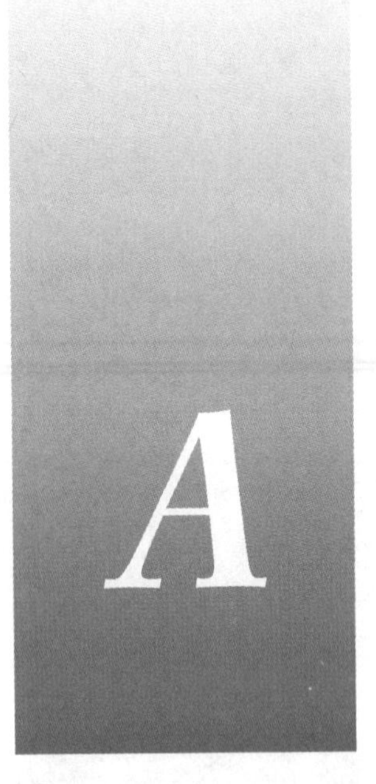

Abortion

Abortion is the spontaneous or induced (therapeutic) expulsion of the products of conception from the uterus before 20 weeks' gestation. Up to 15% of all pregnancies and approximately 30% of first pregnancies end in spontaneous abortion (miscarriage). About 85% of miscarriages occur during the first trimester. (See *Types of spontaneous abortion.*)

Causes

Spontaneous abortion may result from fetal, placental, or maternal factors.

Fetal factors, which usually cause such abortions at up to 12 weeks' gestation, include:

- defective embryologic development resulting from abnormal chromosome division (most common cause of fetal death)
- faulty implantation of the fertilized ovum (such as ectopic pregnancy)
- failure of the endometrium to accept the fertilized ovum.

Placental factors usually cause abortion around the 14th week of gestation, when the placenta takes over the hormone production necessary to maintain the pregnancy. These factors include:

Types of spontaneous abortion

Types of spontaneous abortion include:

- *threatened abortion.* Bloody vaginal discharge occurs during the first half of pregnancy. Approximately 20% of pregnant women have vaginal spotting or actual bleeding early in pregnancy; of these women, about 50% abort.
- *inevitable abortion.* Membranes rupture and the cervix dilates. As labor continues, the uterus expels the products of conception.
- *incomplete abortion.* Uterus retains part or all of the placenta. Before the 10th week of gestation, the fetus and placenta are usually expelled together; after the 10th week, separately. Because part of the placenta may adhere to the uterine wall, bleeding continues. Hemorrhage is possible because the uterus doesn't contract and seal the large vessels that feed the placenta.
- *complete abortion.* Uterus passes all the products of conception. Minimal bleeding usually accompanies complete abortion because the uterus contracts and compresses maternal blood vessels that feed the placenta.
- *missed abortion.* Uterus retains the products of conception for 2 months or more after the death of the fetus. Uterine growth ceases; uterine size may even seem to decrease. Prolonged retention of the dead products of conception may cause coagulation defects, such as disseminated intravascular coagulation, usually after at least 1 month in utero.
- *habitual abortion.* Spontaneous loss of three or more consecutive pregnancies constitutes habitual abortion.
- *septic abortion.* Infection accompanies abortion. This may occur with spontaneous or therapeutic abortions. It's usually related to any remaining fetal or placental tissue in the uterus.

- premature separation of the normally implanted placenta (also known as *abruptio placentae*)
- abnormal placental implantation (also known as *placenta previa*).

Maternal factors usually cause abortion between the 11th and 19th week of gestation and include:

- maternal infection or abnormalities of the reproductive organs (especially an incompetent cervix, in which the cervix dilates painlessly in the second trimester)
- endocrine problems, such as thyroid dysfunction or a luteal phase defect
- trauma
- antiphospholipid antibody syndrome
- blood group incompatibility
- drug ingestion (particularly uterotonic agents).

The goal of *therapeutic abortion* is to preserve the mother's mental or physical health in cases of rape, unplanned pregnancy, or medical conditions, such as moderate or severe cardiac dysfunction.

Signs and symptoms

Prodromal signs of spontaneous abortion may include a pink discharge for several days or a scant brown discharge for several weeks before the onset of cramps and increased vaginal bleeding. For a few hours, the cramps intensify and occur more frequently; then the cervix dilates to expel uterine contents. If the entire contents are expelled, cramps and bleeding subside. However, if any contents remain, cramps and bleeding continue. Infection and sepsis may occur if these contents aren't removed.

Diagnosis

Diagnosis of spontaneous abortion is based on clinical evidence of expulsion of uterine contents, pelvic examination, and laboratory studies. The presence of human chorionic gonadotropin (hCG) in the blood or urine confirms pregnancy; decreased hCG levels suggest spontaneous abortion. Pelvic examination determines the size of the uterus and whether this size is consistent with the length of the pregnancy. Ultrasound visualizes evidence of a gestational sac, size of the fetus, and presence of a heartbeat. Tissue histology indicates evidence of products of conception. Laboratory tests may reflect decreased hemoglobin levels and hematocrit due to blood loss. However, blood loss is rarely excessive in spontaneous abortion.

Treatment

An accurate evaluation of uterine contents is necessary before a treatment plan can be formulated. The progression of spontaneous abortion can't be prevented, except in some cases caused by an incompetent cervix. For those cases where the progression of spotaneous abortion can't be stopped, the patient must be hospitalized to control severe hemorrhage. If bleeding is severe, a transfusion with packed red blood cells or whole blood is required. Initially, the patient receives oxytocin I.V., which stimulates uterine contractions (if given after 20 weeks' gestation because receptors are absent before this gestational age). If any remnants remain in the uterus, dilatation and curettage or dilatation and evacuation (D&E) should be performed to dilate the cervix and remove any remnants.

D&E is also performed in first- and second-trimester therapeutic abortions. In second-trimester therapeutic abortions, the insertion of a prostaglandin vaginal suppository induces labor and the expulsion of uterine contents. When performed competently, second-trimester D&E is a safe procedure and allows for termination of pregnancy without the need for a lengthy induction of labor. Early first-trimester abortion may also be accomplished pharmacologically by using abortifacients, such as mifepristone (RU-486), misoprostol (Cytotec), and methotrexate (Trexall), or surgically by using vacuum aspiration.

SPECIAL NEEDS

After an abortion, whether spontaneous or induced, an Rh-negative female with a negative indirect Coombs' test should receive $Rh_o(D)$ immune globulin (human) to prevent future Rh isoimmunization.

In a habitual aborter, spontaneous abortion may result from an incompetent cervix (a clinical retrospective diagnosis suggested by a history of previous second-trimester losses accompanied by membrane rupture or painless cervical dilation). Treatment involves surgical reinforcement of the cervix (MacDonald or Shirodkar cerclage) 12 to 24 weeks after the last menstrual period. A few weeks before the estimated delivery date, the sutures are removed and the patient awaits the onset of labor. An alternative procedure is to leave the sutures in place and to deliver the infant by cesarean birth. However, cerclage hasn't been shown to be necessarily more effective than bed rest.

Recurrent spontaneous abortions may also result from the presence of antiphospholipid antibodies. Treatment with heparin and aspirin is recommended. (For more details on antiphospholipid antibody syndrome, refer to page 201).

Special considerations

Before induced or therapeutic abortion:

- Explain all procedures thoroughly.
- The patient should *not* have bathroom privileges because she may expel uterine contents without knowing it. After she uses the bedpan, inspect the contents carefully for intrauterine material.

After spontaneous or elective abortion:

- Note the amount, color, and odor of vaginal bleeding. Save and evaluate all the perineal pads the patient uses.
- Administer analgesics and oxytocin, as appropriate.
- Provide perineal care.
- Monitor vital signs.
- Monitor urine output.

Care of the patient who has had a spontaneous abortion includes providing emotional support and counseling during the grieving process. Encourage the patient and her partner to express their feelings. Some couples may want to talk to a member of the clergy or, depending on their religion, may wish to have the fetus baptized.

The patient who has had a therapeutic abortion also benefits from emotional support and counseling. Encourage her and her partner to verbalize their feelings. Remember, she may feel ambivalent about the procedure; intellectual and emotional acceptance of abortion aren't the same. Refer her for counseling, if necessary.

To prepare the patient for discharge:

- Tell the patient to expect vaginal bleeding or spotting and to immediately report any bleeding that lasts longer than 8 to 10 days or that's excessive and bright red.
- Advise the patient to watch for signs of infection, such as a temperature higher than 100.5° F (38° C) or foul-smelling vaginal discharge.
- Encourage the gradual increase of daily activities to include whatever tasks the patient feels comfortable doing, as long as these activities don't increase vaginal bleeding or cause fatigue. Most patients are able to return to work after 24 hours.
- Urge 1 to 2 weeks' abstinence from sexual intercourse, and encourage use of an effective contraceptive method thereafter.
- Instruct the patient to avoid using tampons or douching for 1 to 2 weeks.

- Be sure to inform the patient who desires an elective abortion of all the available alternatives. She needs to know what the procedure involves, what the risks are, and what to expect during and after the procedure, both emotionally and physically. Be sure to ascertain whether the patient is comfortable with her decision to have an elective abortion. Encourage her to verbalize her thoughts when the procedure is performed and at the follow-up visit, usually 2 weeks later. If you identify an inappropriate coping response, refer the patient to a professional counselor.

PREVENTION POINTER

To help decrease the need for a future elective abortion, provide information about effective methods of contraception, including hormonal contraceptives and different barrier methods.

- In cases of spontaneous abortion, stress to the patient that it commonly occurs through no fault of her own and (sometimes) isn't preventable.
- Tell the patient to see her physician in 2 to 4 weeks for a follow-up examination.

PREVENTION POINTER

To minimize the risk of future spontaneous abortions, emphasize the importance of good nutrition and rest and avoidance of alcohol, cigarettes, and drugs. If the patient has a history of habitual spontaneous abortions, suggest that she and her partner each have a thorough physical examination and full laboratory workup. For the woman, this may include premenstrual endometrial biopsy, a hormone assessment (estrogen; progesterone; and thyroid, follicle-stimulating, and luteinizing hormones), a hysterosalpingography and laparoscopy to detect anatomic abnormalities, and blood tests to detect lupus anticoagulant and anticardiolipin antibodies. Genetic counseling may also be indicated.

Acne vulgaris

Acne vulgaris is a chronic inflammatory disease of the sebaceous glands. It's usually associated with a high rate of sebum secretion and occurs on areas of the body that have sebaceous glands, such as the face, neck, chest, back, and shoulders. Excessive sebum is usually secreted into the dilated hair follicles. The sebum joins with the bacteria and keratin in the hair follicles to form a plug. There are two types of acne:

- *inflammatory*, in which the hair follicle is blocked by sebum, causing bacteria to grow and eventually rupture the follicle
- *noninflammatory*, in which the follicle doesn't rupture but remains dilated.

Acne vulgaris develops in approximately 85% of the population, primarily between ages 15 and 18. Although the lesions can appear as early as age 8 or as late as age 58, acne primarily affects adolescents. Although the severity and overall incidence of acne is usually greater in males, it tends to start at an earlier age and last longer in females.

Causes

The cause of acne is multifactorial. Although many myths exist that chocolate or fatty foods may cause acne, studies have shown that diet isn't a precipitating factor. Possible causes of acne include increased activity of sebaceous glands and blockage of the pilosebaceous ducts (hair follicles).

Factors that may predispose one to acne include:

- heredity
- androgen stimulation
- certain drugs, including corticosteroids, corticotropin (ACTH), androgens, iodides, bromides, trimethadione, phenytoin (Dilantin), isoniazid (INH), lithium (Eskalith), and halothane
- cobalt irradiation
- hyperalimentation
- exposure to heavy oils, greases, or tars
- trauma or rubbing from tight clothing
- cosmetics
- emotional stress (although stressful situations may cause acne to flare, stress itself doesn't cause acne)
- tropical climate
- hormonal contraceptive use. (Many females experience acne flare-up during their first few menses after starting or discontinuing hormonal contraceptives.)

Signs and symptoms

The acne plug may appear as:

- a closed comedo, or whitehead (not protruding from the follicle and covered by the epidermis)
- an open comedo, or blackhead (protruding from the follicle and not covered by the epidermis; melanin or pigment of the follicle causes the black color).

Rupture or leakage of an enlarged plug into the epidermis produces inflammation, characteristic acne pustules, papules or, in severe forms, acne cysts or abscesses (chronic, recurring lesions producing acne scars).

In women, signs and symptoms may include increased severity just before or during menstruation when estrogen levels are lowest.

Complications of acne may include:

- acne conglobata
- scarring (with severe cases)
- impaired self-esteem
- abscesses or secondary bacterial infections. (See *How acne develops*, page 166.)

Diagnosis

- Diagnosis is confirmed by characteristic acne lesions, especially in adolescents. Additionally, a culture may be taken to identify a possible secondary bacterial infection, which may present as an exacerbation of pustules or abscesses while on tetracycline or erythromycin drug therapy.

Treatment

Benzoyl peroxide (Benzac 5 or 10) is the treatment of choice for noninflamed lesions; it may also be used for milder forms of inflamed lesions. However, for more severe inflamed acne, treatment should include the application of antibacterial agents, such

How acne develops

The illustrations here show how acne develops.

Excessive sebum production

Acne develops when a hair follicle becomes blocked. The hair follicle becomes blocked when sebaceous glands are stimulated and produce excessive sebum and epithelial cells that line the sebaceous follicles are shed.

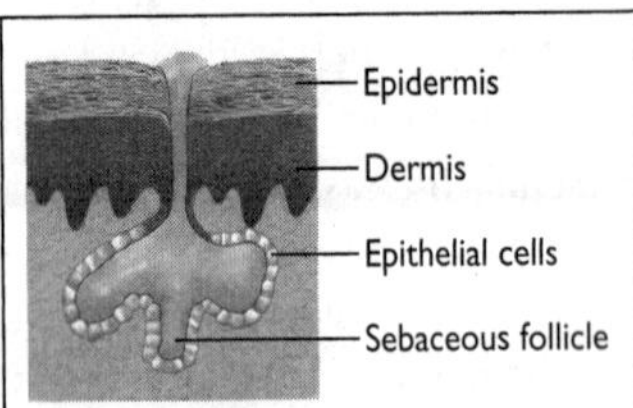

Increased shedding of epithelial cells

Excess sebum and keratin from the epithelial cells form a plug that seals the follicle, and it becomes a favorable environment for bacterial growth. The bacteria produce lipase, an enzyme that interacts with sebum to produce free fatty acids.

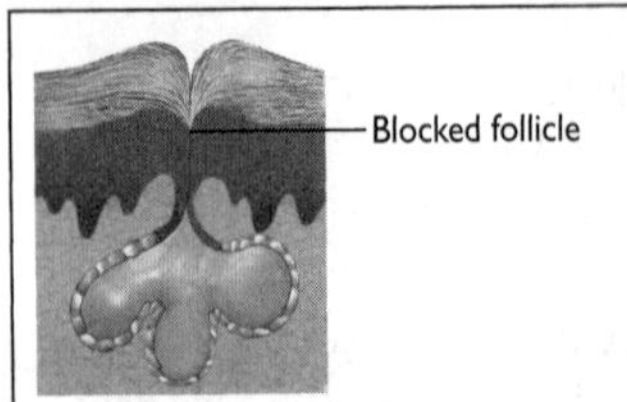

Inflammatory response in follicle

The bacterial growth causes inflammation and the formation of closed or open comedones, which may rupture.

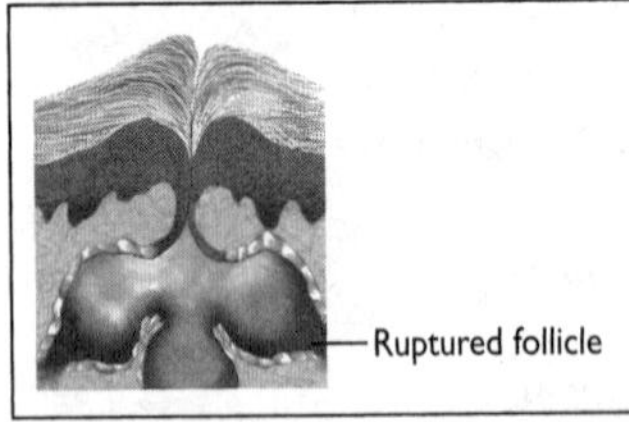

Comedones of acne

Closed comedones (also known as *whiteheads*) don't protrude from follicles and are covered by the epidermis. Open comedones (also known as *blackheads*) protrude from the follicle and are not covered by the epidermis. Melanin or pigment of the follicle causes the black discoloration.

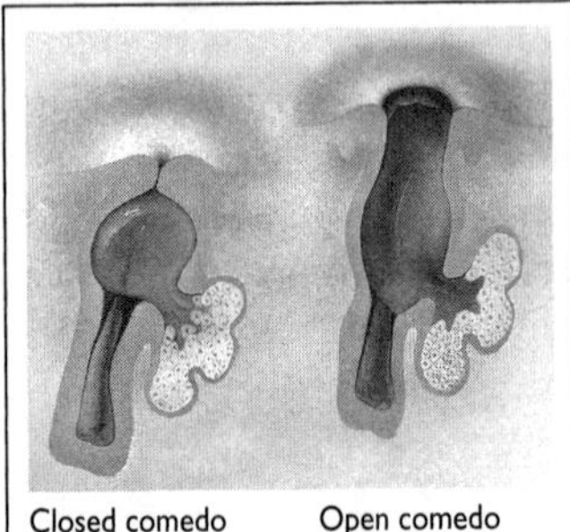

Closed comedo (whitehead) | Open comedo (blackhead)

as clindamycin (Cleocin), or benzoyl peroxide plus erythromycin (Benzamycin) antibacterial agents. These may be applied alone or with tretinoin (Retin-A; retinoic acid), which is a keratolytic. Keratolytic agents, such as benzoyl peroxide and tretinoin, dry and peel the skin in order to help open blocked follicles, moving the sebum up to the skin level.

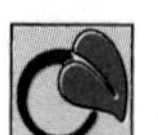

ALTERNATIVE THERAPIES

Natural remedies have also been used successfully in treating acne. Witch hazel has been used as an all-purpose astringent for centuries. Vitamins, such as A, C, and D, have also been used to treat acne.

Systemic therapy consists primarily of:

- antibiotics, usually a tetracycline, to decrease bacterial growth (Dosage is reduced for long-term maintenance when the patient is in remission.)
- oral isotretinoin (Accutane) to inhibit sebaceous gland function and keratinization (Because of its severe adverse effects, a 16- to 20-week course of isotretinoin is limited to patients with severe papulopustular or cystic acne that isn't responding to conventional therapy. This drug is known to cause birth defects; thus, the manufacturer, with Food and Drug Administration approval, recommends the following precautions: pregnancy testing before dispensing; dispensing only a 30-day supply; repeat pregnancy testing throughout the treatment period; effective contraception during treatment; and informed consent. Due to its effects on the liver, a serum triglyceride level should also be drawn before and periodically during isotretinoin treatment.)
- antiandrogens (for females only)
- hormonal contraceptives such as norgestimate/ethinyl estradiol (Ortho Tri-Cyclen)
- antiandrogens and hormonal contraceptives
- spironolactone for short-term treatment only
- cleaning gently with a sponge in order to dislodge superficial comedones (harsh or aggressive scrubbing and washing may increase sebum production and cause more inflammation and scarring)
- surgery to remove comedones and to open and drain pustules (usually performed on an outpatient basis)

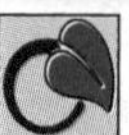

ALTERNATIVE THERAPIES

For severe acne scarring, dermabrasion, with a high-speed metal brush, is an effective treatment to smooth the skin.

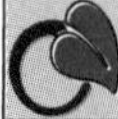

ALTERNATIVE THERAPIES

Bovine collagen injections (into the dermis beneath the scarred area) may be used to fill in affected areas and even out the skin surface (although not recommended by all dermatologists).

Special considerations

The main focus of your care is teaching about the disorder as well as its treatment and prevention:

- Check the patient's drug history because certain medications such as some hormonal contraceptives may cause an acne flare-up.

- Try to identify predisposing factors that may be eliminated or modified.
- Try to identify eruption patterns (seasonal or monthly).
- Explain the causes of acne to the patient and family. Make sure they understand that the prescribed treatment is more likely to improve acne than a strict diet and harsh scrubbing with soap and water. Provide written instructions regarding treatment.
- Describe the importance of not picking at the lesions because it will only further inflame the lesion and may lead to permanent facial scarring. Encourage good personal hygiene in order to prevent secondary infections. Instruct women to remove any makeup daily with a mild cleanser and astringent, especially at bedtime. Also, tell the patient to avoid cosmetics or other oily skin or hair products that block pores and to buy only noncomedogenic cosmetics and skin products.
- Instruct the patient receiving tretinoin to apply it at least 30 minutes after washing her face and at least 1 hour before bedtime. Warn against using it around the eyes or lips. After treatments, the skin should look pink and dry. If it appears red or starts to peel, the preparation may have to be weakened or applied less frequently. Advise the patient to use sunscreen when exposed to sunlight. If the prescribed regimen includes tretinoin and benzoyl peroxide, advise her to avoid skin irritation by using one preparation in the morning and the other at night.
- Instruct the patient to take tetracycline on an empty stomach and not to take it with antacids or milk because it interacts with her metallic ions and will be poorly absorbed.
- Tell the patient who's taking isotretinoin to avoid vitamin A supplements, which can worsen adverse effects. Also, teach the patient how to deal with the dry skin and mucous membranes that usually occur during treatment. Tell the female patient about the severe risk of teratogenicity and to avoid getting pregnant while on isotretinoin therapy. Monitor the patient's liver function and lipid levels.
- Inform the patient that acne may take a long time to clear — possibly even years for complete resolution. Encourage continued and regular local skin care even after acne clears.
- Explain the adverse effects of all drugs.

SPECIAL NEEDS

Pay special attention to the patient's perception of her physical appearance — especially in adolescents because they're still developing their sense of identity and self-esteem — and offer emotional support.

Acute coronary syndromes

Acute coronary syndromes (ACS) describes a group of conditions, including unstable angina, non-Q-wave myocardial infarction, and Q-wave myocardial infarction. ACS are conditions caused by coronary vessel obstruction and thrombotic occlusions from rupture or erosion of plaque.

The *incidence* of ACS is higher in males who are younger than age 70 (although the incidence of angina at 15 years postmenopause is equal to that in men); however, *mortality* after a myocardial infarction (MI) is significantly higher among women than men up to age 75. That's because many prescribers tend to overlook signs and symptoms of ACS in women (of all ages) because of the perceived cardioprotective effect of estrogen.

The higher risk of death among women may be explained partially by differences in medical history (such as diabetes), a lower rate of established treatment use in women, and clinical characteristics. Indeed, among patients under age 50, mortality for women is more than twice that for men. Thus, women are considered a high-risk group. (See *Angina in women.*)

Angina in women

In the past, research on coronary heart disease has been based on data collected from male patients. The symptom of chest tightness or pain is well known as the "hallmark" of angina. Women with angina, however, may report atypical chest pain, such as when the pain radiates to neck, throat, shoulders, or back. Angina in women may also appear as increased shortness of breath, nausea, difficulty breathing, loss of appetite, or weakness. Because of this difference in how angina may present in women, women are commonly misdiagnosed or diagnosed later; therefore, delaying treatment and increasing mortality rates.

Causes

The predominant cause of ACS is due to atherosclerotic plaque disease. Coronary artery vasospasm is a less common cause. The most common cause of unstable angina is coronary artery disease (CAD) due to atherosclerosis. Fatty, fibrous plaques progressively narrow the coronary artery lumina, reducing the volume of blood that can flow through them and leading to myocardial ischemia. (See *Atherosclerotic plaque development*, page 170.)

As atherosclerosis progresses, luminal narrowing is accompanied by vascular changes that constrict the blood vessel and impair blood flow. This causes a precarious balance between myocardial oxygen supply and demand, threatening the myocardium beyond the lesion. When oxygen demand exceeds what the diseased vessel can supply, localized myocardial ischemia results.

Myocardial cells become ischemic within 10 seconds of a coronary artery occlusion. Transient ischemia causes reversible changes at the cellular and tissue levels, depressing myocardial function. Untreated, this can lead to tissue injury or necrosis. Within several minutes, oxygen deprivation forces the myocardium to shift from aerobic to anaerobic metabolism, leading to accumulation of lactic acid and reduction of cellular pH.

Atherosclerotic plaque development

The coronary arteries are made of three layers: intima (the innermost layer), media (the middle layer), and adventitia (the outermost layer).

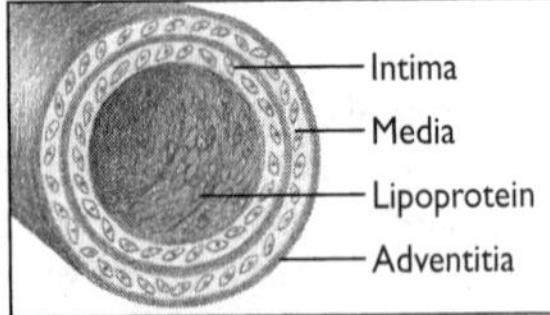

Damaged by risk factors, a fatty streak begins to build up on the intimal layer.

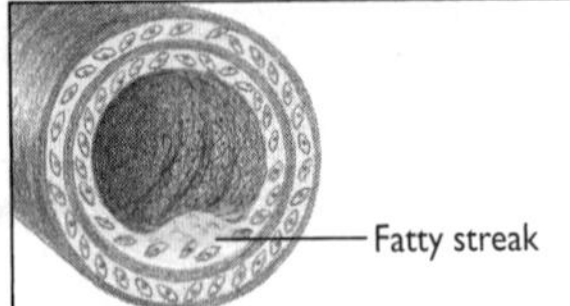

Fibrous plaque and lipids progressively narrow the lumen and impede blood flow to the myocardium.

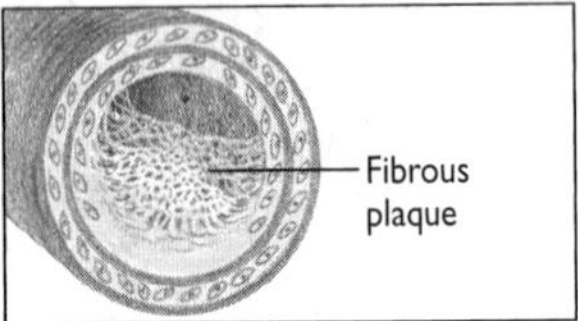

The plaque continues to grow and, in advanced stages, may become a complicated calcified lesion that may rupture.

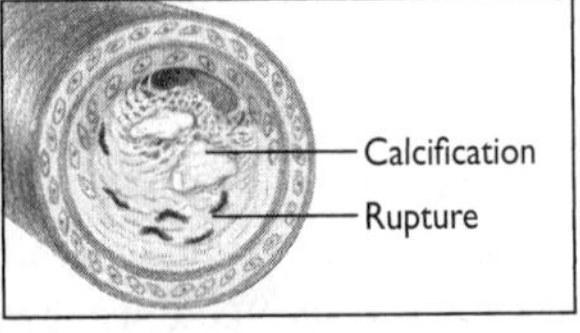

Types of angina

There are four types of angina:

- *stable angina*—pain that's predictable in frequency and duration and relieved by rest and nitroglycerin
- *unstable angina*—pain that increases in frequency and duration and is more easily induced, which indicates a worsening of coronary artery disease that may progress to myocardial infarction
- *Prinzmetal's* or *variant angina*—pain that's caused by spasm of the coronary arteries, which may occur spontaneously and may not be related to physical exercise or emotional stress
- *microvascular angina*—impairment of vasodilator reserve that causes angina-like chest pain in a person with normal coronary arteries.

The combination of hypoxia, reduced energy availability, and acidosis rapidly impairs left ventricular function. The strength of contractions in the affected myocardial region is reduced as the fibers shorten inadequately, resulting in less force and velocity. Moreover, wall motion is abnormal in the ischemic area, resulting in less blood being ejected from the heart with each contraction. Restoring blood flow through the coronary arteries restores aerobic metabolism and contractility. However, if blood flow isn't restored, MI results. (See *Types of angina.*)

Other causes of MI include:

CAD IN WOMEN

Coronary artery disease (CAD) results from the narrowing of the coronary arteries over time due to atherosclerosis. The primary effect of CAD is the loss of oxygen and nutrients to myocardial tissue because of diminished coronary blood flow. As the population ages, the prevalence of CAD is increasing, especially in women who smoke or take hormonal contraceptives. Although women are typically 10 years older than men when their risk of CAD increases, CAD is the leading cause of death in women.

CAD may be asymptomatic in the older adult because of a decrease in sympathetic response. Dyspnea and fatigue are two key signals of ischemia in an active, older adult.

Signs and symptoms

Signs and symptoms of CAD may include:

- angina—the classic sign of CAD—which results from a reduced supply of oxygen to the myocardium and may be described as burning, squeezing, or tightness in the chest possibly radiating to the left arm, neck, jaw, or shoulder blade
- nausea and vomiting as a result of reflex stimulation of the vomiting centers by pain
- cool extremities and pallor caused by sympathetic stimulation
- diaphoresis due to sympathetic stimulation
- xanthelasma (fat deposits on the eyelids) occurring secondary to hyperlipidemia and atherosclerosis.

- ventricular hypertrophy due to hypertension, valvular disease, or cardiomyopathy
- embolic occlusion of the coronary arteries
- hypoxia, as in carbon monoxide poisoning or acute pulmonary disorders
- cocaine and amphetamines, which increase myocardial oxygen demand and may cause coronary vasospasm
- underlying coronary artery disease, which may be masked by severe anemia (see *CAD in women*)
- inflammation of epicardial arteries.

Predisposing risk factors for MI include:

- positive family history
- gender (men and postmenopausal women are more susceptible to MI than premenopausal women, although the incidence is increasing among women, especially those who smoke and take hormonal contraceptives)
- hypertension
- smoking
- elevated serum triglyceride, total cholesterol, and low-density lipoprotein levels (see *Hyperlipidemia in women*, page 172)
- obesity
- excessive intake of saturated fats
- sedentary lifestyle
- aging
- stress or type A personality
- drug use, especially cocaine and amphetamines.

MI results from occlusion of one or more of the coronary arteries. Occlusion can stem from atherosclerosis,

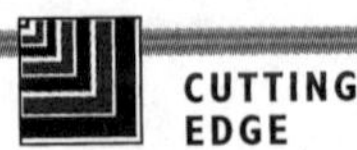

Hyperlipidemia in women

Hyperlipidemia has been undertreated in women. Perhaps the reliance on hormone replacement therapy (HRT) in the past has contributed to this. Recent studies, however, have alerted us that HRT has no benefit for prevention of coronary events. Women with hyperlipidemia should be counseled about lifestyle changes, such as diet and exercise, to decrease cholesterol. If drug therapy is warranted, statins should be used as first-line therapy.

thrombosis, platelet aggregation, or coronary artery stenosis or spasm. If coronary artery occlusion causes ischemia lasting longer than 30 to 45 minutes, irreversible myocardial cell damage and muscle death occur. The site of the MI depends on the vessels involved. Occlusion of the circumflex branch of the left coronary artery causes a lateral wall infarction; occlusion of the anterior descending branch of the left coronary artery causes an anterior wall infarction. True posterior or inferior wall infarctions generally result from occlusion of the right coronary artery or one of its branches.

Right ventricular infarctions may also result from right coronary artery occlusion, can accompany inferior infarctions, and may cause right-sided heart failure. In Q-wave (transmural) MI, tissue damage extends through all myocardial layers; in non-Q-wave (subendocardial) MI, damage occurs only in the innermost and, possibly, middle layers.

All infarcts have a central area of necrosis or infarction surrounded by an area of potentially viable hypoxic injury. This zone may be salvaged if circulation is restored or it may progress to necrosis. The zone of injury, in turn, is surrounded by an area of viable ischemic tissue. (See *Zones of myocardial infarction.*) Although ischemia begins immediately, the size of the infarct can be limited if circulation is restored within 6 hours.

Signs and symptoms

The symptoms of ACS are due to myocardial ischemia, the underlying cause of which is an imbalance between supply and demand of myocardial oxygenation. Typically, angina is a symptom of myocardial ischemia. It is usually described as a sensation of chest pressure, tightness, or heaviness that's produced by activities or conditions that increase myocardial oxygen demand. However, not all patients will experience chest pains. Some patients will present with neck, jaw, ear, arm, or epigastric pain. Others may experience shortness of breath, lightheadedness or dizziness, nausea and vomiting, diaphoresis, or severe weakness, which may represent anginal equivalent symptoms. (See *Complications of angina.*)

Diagnosis

The initial diagnosis of ACS is based almost entirely on the patient's medical and family history, risk factors

Zones of myocardial infarction

Myocardial infarction has a central area of necrosis surrounded by a zone of injury that may recover if revascularization occurs. An outer ring of reversible ischemia surrounds this zone of injury. Characteristic electrocardiographic changes are associated with each zone.

Myocardial ischemia
- T-wave inversion
- ST-segment depression

Myocardial injury
- ST-segment elevation
- T-wave inversion

Myocardial infarction
- Q waves
- ST-segment elevation
- T-wave inversion

Complications of angina

Complications of angina include:
- acute MI
- cardiogenic shock
- ischemic mitral insufficiency
- arrhythmias
- atrioventricular nodal blockade.

Complications of MI include:
- arrhythmias
- cardiogenic shock
- heart failure causing pulmonary edema
- pericarditis
- rupture of the atrial or ventricular septum, ventricular wall, or valves
- mural thrombi causing cerebral or pulmonary emboli
- ventricular aneurysms
- myocardial rupture
- extensions of the original infarction.

and, to a lesser extent, an electrocardiogram (ECG). ECG is the most important diagnostic test for angina. It may show changes during symptoms and in response to treatment. It may also show preexisting structural or ischemic heart disease (left ventricular hypertrophy, Q waves). An ECG may be normal between anginal episodes. A normal ECG or one that remains unchanged from baseline doesn't exclude the possibility that chest pain is ischemic in origin. Changes that may be seen during anginal episodes include:
- transient ST segment elevations (ST-segment elevation suggests either MI or Prinzmetal's angina)
- dynamic T-wave changes
- ST depression.

A diagnosis of CAD is determined using the following tests:
- Ultra-fast CT scan may be used to identify calcium deposits in coronary arteries. Calcium scoring correlates with the degree of CAD.
- Stress testing may be performed to detect ST-segment changes during exercise or pharmacologic stress, indicating ischemia, and to determine a safe exercise prescription.
- Coronary angiography reveals the location and degree of coronary artery stenosis or obstruction, collateral circulation, and the condition of the artery beyond the narrowing.

- Intravascular ultrasound may be used to further define coronary anatomy and luminal narrowing.
- Myocardial perfusion imaging with thallium-201 may be performed during treadmill exercise to detect ischemic areas of the myocardium; they appear as "cold spots," which normalize during rest, indicating viable tissue.
- Stress echocardiography may show abnormal wall motion in ischemic areas.
- Rest perfusion imaging with sestamibi may be used to rule out myocardial ischemia in the patient with a chest pain syndrome that isn't clearly cardiac in nature.

A diagnosis of MI is determined using the following tests:

- Serial 12-lead ECG may reveal characteristic changes, such as serial ST-segment depression in non-Q-wave MI (a more limited area of damage insufficient to cause changes in the pattern of ventricular depolarization) and ST-segment elevation in Q-wave MI (a larger area of damage, which causes permanent change in the pattern of ventricular depolarization). An ECG can also identify the location of MI, arrhythmias, hypertrophy, and pericarditis.
- Serial creatine kinase fraction (CK-MB) is the standard test for diagnosing MI.
- Serial cardiac enzymes and proteins may show a characteristic rise and fall — specifically, CK-MB, the proteins troponin T and I, and myoglobin — that confirm the diagnosis of MI.
- Laboratory testing may reveal elevated white blood cell count, C-reactive protein level, and erythrocyte sedimentation rate due to inflammation, and increased glucose levels following the release of catecholamines.
- Echocardiography may show ventricular wall motion abnormalities and may detect septal or papillary muscle rupture.
- Chest X-rays may show left-sided heart failure or cardiomegaly due to ventricular dilation. They may also show complications of ischemia such as pulmonary edema, or provide clues to alternative causes of symptoms, such as thoracic aneurysm or pneumonia.
- Nuclear imaging scanning using sestamibi, thallium-201, and technetium 99m may be used to identify areas of infarction and viable muscle cells.
- Cardiac catheterization may be used to identify the involved coronary artery as well as to provide information on ventricular function, pressures, and volumes within the heart.

Differential diagnosis must rule out:

- anxiety
- aortic stenosis
- asthma
- dilated cardiomyopathy
- esophagitis
- gastroenteritis
- gastroesophageal reflux disease
- hypertensive crisis
- myocardial infarction
- myocarditis
- pericarditis and cardiac tamponade
- pneumothorax

- pulmonary embolism.

Treatment

The goals of treatment are to preserve patency of the coronary artery, increase blood flow through stenosed lesions, and reduce myocardial oxygen demand. Patients with severe unstable angina and ECG changes should be admitted to a telemetry unit. All patients should receive antiplatelet agents, and patients with ongoing ischemia should receive aggressive medical intervention until signs of ischemia resolve, as indicated on ECG and by lack of signs and symptoms.

The following drugs have been used to treat ACS:

- Antiplatelets have been shown to reduce mortality by reducing the risk of fatal strokes and MIs.
- Nitrates oppose coronary artery spasm and reduce myocardial oxygen demand by reducing preload and afterload.
- Analgesics reduce pain, which decreases sympathetic stress and reduces preload.
- Anticoagulants prevent recurrence of clot after spontaneous fibrinolysis.
- Beta-adrenergic blockers (antiarrhythmic and antihypertensive) reduce ischemia, afterload, and wall stress. In patients with acute MI, they decrease infarct size and short- and long-term mortality, which is a function of their anti-ischemic and antiarrhythmic properties.
- Glycoprotein IIB/IIA inhibitors prevent the binding of fibrinogen, thereby blocking platelet aggregation. Studies suggest that adding I.V. glycoprotein IIB/IIA inhibitors to aspirin and heparin early in treatment improve early and late outcomes, including mortality, Q-wave MI, need for revascularization procedures, and length of hospital stay.
- IIB/IIA antagonists with aspirin are standard antiplatelet therapy for a patient at high risk for unstable angina. Adenosine diphosphate (ADP) antagonists aren't considered standard therapy but may be useful in a patient who can't tolerate aspirin.

Treatment of an MI typically involves following the treatment guidelines recommended by the American College of Cardiology/American Heart Association (ACC/AHA) Task Force on Practice Guidelines. These include:

- assessment of the patient with chest pain in the emergency department within 10 minutes of symptom onset because at least 50% of deaths take place within 1 hour of the onset of symptoms (Moreover, thrombolytic therapy is most effective when started within the first 3 hours after the onset of symptoms.)
- oxygen by nasal cannula for 2 to 3 hours to increase blood oxygenation
- nitroglycerin sublingually or I.V. to relieve chest pain, unless systolic blood pressure is less than 90 mm Hg or heart rate is less than 50 or greater than 100 beats/minute
- morphine or meperidine (Demerol) for analgesia because pain stimulates the sympathetic nervous system, leading to an increase in heart rate and vasoconstriction
- aspirin every day indefinitely to inhibit platelet aggregation

- continuous cardiac monitoring to detect arrhythmias and ischemia
- I.V. fibrinolytic therapy for the patient experiencing chest pain for at least 30 minutes who reaches the hospital within 12 hours of the onset of symptoms (unless contraindications exist) and whose ECG shows new left bundle-branch block (LBBB) or ST-segment elevation of at least 1 to 2 mm in two or more ECG leads (The greatest benefit of such reperfusion therapy, however, occurs when reperfusion takes place within 3 hours of the onset of chest pain.)
- I.V. heparin for the patient who has received fibrinolytic therapy to increase the chances of patency in the affected coronary artery
- percutaneous transluminal coronary angioplasty (PTCA), which is superior to fibrinolytic therapy if it can be performed in a timely manner in a facility with personnel skilled in the procedure
- glycoprotein IIB/IIIA receptor blocking agents, which strongly inhibit platelet aggregation (They're indicated as adjunct therapy with PTCA in acute ST-segment elevation MI and as a primary therapy in non-ST-segment elevation MI. Their use in combination with fibrinolytic agents is controversial.)
- limitation of physical activity for the first 12 hours to reduce cardiac workload, thereby limiting the area of necrosis
- keeping atropine, amiodarone, transcutaneous pacing patches or a transvenous pacemaker, a defibrillator, and epinephrine readily available to treat arrhythmias (The ACC/AHA doesn't recommend the prophylactic use of antiarrhythmic drugs during the first 24 hours.)
- I.V. nitroglycerin for 24 to 48 hours in the patient without hypotension, bradycardia, or excessive tachycardia to reduce afterload and preload and relieve chest pain
- early I.V. beta-adrenergic blockers to the patient with an evolving acute MI followed by oral therapy (as long as there are no contraindications) to reduce heart rate and myocardial contractile force, thereby reducing myocardial oxygen requirements
- angiotensin-converting enzyme inhibitors in the patient with an evolving MI with ST-segment elevation or LBBB (but without hypotension or other contraindications) to reduce afterload and preload and prevent remodeling
- magnesium sulfate for 24 hours to correct hypomagnesemia, if needed
- angiography and possible percutaneous or surgical revascularization for the patient with spontaneous or provoked myocardial ischemia following an acute MI
- exercise testing before discharge to determine the adequacy of medical therapy and to obtain baseline information for an appropriate exercise prescription (Exercise testing can also determine functional capacity and decrease the patient's risk of a subsequent cardiac event.)
- reducing cardiac risk through a program of weight control; a low-fat, low-cholesterol diet; smoking cessation; and regular exercise

- lipid-lowering agents, as indicated by the fasting lipid profile. (See *Treating myocardial infarction*, pages 178 and 179.)

Treatment of CAD may involve:

- nitrates, such as nitroglycerin (given sublingually, orally, transdermally, or topically in ointment form), isosorbide dinitrate (given sublingually or orally), or isosorbide mononitrate (given orally) to reduce myocardial oxygen consumption
- beta-adrenergic blockers to reduce the heart's workload and oxygen demands by reducing heart rate and peripheral resistance to blood flow
- calcium channel blockers to prevent coronary artery spasm
- antiplatelet drugs to minimize platelet aggregation and the risk of coronary occlusion
- antilipemic drugs to reduce serum cholesterol or triglyceride levels
- antihypertensive drugs to control hypertension
- estrogen replacement therapy to reduce the risk of CAD in postmenopausal women
- coronary artery bypass graft (CABG) surgery to restore blood flow by bypassing an occluded artery using another vessel
- "key-hole" or minimally invasive surgery, an alternative to traditional CABG using fiber-optic cameras inserted through small incisions in the chest, to correct blockages in one or two accessible arteries
- angioplasty, to relieve occlusion in patients with partial occlusion but without calcification
- laser angioplasty to correct occlusion by vaporizing fatty deposits
- rotational atherectomy to remove arterial plaque with a high-speed burr
- stent placement in a reopened artery to hold the artery open
- drug-eluting stent placement, currently under clinical trials, to hold a reopened artery open and to minimize the risk of in-stent restenosis
- lifestyle modifications to reduce further progression of CAD; these include smoking cessation, regular exercise, stress management, maintaining an ideal body weight, and following a low-fat, low-sodium diet.

Special considerations

Care for the patient who has suffered an ACS is directed toward detecting complications, preventing further myocardial damage, and promoting comfort, rest, and emotional well-being. Commonly, the patient with an MI receives treatment in the intensive care unit (ICU), where he's under constant observation for complications. Other considerations include:

- On admission to the ICU, monitor and record the patient's ECG, blood pressure, temperature, and heart and breath sounds.
- Assess and record the severity and duration of pain, and administer analgesics. Avoid I.M. injections; absorption from the muscle is unpredictable, and bleeding is likely if the patient is receiving fibrinolytic therapy.
- Check the patient's blood pressure after giving nitroglycerin, especially the first dose.

(Text continues on page 180.)

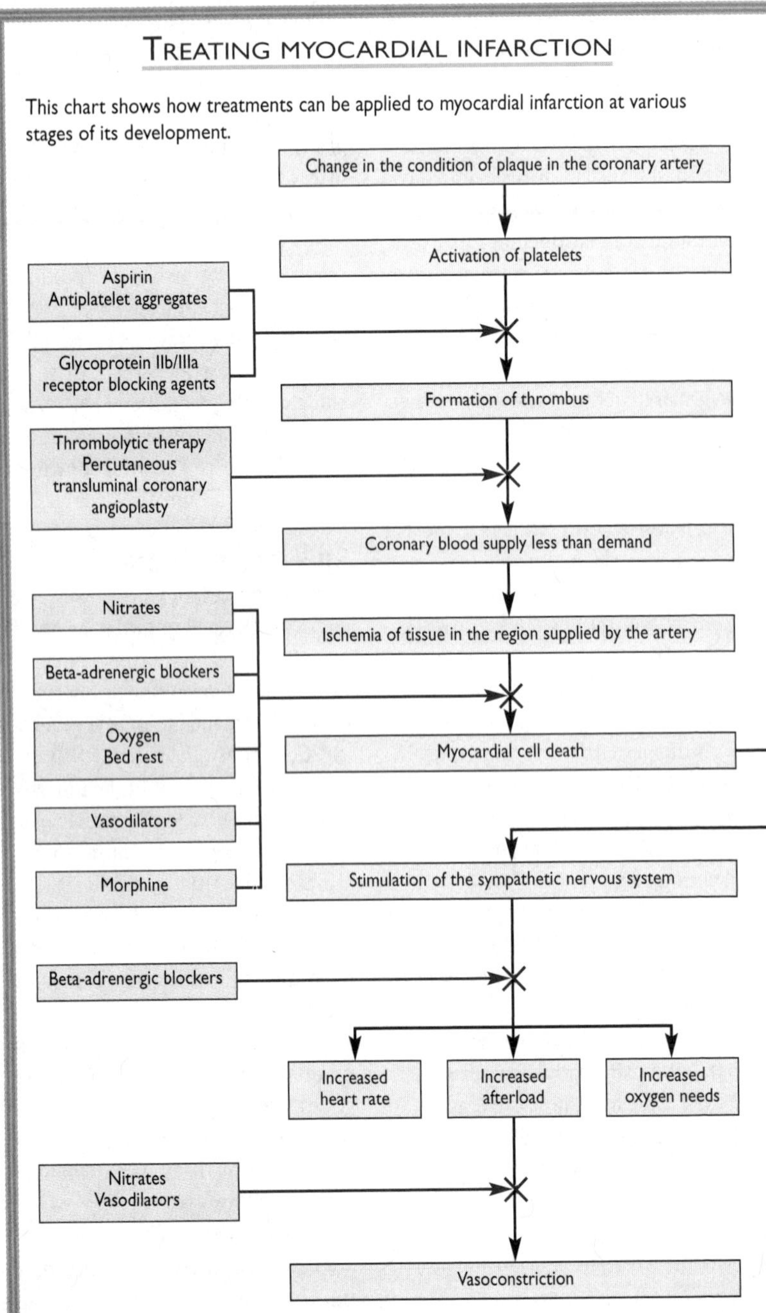
Treating myocardial infarction
This chart shows how treatments can be applied to myocardial infarction at various stages of its development.
Change in the condition of plaque in the coronary artery
Activation of platelets
Aspirin
Antiplatelet aggregates
Glycoprotein IIb/IIIa receptor blocking agents
Formation of thrombus
Thrombolytic therapy
Percutaneous transluminal coronary angioplasty
Coronary blood supply less than demand
Ischemia of tissue in the region supplied by the artery
Nitrates
Beta-adrenergic blockers
Oxygen
Bed rest
Vasodilators
Morphine
Myocardial cell death
Stimulation of the sympathetic nervous system
Beta-adrenergic blockers
Increased heart rate
Increased afterload
Increased oxygen needs
Nitrates
Vasodilators
Vasoconstriction

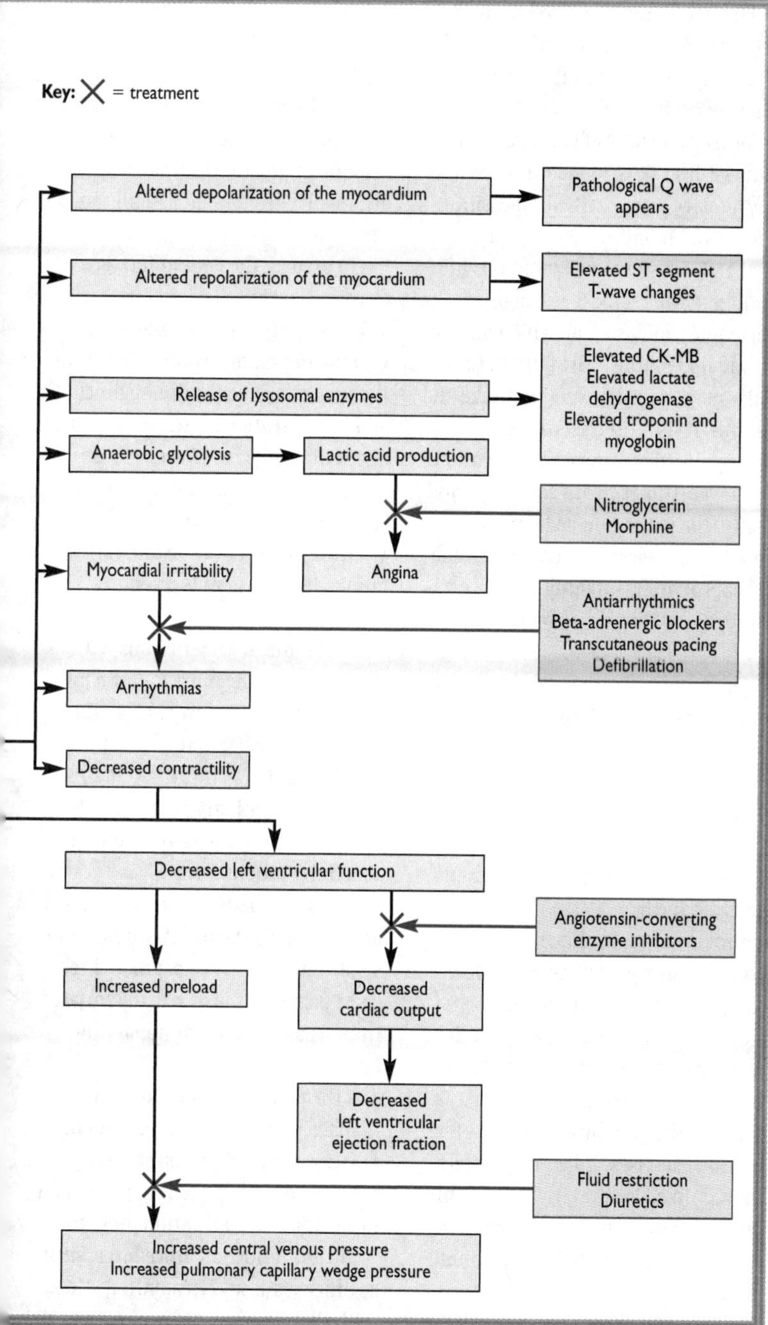
Key: ✕ = treatment
Altered depolarization of the myocardium
Pathological Q wave appears
Altered repolarization of the myocardium
Elevated ST segment
T-wave changes
Release of lysosomal enzymes
Elevated CK-MB
Elevated lactate dehydrogenase
Elevated troponin and myoglobin
Anaerobic glycolysis
Lactic acid production
Nitroglycerin
Morphine
Myocardial irritability
Angina
Antiarrhythmics
Beta-adrenergic blockers
Transcutaneous pacing
Defibrillation
Arrhythmias
Decreased contractility
Decreased left ventricular function
Angiotensin-converting enzyme inhibitors
Increased preload
Decreased cardiac output
Decreased left ventricular ejection fraction
Fluid restriction
Diuretics
Increased central venous pressure
Increased pulmonary capillary wedge pressure

- Frequently monitor the ECG to detect rate changes or arrhythmias. Place rhythm strips in the patient's chart periodically for evaluation.
- During episodes of chest pain, obtain 12-lead ECG, blood pressure, and pulmonary artery catheter measurements and monitor them for changes.
- Watch for signs and symptoms of fluid retention (crackles, cough, tachypnea, and edema), which may indicate impending heart failure. Carefully monitor daily weight, intake and output, respirations, serum enzyme levels, and blood pressure. Auscultate for adventitious breath sounds periodically (the patient on bed rest commonly has atelectatic crackles, which disappear after coughing), for S_3 or S_4 gallops, and for new-onset heart murmurs.
- Organize patient care and activities to maximize periods of uninterrupted rest.
- Ask the dietary department to provide a clear liquid diet until nausea subsides. A low-cholesterol, low-sodium, low-fat, high-fiber diet may be prescribed.
- Provide a stool softener to prevent straining during defecation, which causes vagal stimulation and may slow the heart rate. Allow the patient to use a bedside commode, and provide as much privacy as possible.
- Assist the patient with range-of-motion exercises. If he's completely immobilized by a severe MI, turn him often. Antiembolism stockings help prevent venostasis and thrombophlebitis.
- Provide emotional support to the patient, and help reduce stress and anxiety; administer tranquilizers as needed. Explain procedures and answer questions. Explain the ICU's environment and routine to ease anxiety. Involve the patient's family in her care as much as possible.

To prepare the patient for discharge:

- Thoroughly explain dosages and therapy to promote compliance with the prescribed medication regimen and other treatment measures. Warn about drug adverse effects, and advise the patient to watch for and report signs of toxicity (anorexia, nausea, vomiting, and yellow vision, for example, if the patient is receiving digoxin).
- Review dietary restrictions with the patient. If she must follow a low-sodium or low-fat, low-cholesterol diet, provide a list of foods that she should avoid. Ask the dietitian to speak to the patient and her family.
- Counsel the patient to resume sexual activity progressively.
- Advise the patient to report typical or atypical chest pain. Postinfarction syndrome may develop, producing chest pain that must be differentiated from recurrent MI, pulmonary infarct, or heart failure.
- If the patient has a Holter monitor in place, explain its purpose and use.
- Stress the need to stop smoking.
- Encourage the patient to participate in a cardiac rehabilitation program.
- Review follow-up procedures, such as office visits and treadmill testing, with the patient.

Alopecia

Alopecia, the partial or complete loss of hair, most commonly occurs on the scalp as well as bearded areas, eyebrows, and eyelashes. Hair loss elsewhere on the body is less common and less conspicuous. In the nonscarring form of this disorder (noncicatricial alopecia), the hair follicle can generally regrow hair. However, scarring alopecia usually destroys the hair follicle, making hair loss irreversible. Both men and women lose hair density as they age, but in different patterns — male-pattern baldness and female-pattern baldness.

Male-pattern baldness is characterized by a gradual recession of the hairline to form an "M" shape and is caused by hormones and genetic predisposition. The existing hair may be finer and may not grow as long as it formerly did. The hair at the crown also begins to thin, and eventually the top points of the hairline "M" meet the thinned crown, leaving a horseshoe pattern of hair around the sides of the head. Unlike the gradual recession of the hairline in male-pattern baldness, female-pattern baldness is an overall thinning that maintains the normal hairline.

Causes

The most common form of nonscarring alopecia in men and women is androgenetic alopecia, which is hair loss mediated by a chemical known as dihydrotestosterone (DHT). This hair loss appears to be related to androgen levels and to aging. Genetic predisposition commonly influences time of onset, degree of baldness, speed with which it spreads, and pattern of hair loss.

Hormones, aging, and genetic predisposition cause female-pattern baldness, which may be more noticeable after a woman reaches menopause. Estrogen in a woman's body counteracts the small amount of testosterone that's converted to DHT. After menopause, a woman no longer has the estrogen to counteract the conversion of DHT. Other reasons for alopecia in women include:

- temporary shedding of hair (telogen effluvium), which is more common in women
- breaking of hair from such things as styling treatments and twisting and pulling of hair
- patchy areas of hair loss (alopecia areata), an immune disorder causing temporary hair loss
- some medications (such as chemotherapy)
- certain skin diseases.

Other forms of nonscarring alopecia include:

- *physiologic alopecia* (usually temporary) — sudden hair loss in infants, loss of straight hairline in adolescents, and diffuse hair loss after childbirth
- *alopecia areata* (idiopathic form) — generally reversible and self-limiting; occurs most commonly in young and middle-age adults of both sexes. (See *Alopecia areata*, page 182.)

Predisposing factors of nonscarring alopecia also include radiation, many types of drug therapies and drug reactions, bacterial and fungal

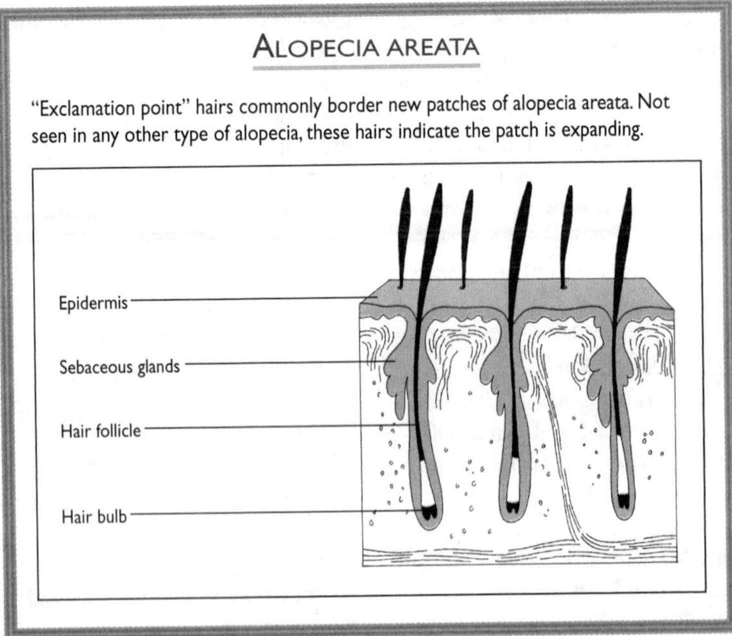

infections, psoriasis, seborrhea, and endocrine disorders, such as thyroid, parathyroid, and pituitary dysfunctions.

Scarring alopecia causes irreversible hair loss. It may result from physical or chemical trauma or chronic tension on a hair shaft, as occurs in braiding. Diseases that produce alopecia include destructive skin tumors; granulomas; lupus erythematosus; scleroderma; follicular lichen planus; and severe fungal, bacterial, or viral infections, such as kerion, folliculitis, or herpes simplex. Hair loss in patches, diffuse shedding of hair, breaking of hair shafts, or hair loss associated with redness, scaling, pain, or rapid progression could be caused by these or other underlying conditions.

Signs and symptoms

In androgenetic alopecia, hair loss is gradual and usually affects the thinner, shorter, and less pigmented hairs of the frontal and parietal portions of the scalp. In women, hair loss is generally more diffuse and mainly affects the top of the scalp; completely bald areas are uncommon but may occur. Also, the frontal hairline is maintained. However, hair loss of female-pattern baldness is permanent.

Alopecia areata affects small patches of the scalp, but may also occur as alopecia totalis, which involves the entire scalp, or as alopecia universalis, which involves the entire body. Although mild erythema may occur initially, affected areas of scalp or skin appear normal. "Exclamation point" hairs (loose hairs with dark, rough, brushlike tips on narrow, less pigmented shafts) occur at the periphery of new patches. Regrowth initially appears as fine, white, dry hair, which is replaced by normal hair.

Diagnosis

Physical examination alone is usually sufficient to confirm the diagnosis of alopecia. Diagnosis, however, must also identify any underlying disorder.

Treatment

Topical application of minoxidil, a peripheral vasodilator more typically used as an oral antihypertensive, is the preferred treatment of androgenetic alopecia. It's the only FDA-approved treatment for hair loss in women. It's available over the counter and is applied twice daily to the scalp. It may take at least 4 months for results to be seen and must be used continuously. Any interruption in treatment will cause extra hair to be lost. Minoxidil has been shown to be effective in only 30% to 40% of users.

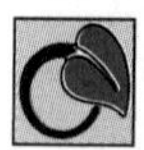

ALTERNATIVE THERAPIES

An alternative treatment for alopecia is hair transplant. Hair transplant consists of removing tiny plugs of hair from areas where the hair is continuing to grow and placing them in areas that are balding. Undergoing this procedure may cause scarring at the donor sites and carries a modest risk of infection. The procedure usually requires multiple sessions and is expensive; however, the result is excellent and permanent.

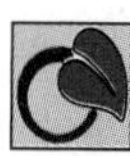

ALTERNATIVE THERAPIES

An alternative, cheaper, and safer solution for alopecia is using hair weaves and wigs, which come in a variety of styles, colors, and textures. They may be bought at a boutique specializing in wigs and hair pieces and can effectively and safely disguise a woman's hair loss and improve her self-image.

In alopecia areata, minoxidil is more effective, although treatment is commonly unnecessary because spontaneous regrowth is common. Intralesional corticosteroid injections are beneficial for small patches and may produce regrowth in 4 to 6 weeks. Anthralin, topical cyclosporine, oral inosiplex, and topical nitrogen mustard have all been used in treating alopecia areata. Hair loss that persists for more than 1 year has a poor prognosis for regrowth.

In the obsessive-compulsive disorder trichotillomania (pulling of one's own hair), an occlusive dressing may promote normal hair growth simply by preventing the patient from hair pulling. Clomipramine may be effective for short-term treatment.

Treatment of other types of alopecia varies according to the underlying cause.

Special considerations

- Reassure a woman with female-pattern alopecia that it doesn't lead to total baldness. Most forms of female-pattern baldness are mild. Suggest that she wear a wig.

- If the patient has alopecia areata, explain the disorder and reassure her that complete regrowth is possible.
- There's no known prevention for female-pattern baldness. Provide the woman with emotional support as female-pattern baldness may affect self-esteem and cause psychological stress and anxiety due to changes in her appearance.

Alzheimer's disease

Alzheimer's disease is the most common form of dementia. It's a degenerative disorder of the cerebral cortex, especially the frontal lobe, which accounts for more than half of all cases of dementia. Although primarily found in the elderly population, 1% to 10% of cases have their onset in middle age. Because this is primarily a slow but progressive dementia, the prognosis for a patient with this disease is poor. The course of the disease varies in each person, but on average, patients with the disease live from 8 to 10 years after diagnosis.

The prevalence of Alzheimer's disease usually begins after age 60 and increases dramatically with age. Its prevalence is highest among those who are age 85 and older. Because women make up 72% of the U.S. population over age 85 and usually live longer than men, they're more likely to develop Alzheimer's disease.

SPECIAL NEEDS

Alzheimer's disease also appears to be more prevalent among Blacks. Various studies have found the prevalence rate to be 14% to 100% higher in Blacks than in Whites.

Causes

The exact cause of Alzheimer's disease is unknown. Factors that have been associated with its development include:

- *neurochemical* — deficiencies in the neurotransmitters acetylcholine, somatostatin, substance P, and norepinephrine
- *environmental* — repeated head trauma; exposure to aluminum or manganese
- *genetic* — Aprolipoprotein E gene, the autosomal dominant form of Alzheimer's disease associated with early onset and death, as well as family history of the disease or the presence of Down syndrome in the patient.

Other risk factors include:

- age
- vascular disease (Those with hypertension or high cholesterol have been found twice as likely to get Alzheimer's disease, and those with both risk factors are four times as likely to develop dementia.)
- use of hormone replacement therapy in postmenopausal women. (See *Dementia and CHT.*)

The brain tissue of patients with Alzheimer's disease exhibits three distinct and characteristic features:

- neurofibrillatory tangles (fibrous proteins)
- neuritic plaques (composed of degenerating axons and dendrites)
- granulovascular changes.

Additional structural changes include cortical atrophy, ventricular dilation, deposition of amyloid (a glycoprotein) around the cortical blood vessels, and reduced brain volume. A selective loss of cholinergic neurons in the pathways to the frontal lobes and hippocampus, areas that are important for memory and cognitive functions, are also found. Examination of the brain after death commonly reveals an atrophic brain, usually weighing less than 1,000 g (where normal is 1,380 g).

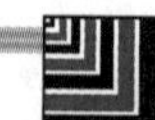

CUTTING EDGE

Dementia and CHT

In May of 2003, the Women's Health Initiative Memory Study (WHIMS) performed a study with 4,500 women ages 65 and older to measure whether combination hormone therapy (CHT) decreased the risk of dementia. Surprisingly, the study concluded that those women who took combination estrogen plus progesterone hormone therapy, particularly Prempro, were at increased risk for dementia. The study showed these women had twice the risk of dementia compared to the placebo group.

In another study in July of 2002, researchers found that CHT also increased the risk of breast cancer, heart disease, stroke, and blood clots, which outweighed its benefits for hip fractures, bone density, and colorectal cancer. In addition to these recent findings, women of any age should consult with their physician about the individual risks and benefits of CHT.

Signs and symptoms

Typical signs and symptoms of Alzheimer's disease reflect neurologic abnormalities associated with the disease and include:

- gradual loss of recent and remote memory, loss of sense of smell, and flattening of affect and personality
- difficulty with learning new information
- deterioration in personal hygiene
- inability to concentrate
- increasing difficulty with abstraction and judgment
- impaired communication
- severe deterioration in memory, language, and motor function
- loss of coordination
- inability to write or speak
- personality changes, wandering
- nocturnal awakenings
- loss of eye contact and fearful look
- signs of anxiety such as wringing of hands
- acute confusion, agitation, compulsiveness, or fearfulness when overwhelmed with anxiety
- disorientation and emotional lability
- progressive deterioration of physical and intellectual ability.

The most common complications include:

- injury secondary to violent behavior, confusion, or wandering
- pneumonia and other infections
- malnutrition
- dehydration
- aspiration
- death.

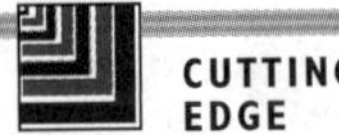

CUTTING EDGE

Namenda approval

In October of 2003, the Food and Drug Administration approved memantine (Namenda), the first drug for the treatment of patients with moderate to severe Alzheimer's disease. Previous treatments have been for patients with mild to moderate Alzheimer's disease.

Namenda's mechanism of action is different from other available drugs. It blocks the activation of N-methyl-D-aspartate receptors, which are thought to contribute to the symptoms of Alzheimer's.

Although the drug doesn't stop or slow the underlying neurodegeneration of the disease, it's been found effective at reducing symptoms and has a low incidence of adverse effects.

Diagnosis

Alzheimer's disease is diagnosed by exclusion; that is, by ruling out other disorders as the cause for the patient's signs and symptoms. The only true way to confirm Alzheimer's disease is by finding pathologic changes in the brain at autopsy. However, the following diagnostic tests may be useful:

- Positron emission tomography shows changes in the metabolism of the cerebral cortex.
- Computed tomography (CT) scan shows evidence of early brain atrophy in excess of that which occurs in normal aging.
- Magnetic resonance imaging (MRI) shows no lesion as the cause of the dementia.
- EEG shows evidence of slowed brain waves in the later stages of the disease.
- Cerebral blood flow studies show abnormalities in blood flow.

Treatment

No cure or definitive treatment exists for Alzheimer's disease. Rather, treatment is symptomatic.

Treatment of cognitive symptoms includes:

- N-methyl-D-aspartate (NMDA) receptor antagonist (such as memantine [Namenda]) to treat moderate to severe symptoms of Alzheimer's disease (see *Namenda approval*)
- cholinesterase inhibitors (such as donepezil [Aricept], rivastigmine [Exelon], galantamine [Reminyl], and tacrine [Cognex]) to help improve memory deficits
- hyperbaric oxygen to increase oxygenation to the brain
- vitamin E supplements to prevent red blood cell destruction, thereby maintaining oxygen blood flow to the brain
- cerebral vasodilators (such as ergoloid mesylates, isoxsuprine, and cyclandelate) to enhance cerebral circulation
- choline salts, lecithin, physostigmine, or an experimental agent (such as deanol, enkephalins, and naloxone) to attempt to slow the disease process.

Treatment for agitation includes:

- antidepressants, if depression appears to exacerbate dementia
- anxiolytics to decrease anxiety
- psychostimulants (such as methylphenidate) to enhance the patient's mood.

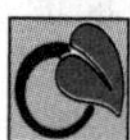

ALTERNATIVE THERAPIES

There are many alternative treatments proven or purported to treat Alzheimer's disease. However, herbal and dietary supplements haven't been approved by the FDA and, therefore, their safety and effectiveness remain unknown. Some of these alternative treatments include:

- ginkgo biloba — a plant extract with antioxidant and anti-inflammatory properties that may protect cell membranes and regulate neurotransmitter function and, in turn, may improve a patient's cognition, social behavior, and ability to carry out activities of daily living
- huperzine A — a moss extract that has been used in traditional Chinese medicine for centuries that has similar properties to those of FDA-approved Alzheimer's disease medications and found to be effective in treating Alzheimer's disease
- phosphatidylserine — a lipid that's found in the cell membranes of neurons used to protect cells from degenerating as they do in Alzheimer's disease and similar disorders.

Special considerations

Overall care is focused on supporting the patient's remaining abilities and compensating for those she's lost.

- Establish an effective communication system with the patient and family to help them adjust to the patient's altered cognitive abilities.
- Offer emotional support to the patient and family members. Caring for a person with Alzheimer's is life-altering. Behavior problems may be worsened by excess stimulation or change in established routine. Teach them about the disease, and refer them to social services and community resources for legal and financial advice and support.
- Anxiety may cause the patient to become agitated or fearful. Intervene by helping her focus on another acivity.
- Provide the patient with a safe environment. Encourage her to exercise, as ordered, to help maintain mobility.

Amenorrhea

Amenorrhea is the abnormal absence or suppression of menstruation. Absence of menstruation is normal before puberty, after menopause, or during pregnancy and lactation; it's abnormal and, therefore, pathologic at any other time. Primary amenorrhea is the absence of menarche in an adolescent (age 16 and older). Secondary amenorrhea is the failure of menstruation for at least 3 months after the normal onset of menarche. Primary amenorrhea occurs in 1% of women; secondary amenorrhea is seen in about 4% of women. Prognosis varies depending on the specific cause. Surgical correction of outflow tract obstruction is usually curative.

Causes

Amenorrhea usually results from:

- anovulation due to hormonal abnormalities, such as decreased secretion of estrogen, gonadotropins, luteinizing hormone, and follicle-stimulating hormone (FSH)

- lack of ovarian response to gonadotropins
- constant presence of progesterone or other endocrine abnormalities.

Amenorrhea may also result from:

- absence of a uterus
- endometrial damage
- ovarian, adrenal, or pituitary tumors
- emotional disorders (common in patients with severe disorders, such as depression and anorexia nervosa), mild emotional disturbances tending to distort the ovulatory cycle, severe psychic trauma abruptly changing the bleeding pattern or completely suppressing one or more full ovulatory cycles
- malnutrition and intense exercise, causing an inadequate hypothalamic response.

The pathogenic mechanism varies depending on the cause and whether the defect is structural, hormonal, or both. Women who have adequate estrogen levels but a progesterone deficiency don't ovulate and are, thus, infertile. In primary amenorrhea, the hypothalamic-pituitary-ovarian axis is dysfunctional. Because of anatomical defects of the central nervous system, the ovary doesn't receive the hormonal signals that normally initiate the development of secondary sex characteristics and the beginning of menstruation.

Secondary amenorrhea can result from several central factors (hypogonadotropic hypoestrogenic anovulation) or uterine factors (as with Asherman's syndrome, in which the endometrium is sufficiently scarred that no functional endometrium exists) as well as cervical stenosis and premature ovarian failure, among others.

Signs and symptoms

Because amenorrhea may result from one of several disorders, signs and symptoms depend on the specific cause. Signs and symptoms may include:

- absence of menstruation
- vasomotor flushes, vaginal atrophy, hirsutism (abnormal hairiness), and acne (secondary amenorrhea).

Complications of amenorrhea include:

- infertility
- endometrial adenocarcinoma (amenorrhea associated with anovulation that gives rise to unopposed estrogen stimulation of the endometrium).

Diagnosis

Diagnosis of amenorrhea is based on:

- history of failure to menstruate in females age 16 and older, if consistent with bone age (confirms primary amenorrhea)
- absence of menstruation for 3 months in a previously established menstrual pattern (secondary amenorrhea)
- physical and pelvic examination and sensitive pregnancy test ruling out pregnancy as well as anatomic abnormalities (such as cervical stenosis) that may cause false amenorrhea (cryptomenorrhea), in which menstruation occurs without external bleeding

- onset of menstruation (spotting) within 1 week after giving pure progestational agents such as medroxyprogesterone (Provera), indicating enough estrogen to stimulate the lining of the uterus (if menstruation doesn't occur, special diagnostic studies, such as gonadotropin levels, are indicated)
- blood and urine studies showing hormonal imbalances, such as lack of ovarian response to gonadotropins (elevated pituitary gonadotropin levels), failure of gonadotropin secretion (low pituitary gonadotropin levels), and abnormal thyroid levels (Without suspicion of premature ovarian failure or central hypogonadotropism, gonadotropin levels aren't clinically meaningful because they're released in a pulsatile fashion; at a given time of day, levels may be elevated, low, or average.)
- complete medical workup, including appropriate X-rays, laparoscopy, and a biopsy, to identify ovarian, adrenal, and pituitary tumors.

Tests to identify dominant or missing hormones include:

- "ferning" of cervical mucus on microscopic examination (an estrogen effect)
- vaginal cytologic examination
- endometrial biopsy
- serum progesterone level
- serum androgen levels
- elevated urinary 17-ketosteroid levels with excessive androgen secretions
- plasma FSH level more than 50 IU/L, depending on the laboratory (suggests primary ovarian failure); or normal or low FSH level (possible hypothalamic or pituitary abnormality, depending on the clinical situation).

Treatment

Treatment of amenorrhea may include:

- appropriate hormone replacement to reestablish menstruation
- treatment of the cause of amenorrhea not related to hormone deficiency (for example, surgery for amenorrhea due to a tumor or obstruction)
- inducing ovulation (With an intact pituitary gland, clomiphene [Clomid] may induce ovulation in women with secondary amenorrhea due to gonadotropin deficiency, polycystic ovarian disease, or excessive weight loss or gain.)
- FSH and human menopausal gonadotropins (Pergonal) for women with pituitary disease
- improving nutritional status
- modification of exercise routine.

Special considerations

- Explain all diagnostic procedures.
- Provide reassurance and emotional support. Psychiatric counseling may be necessary if amenorrhea results from emotional disturbances.
- After treatment, teach the patient how to keep an accurate record of her menstrual cycles to aid in early detection of recurrent amenorrhea.

Anemia, folic acid deficiency

Folic acid deficiency anemia is a common, slowly progressive, megaloblastic anemia. It commonly occurs in in-

FOODS HIGH IN FOLIC ACID

Folic acid (pteroylglutamic acid, folacin) is found in most body tissues, where it acts as a coenzyme in metabolic processes involving one carbon transfer. It's essential for formation and maturation of red blood cells and for synthesis of deoxyribonucleic acid. Although its body stores are relatively small (about 70 mg), this vitamin is plentiful in most well-balanced diets.

Even so, because folic acid is water-soluble and heat-labile, cooking easily destroys it. In addition, approximately 20% of folic acid intake is excreted unabsorbed. Insufficient daily folic acid intake (less than 50 mcg/day) usually induces folic acid deficiency within 4 months. At right is a list of foods high in folic acid content.

Food	mcg/100 g
Asparagus spears	109
Beef liver	294
Broccoli spears	54
Collards (cooked)	102
Mushrooms	24
Oatmeal	33
Peanut butter	57
Red beans	180
Wheat germ	305

fants, adolescents, pregnant and lactating females, alcoholics, elderly people, and people with malignant or intestinal diseases.

Causes

Folic acid deficiency anemia may result from:

- alcohol abuse (alcohol may suppress metabolic effects of folate)
- poor diet (common in alcoholics, elderly people living alone, and infants, especially those with infections or diarrhea)
- impaired absorption (due to intestinal dysfunction from bowel resection or such disorders as celiac disease, tropical sprue, and regional jejunitis)
- bacteria competing for available folic acid
- excessive cooking, which can destroy a high percentage of folic acid in foods (see *Foods high in folic acid*)
- limited storage capacity in infants
- prolonged drug therapy (anticonvulsants and estrogens)
- increased folic acid requirements during pregnancy, during rapid growth in infancy (common because of recent increase in survival of premature infants), during childhood and adolescence (because of general use of cow's milk, which is a poor source of folate), and in patients with neoplastic diseases and some skin diseases (chronic exfoliative dermatitis).

Signs and symptoms

Folic acid deficiency anemia gradually produces clinical features characteristic of other megaloblastic anemias,

without the neurologic manifestations, including:
- progressive fatigue
- shortness of breath
- palpitations
- weakness
- glossitis
- nausea
- anorexia
- headache
- fainting
- irritability
- forgetfulness
- pallor or slight jaundice.

Folic acid deficiency anemia doesn't cause neurologic impairment unless it's associated with vitamin B_{12} deficiency, as in pernicious anemia.

SPECIAL NEEDS

Folic acid deficiency in pregnancy has been strongly associated with neural tube defects in infants.

Diagnosis

The Schilling test and a therapeutic trial of vitamin B_{12} injections distinguish between folic acid deficiency anemia and other types of anemia, such as pernicious anemia. Significant findings include macrocytosis, decreased reticulocyte count, abnormal platelets, and serum folate less than 4 mg/ml. (See *Tests for blood composition, production, and function*, page 192.)

Treatment

Treatment of folic acid deficiency anemia consists primarily of folic acid supplements and elimination of contributing causes. Folic acid supplements are recommended for *all* pregnant women. They may be given orally (usually 1 to 5 mg/day) or parenterally (to patients who are severely ill, have malabsorption, or are unable to take oral medication). Many patients respond favorably to a well-balanced diet. If the patient has combined B_{12} and folate deficiencies, folic acid replenishment alone may aggravate neurologic dysfunction.

Special considerations

- Teach the patient to meet daily folic acid requirements by including a food from each food group in every meal. If the patient has a severe deficiency, explain that diet only reinforces folic acid supplementation and isn't therapeutic by itself. Urge compliance with the prescribed course of therapy. Advise the patient not to stop taking the supplements when she begins to feel better.
- If the patient has glossitis, emphasize the importance of good oral hygiene. Suggest regular use of mild or diluted mouthwash and a soft toothbrush.
- Watch fluid and electrolyte balance, particularly in the patient who has severe diarrhea and is receiving parenteral fluid replacement therapy.
- Because anemia causes severe fatigue, schedule regular rest periods until the patient can resume normal activity.

Tests for blood composition, production, and function

Below are lists of blood tests used to evaluate overall composition and red blood cell (RBC) function.

Overall composition

- *Peripheral blood smear* shows maturity and morphologic characteristics of blood elements and determines qualitative abnormalities.
- *Complete blood count* determines the actual number of blood elements in relation to volume and quantifies abnormalities.
- *Bone marrow aspiration or biopsy* allows evaluation of hematopoiesis by showing blood elements and precursors and abnormal or malignant cells.

RBC function

- *Hematocrit,* or packed cell volume (PCV), measures the percentage of RBCs per fluid volume of whole blood.
- *Hemoglobin* measures the amount (grams) of hemoglobin per deciliter of blood to determine oxygen-carrying capacity.
- *Reticulocyte count* assesses RBC production by determining concentration of this erythrocyte precursor.
- *Schilling test* determines absorption of vitamin B_{12} (necessary for erythropoiesis) by measuring excretion of radioactive B_{12} in the urine.
- *Mean corpuscular volume* describes the RBC in terms of size.
- *Mean corpuscular hemoglobin* determines average amount of hemoglobin per RBC.
- *Mean corpuscular hemoglobin concentration* establishes average hemoglobin concentration in 1 dl of packed RBCs.
- *Sucrose hemolysis test* assesses the susceptibility of RBCs to hemolyze with complement.
- *Direct Coombs' test* demonstrates the presence of immunoglobulin (Ig) G antibodies (such as antibodies to Rh factor) and complement on circulating RBCs.
- *Indirect Coombs' test,* a two-step test, detects the presence of IgG antibodies in the serum.
- *Sideroblast test* detects stainable iron (available for hemoglobin synthesis) in normoblastic RBCs.
- *Hemoglobin electrophoresis* demonstrates abnormal hemoglobin such as sickle cell.

PREVENTION POINTER

To prevent folic acid deficiency anemia, emphasize the importance of a well-balanced diet high in folic acid. Identify alcoholics with poor dietary habits, and try to arrange for appropriate counseling. Instruct mothers who aren't breast-feeding to use commercially prepared infant formulas.

Anemia, iron deficiency

Iron deficiency anemia is caused by an inadequate supply of iron for optimal formation of red blood cells (RBCs), resulting in smaller (microcytic) cells with less color on staining. Body stores of iron, including plasma iron, decrease, as do levels of transferrin, which binds with and transports iron. Insufficient body stores of iron lead to a depleted RBC mass and, in turn, to a decreased hemoglobin concentration (hypochromia) and decreased oxygen-carrying capacity of the blood. (See *Absorption and storage of iron.*)

A common disease worldwide, iron-deficiency anemia affects 20% of women of childbearing age and 2% of adult men in the United States. Iron-deficiency anemia occurs most commonly in premenopausal women, infants (particularly premature or low-birth-weight infants), children, and adolescents (especially girls).

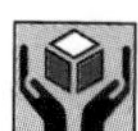

SPECIAL NEEDS

Iron deficiency is also common among persons of low socioeconomic status due to the high cost of a well-balanced diet that includes foods rich in iron.

Absorption and storage of iron

Iron, which is essential to erythropoiesis, is abundant throughout the body. Two-thirds of total body iron is found in hemoglobin; the other third, mostly in the reticuloendothelial system (liver, spleen, bone marrow), with small amounts in muscle, blood serum, and body cells.

Adequate dietary ingestion of iron and recirculation of iron released from disintegrating red cells maintain iron supplies. The duodenum and upper part of the small intestine absorb dietary iron. Such absorption depends on gastric acid content, the amount of reducing substances (ascorbic acid, for example) present in the alimentary canal, and dietary iron intake. If iron intake is deficient, the body gradually depletes its iron stores, causing decreased hemoglobin levels and, eventually, symptoms of iron deficiency anemia.

Causes

The principal cause of iron deficiency anemia in premenopausal women is blood loss from menses. However, iron deficiency anemia may result from various other causes:

- inadequate dietary intake of iron (less than 1 to 2 mg/day), as in prolonged, unsupplemented breast-feeding or bottle-feeding of infants or during periods of stress such as rapid growth in children and adolescents
- iron malabsorption, as in chronic diarrhea, partial or total gastrectomy, chronic diverticulosis, and malabsorption syndromes, such as celiac disease and pernicious anemia
- blood loss secondary to drug-induced GI bleeding (from anticoagulants, aspirin, and steroids) or due to heavy menses, hemorrhage from trauma, GI ulcers, esophageal varices, or cancer
- pregnancy, which diverts maternal iron to the fetus for erythropoiesis
- intravascular hemolysis-induced hemoglobinuria or paroxysmal nocturnal hemoglobinuria
- mechanical erythrocyte trauma caused by a prosthetic heart valve or vena cava filters.

Signs and symptoms

Because of the gradual progression of iron deficiency anemia, many patients are initially asymptomatic except for symptoms of an underlying condition. They tend not to seek medical treatment until anemia is severe. At advanced stages, decreased hemoglobin levels and the subsequent decrease in the blood's oxygen-carrying capacity cause the patient to develop dyspnea on exertion, fatigue, listlessness, pallor, inability to concentrate, irritability, headache, and a susceptibility to infection. Decreased oxygen perfusion causes the heart to compensate with increased cardiac output and tachycardia.

In chronic iron deficiency anemia, nails become spoon-shaped and brittle, the corners of the mouth crack, the tongue turns smooth, and the patient complains of dysphagia or may develop pica. Associated neuromuscular effects include vasomotor disturbances, numbness and tingling of the extremities, and neuralgic pain.

Diagnosis

Diagnosis of iron deficiency anemia must rule out other forms of anemia, such as those that result from thalassemia minor, cancer, and chronic inflammatory, hepatic, and renal disease. Bone marrow studies reveal depleted or absent iron stores (done by staining) and normoblastic hyperplasia. Blood studies (serum iron levels, total iron-binding capacity, and ferritin levels) and stores in bone marrow may confirm iron deficiency anemia. However, the results of these tests can be misleading because of complicating factors, such as infection, pneumonia, blood transfusion, or iron supplements. Characteristic blood test results include:

- low hemoglobin levels (in males, less than 12 g/dl; in females, less than 10 g/dl)
- low hematocrit (males, less than 47 ml/dl; females, less than 42 ml/dl)
- low serum iron levels, with high binding capacity
- low serum ferritin levels
- low RBC count, with microcytic and hypochromic cells (in early stages, RBC count may be normal, except in infants and children)
- decreased mean corpuscular hemoglobin in severe anemia.

Treatment

The priority of treatment is to determine the underlying cause of anemia. Once this is determined, iron replacement therapy can begin. The preferred treatment is an oral preparation of iron or a combination of iron and ascorbic acid (which enhances iron absorption). However, in some cases, iron may have to be administered parenterally — for instance, if the patient is noncompliant to the oral preparation, if she needs more iron than she can take orally, if malabsorption prevents adequate iron absorption, or if a maximum rate of hemoglobin regeneration is desired.

Because total dose I.V. infusion of supplemental iron is painless and requires fewer injections, it's usually preferred to I.M. administration. Pregnant patients and geriatric patients with severe anemia, for example, should receive a total dose infusion of iron dextran in normal saline solution

Supportive management of anemia patients

Supportive management of anemia patients includes attention to nutritional needs, activity limits, infection risk, and complication prevention.

Nutritional needs

To meet the anemic patient's nutritional needs:

- If the patient is fatigued, urge her to eat small, frequent meals throughout the day.
- If she has oral lesions, suggest soft, cool, bland foods.
- If she has dyspepsia, eliminate spicy foods, and include milk and dairy products in her diet.
- If the patient is anorexic and irritable, encourage her family to bring her favorite foods from home (unless her diet is restricted) and to keep her company during meals, if possible.

Activity limits

To set limitations on activities:

- Assess the effect of a specific activity by monitoring pulse rate during the activity. If the patient's pulse accelerates rapidly and she develops hypotension with hyperpnea, diaphoresis, light-headedness, palpitations, shortness of breath, or weakness, the activity is too strenuous.
- Tell the patient to pace her activities and allow for frequent rest periods.

Infection risk

To decrease susceptibility to infection:

- Use strict sterile technique.
- Isolate the patient from infectious persons.
- Instruct the patient to avoid crowds and other sources of infection. Encourage her to practice good hand-washing technique. Stress the importance of receiving necessary immunizations and prompt medical treatment for any sign of infection.

Complication prevention

To prevent complications:

- Observe for signs of bleeding that may exacerbate anemia. Check stool for occult bleeding. Assess for ecchymoses, gingival bleeding, and hematuria. Monitor vital signs frequently.
- If the patient is confined to strict bed rest, assist with range-of-motion exercises and frequent turning, coughing, and deep breathing.
- If blood transfusions are needed for severe anemia (hemoglobin level less than 5 g/dl), give washed red blood cells as ordered, in partial exchange if evidence of pump failure is present. Carefully monitor for signs of circulatory overload or transfusion reaction. Watch for a change in pulse rate, blood pressure, or respiratory rate, or onset of fever, chills, pruritus, or edema. If any of these signs develop, stop the transfusion and notify the physician.
- Warn the patient to move about or change positions slowly to minimize dizziness induced by cerebral hypoxia.

over 8 hours. To minimize the risk of an allergic reaction to iron, an I.V. test dose of 0.5 ml should be given first. (For more patient care information, see *Supportive management of anemia patients.*)

Special considerations

- Monitor the patient's compliance with the prescribed iron supplement therapy. Advise the patient not to stop therapy even if she feels better be-

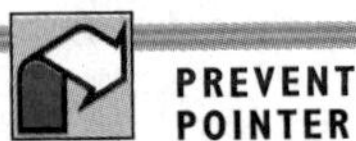

PREVENTION POINTER

Preventing iron deficiency anemia

Health professionals can play a vital role in preventing iron deficiency anemia by:

- teaching the basics of a nutritionally balanced diet — red meats, green vegetables, eggs, whole wheat products, and iron-fortified bread (However, no food in itself contains enough iron to *treat* iron deficiency anemia; an average-sized person with anemia would have to eat at least 10 lb of steak daily to receive therapeutic amounts of iron.)
- emphasizing the need for high-risk individuals, such as premature infants, children under age 2, and pregnant women, to receive prophylactic oral iron, as ordered by a physician (Children under age 2 should also receive supplemental cereals and formulas high in iron.)
- assessing a family's dietary habits for iron intake and noting the influence of childhood eating patterns, cultural food preferences, and family income on adequate nutrition
- encouraging families with deficient iron intake to eat meat, fish, or poultry; whole or enriched grains; and foods high in ascorbic acid
- instructing the patient to drink liquid supplemental iron through a straw to prevent staining her teeth
- telling the patient to report reactions to iron medications, such as nausea, vomiting, diarrhea, constipation, fever, or severe stomach pain, which may require a dosage adjustment
- monitoring the infusion rate carefully in a patient receiving I.V. iron and observing for an allergic reaction as well as dizziness, headache, and thrombophlebitis around the I.V. site (Stop the infusion and begin supportive treatment immediately if the patient shows signs of an adverse reaction.)
- using the Z-track injection method when administering iron I.M. to prevent skin discoloration, scarring, and irritating iron deposits on the skin
- cautioning the patient that an iron deficiency may recur and regular checkups and blood studies should be conducted.

cause replacement of iron stores takes time.

- Tell the patient that she may take iron supplements with a meal to decrease gastric irritation. Advise her to avoid milk, milk products, and antacids because they interfere with iron absorption; however, vitamin C can increase absorption.
- Warn the patient that iron supplements may result in dark green or black stools and can cause constipation.
- Carefully assess a patient's drug history because certain drugs, such as pancreatic enzymes and vitamin E, may interfere with iron metabolism and absorption and aspirin, steroids, and other drugs may cause GI bleeding. (Teach the patient who must take gastric irritants to take these medications with meals.)
- Explain to the patient how she can maintain a healthy iron level. (See *Preventing iron deficiency anemia.*)

Anorexia nervosa

The key feature of anorexia nervosa is self-imposed starvation, resulting from a distorted body image and an intense, irrational fear of gaining weight. An anorexic patient is preoccupied with her body size, describes herself as "fat," and commonly expresses dissatisfaction with a particular aspect of her physical appearance. Although the term *anorexia* suggests that the patient's weight loss is associated with a loss of appetite, this is rare. Indeed, anorexia nervosa and bulimia nervosa can occur simultaneously (See "Bulimia nervosa," page 225.) In anorexia nervosa, the refusal to eat may be accompanied by compulsive exercising, self-induced vomiting, or abuse of laxatives or diuretics.

Anorexia occurs in 1% to 2% of the female population and in 0.1% to 0.2% of the male population. This disorder occurs primarily in adolescents and young adults but may also affect older women. The occurrence among males is rising, but this disorder remains more prevalent in females. The prognosis varies but improves if the patient is diagnosed early, or if she wants to overcome the disorder and voluntarily seeks help. Mortality ranges from 5% to 15% — one-third of these deaths can be attributed to suicide.

Causes

No one knows what causes anorexia nervosa. Researchers in neuroendocrinology are seeking a physiologic cause but have found nothing definite. Clearly, social attitudes that equate slimness with beauty play some role in provoking this disorder; family factors are also implicated. Most theorists believe that refusing to eat is a subconscious effort to exert personal control over one's life.

Signs and symptoms

The patient's history usually reveals a 25% or greater weight loss for no organic reason, coupled with a morbid dread of being fat and a compulsion to be thin. Such a patient tends to be angry and ritualistic. She may report amenorrhea, infertility, loss of libido, fatigue, sleep alterations, intolerance to cold, and constipation.

Hypotension and bradycardia may be present. Inspection may reveal an emaciated appearance, with skeletal muscle atrophy, loss of fatty tissue, atrophy of breast tissue, blotchy or sallow skin, lanugo on the face and body, and dryness or loss of scalp hair. If the patient is also bulimic, inspection may reveal calluses on the knuckles and abrasions and scars on the dorsum of the hand, resulting from tooth injury during self-induced vomiting. Other signs of vomiting include dental caries and oral or pharyngeal abrasions. (See *Complications of anorexia nervosa,* page 198.)

Palpation may disclose painless salivary gland enlargement and bowel distention. Slowed reflexes may occur on percussion. Oddly, the patient usually demonstrates hyperactivity and vigor (despite malnourishment). She may exercise avidly without apparent fatigue.

Complications of Anorexia Nervosa

Serious medical complications can result from the malnutrition, dehydration, and electrolyte imbalances caused by prolonged starvation, frequent vomiting, or laxative abuse typical in anorexia nervosa.

Malnutrition and related problems

Malnutrition may cause hypoalbuminemia and subsequent edema or hypokalemia, leading to ventricular arrhythmias and renal failure.

Poor nutrition and dehydration coupled with laxative abuse produce changes in the bowel similar to those in chronic inflammatory bowel disease. Frequent vomiting can cause esophageal erosion, ulcers, tears, and bleeding as well as tooth and gum erosion and dental caries.

Cardiovascular consequences

Cardiovascular complications, which can be life-threatening, include decreased left ventricular muscle mass, chamber size, and myocardial oxygen uptake; reduced cardiac output; hypotension; bradycardia; electrocardiographic changes, such as a nonspecific ST interval, T-wave changes, and a prolonged PR interval; heart failure; and sudden death, possibly caused by ventricular arrhythmias.

Infection and amenorrhea

Anorexia nervosa may increase the patient's susceptibility to infection.

In addition, amenorrhea, which may occur when the patient loses 25% of her normal body weight, is usually associated with anemia. Possible complications of prolonged amenorrhea include estrogen deficiency (increasing the risk of calcium deficiency and osteoporosis) and infertility. Menses usually return to normal when the patient weighs at least 95% of her normal weight.

During psychosocial assessment, the anorexic patient may express a morbid fear of gaining weight and an obsession with her physical appearance. Paradoxically, she may also be obsessed with food, preparing elaborate meals for others. Social regression, including poor sexual adjustment and fear of failure, is common. Like bulimia nervosa, anorexia nervosa is commonly associated with depression. The patient may report feelings of despair, hopelessness, and worthlessness as well as suicidal thoughts.

Diagnosis

For characteristic findings in patients with anorexia nervosa, see *Diagnosing anorexia nervosa.*

In addition, laboratory tests help to identify various disorders and deficiencies and rule out endocrine, metabolic, and central nervous system abnormalities; cancer; malabsorption syndrome; and other disorders that cause physical wasting.

Abnormal findings that may accompany a weight loss exceeding 30% of normal body weight include:

- low hemoglobin level, platelet count, and white blood cell count

- prolonged bleeding time due to thrombocytopenia
- decreased erythrocyte sedimentation rate
- decreased levels of serum creatinine, blood urea nitrogen, uric acid, cholesterol, total protein, albumin, sodium, potassium, chloride, calcium, and fasting blood glucose (resulting from malnutrition)
- elevated levels of alanine aminotransferase and aspartate aminotransferase in severe starvation states
- elevated serum amylase levels when pancreatitis isn't present
- in females, decreased levels of serum luteinizing hormone and follicle-stimulating hormone
- decreased triiodothyronine levels resulting from a lower basal metabolic rate
- dilute urine caused by the kidneys' impaired ability to concentrate urine
- nonspecific ST interval, prolonged PR interval, and T-wave changes on the electrocardiogram, with ventricular arrhythmias possibly present as well.

Diagnosing anorexia nervosa

A diagnosis of anorexia nervosa is made when the patient meets the following criteria put forth in *Diagnostic and Statistical Manual of Mental Disorders,* Fourth Edition, Text Revision:

- The patient refuses to maintain body weight over a minimal normal weight for age and height (for instance, weight loss leading to maintenance of body weight 15% below that expected) or failure to achieve expected weight gain during a growth period, leading to body weight 15% below that expected.
- The patient experiences intense fear of gaining weight or becoming fat, despite her underweight status.
- The patient has a distorted perception of body weight, size, or shape. (That is, the person claims to feel fat even when emaciated or believes that one body area is too fat even when it's obviously underweight).
- The patient has missed at least three consecutive menstrual cycles when otherwise expected to occur.

Treatment

Appropriate treatment aims to promote weight gain or control the patient's compulsive binge eating and purging. Malnutrition and the underlying psychological dysfunction must be corrected. Hospitalization in a medical or psychiatric unit may be required to improve the patient's precarious physical condition. The hospital stay may be as brief as 2 weeks or may stretch from a few months to 2 years or longer.

A team approach to care — combining aggressive medical management, nutritional counseling, and individual, group, or family psychotherapy or behavior modification therapy — is the most effective treatment for anorexia nervosa. Even so, treatment results may be discouraging. Many clinical centers are developing inpatient and outpatient programs specifically aimed at managing eating disorders.

Treatment may include behavior modification (privileges depend on weight gain); curtailed activity for physical reasons (such as arrhythmias); vitamin and mineral supplements; a reasonable diet with or without liquid supplements; subclavian, peripheral, or enteral hyperalimentation (enteral and peripheral routes carry less risk of infection); and group, family, or individual psychotherapy.

All forms of psychotherapy, from psychoanalysis to hypnotherapy, have been used in treating anorexia nervosa, with varying success. To be successful, psychotherapy should address the underlying problems of low self-esteem, guilt, anxiety, feelings of hopelessness and helplessness, and depression.

Special considerations

- During hospitalization, regularly monitor vital signs, nutritional status, and intake and output. Weigh the patient daily — before breakfast if possible. Because the patient fears being weighed, vary the weighing routine. Keep in mind that weight should increase from morning to night.
- Help the patient establish a target weight, and support her efforts to achieve this goal.
- Negotiate an adequate food intake with the patient. Make sure she understands that she'll need to comply with this contract or lose privileges. Frequently offer small portions of food or drinks if the patient wants them. Allow the patient to maintain control over the types and amounts of food she eats, if possible.
- Maintain one-on-one supervision of the patient during meals and for 1 hour afterward to ensure compliance with the dietary treatment program. For the hospitalized anorexic patient, food is considered a medication.
- During an acute anorexic episode, nutritionally complete liquids are more acceptable than solid food because they eliminate the need to choose between foods — something many anorexic patients find difficult. If tube feedings or other special feeding measures become necessary, fully explain these measures to the patient, and be ready to discuss her fears or reluctance; limit the discussion about food itself.
- Expect a weight gain of about 1 lb (0.5 kg) per week.
- If edema or bloating occurs after the patient has returned to normal eating behavior, reassure her that this phenomenon is temporary. She may fear that she is becoming fat and stop complying with the plan of treatment.
- Encourage the patient to recognize and express her feelings freely. If she understands that she can be assertive, she gradually may learn that expressing her true feelings won't result in her losing control or love.
- If a patient receiving outpatient treatment must be hospitalized, maintain contact with her treatment team to facilitate a smooth return to the outpatient setting.
- Remember that the anorexic patient uses exercise, preoccupation with food, ritualism, manipulation, and lying as mechanisms to preserve the

only control she thinks that she has in her life.

- Because the patient and her family may need therapy to uncover and correct dysfunctional patterns, refer them to Anorexia Nervosa and Related Eating Disorders, a national information and support organization. This organization may help them understand what anorexia is, convince them that they need help, and help them find a psychotherapist or medical physician who is experienced in treating this disorder.
- Teach the patient how to keep a food journal, including the types of food eaten, eating frequency, and feelings associated with eating and exercise.
- Advise family members to avoid discussing food with the patient.

Antiphospholipid antibody syndrome

Antiphospholipid antibody syndrome is perhaps one of the most confounding immunologic disorders. It's an acquired autoimmune disorder defined by the presence of antibodies against phospholipids. It's characterized by vascular thrombosis and recurrent pregnancy loss.

Primary antiphospholipid antibody syndrome occurs when the syndrome exists in the absence of other major autoimmune disorders such as systemic lupus erythematosus (SLE). Antiphospholipid antibody syndrome is classified as *secondary* when it occurs in the presence of such a disorder as SLE. One-third of patients with SLE also have antiphospholipid antibodies, and approximately one-third of those with antibodies have clinical signs of antiphospholipid antibody syndrome. Rarely, a patient will have *catastrophic* antiphospholipid antibody syndrome, or multiorgan system failure resulting from widespread formation of microthrombi. (See *Complications of antiphospholipid antibody syndrome.*)

Because antiphospholipid antibodies are known to occur more frequent-

COMPLICATIONS OF ANTIPHOSPHOLIPID ANTIBODY SYNDROME

In addition to the presence of antiphospholipid antibody syndrome in women with recurrent spontaneous abortions, pregnant women with antiphospholipid antibodies can suffer other obstetric complications, including:

- thrombosis
- fetal death in utero
- thrombocytopenia
- intrauterine growth retardation
- stillbirth
- preeclampsia
- preterm delivery
- abruptio placentae
- uteroplacental insufficiency.

Patients with catastrophic antiphospholipid syndrome may experience the following conditions:

- thrombocytopenia
- acute respiratory distress syndrome
- kidney failure
- encephalopathy
- heart failure
- livedo reticularis.

ly in women, one must be especially alert to the concerns of thromboembolism. Women are more likely to experience periods of higher risk for thromboembolism in their lifetime, such as through hormonal therapy and pregnancy. Combine these factors with the presence of antiphospholipid antibodies, and the risks increase even more.

Causes

The lupus anticoagulant and anticardiolipin antibodies are types of antiphospholipid antibodies that are present in antiphospholipid antibody syndrome. These antibodies target platelets and vascular endothelium, causing thrombosis. The antibodies also block the formation of prostacyclin, which leads to thrombosis and vasoconstriction.

The mechanism of pregnancy loss and thrombosis in the antiphospholipid antibody syndrome remains unclear, although several theories do exist. The consensus is that thrombosis leading to placental insufficiency is the central mechanism. Placental vessel thrombosis and ischemia, a process that almost certainly starts from the very earliest time in pregnancy and leads to a progressive decrease in fetal circulation, is the most common belief. Early pregnancy loss may also be due to uteroplacental thrombosis and vasoconstriction that results from binding of the immunoglobulins to both platelet and endothelial membrane phospholipids.

Antiphospholipid antibodies are also considered by some to be cytotoxic to the trophoblast or fetus tissues when passing through the placenta. This mechanism could explain a relationship between antiphospholipid antibodies and neonate thrombocytopenia, congenital heart block, and neonatal lupus syndrome.

Signs and symptoms

In antiphospholipid antibody syndrome, blood clots can affect any part of the body. Clinical features may include:

- stroke and transient ischemic attack
- myocardial infarction
- kidney disease
- livedo reticularis (red-blue, netlike mottling of the skin)
- pulmonary hypertension
- leg ulcers
- recurrent spontaneous abortion.

Other features include:

- labile hypertension
- migraine
- epilepsy
- transverse myelopathy
- thrombocytopenia
- valvular heart disease
- ocular ischemia.

Diagnosis

Currently, no single test is available to diagnosis antiphospholipid antibody syndrome. The diagnosis is difficult because a patient may show isolated, transient, or borderline laboratory changes. Testing should include evaluating for the presence of lupus anticoagulant or specified levels of anticardiolipin antibodies, in combination with one or more characteristic clinical events.

Forms of lupus anticoagulant testing include:
- dilute Russell's viper venom time (dRVVT)
- partial thromboplastin time (PTT)
- kaolin clotting time
- tissue thromboplastin inhibition test
- hexagonal phase phospholipid
- textarin/ecarin test.

The presence of anticardiolipin antibodies is determined by an enzyme-linked immunosorbent assay (ELISA). Antiphospholipid antibody syndrome has been seen mainly with elevated levels of immunoglobulin G. Other laboratory testing may include evaluation of phosphatidylserine and beta$_2$-glycoprotein (ß$_2$GPI).

Treatment

Available studies recommend treatment of acute thrombosis in the same way as thrombosis resulting from other etiologies. This treatment may include anticoagulation with heparin or warfarin. Treatment of asymptomatic patients may be considered for those with SLE, family history of thromboembolism, or significant laboratory abnormalities.

Patients with catastrophic antiphospholipid antibody syndrome may benefit from aggressive treatment with immunosuppression via plasmapheresis and I.V. cyclophosphamide. Immediate supportive therapy is crucial in these patients for resolution of organ failure.

Several investigators have proposed various treatments for the treatment of antiphospholipid antibody syndrome during pregnancy. Treatment alternatives have included prednisone, aspirin, heparin, immunoglobulins, azathioprine, plasma exchange, and others. These treatments are thought to affect the immune and coagulation systems to counteract the adverse actions of antiphospholipid antibodies. A favored therapeutic option consists of combining antiplatelet therapy (low-dose aspirin) with either immunosuppression (prednisone) or anticoagulation (heparin). Low-dose aspirin therapy is considered safe in pregnancy and generally free of adverse effects, but prednisone and heparin can cause serious maternal complications, such as cataract formation, osteoporosis, bleeding, and peptic ulcer disease. Therefore, demonstration of a measurable benefit of combination therapy is necessary to justify prednisone or heparin administration.

Special considerations

Primary care providers must be aware that antiphospholipid antibody syndrome exists. Screening for antiphospholipid antibodies should be part of the investigation of women with recurrent spontaneous abortions. Awareness of available treatment options and patient education is also critical.

The decision to screen for antiphospholipid antibodies is sometimes difficult as they can be present in the normal population. However, by identifying the patient with this condition, treatment options can be offered to aid in the prevention of a thrombo-

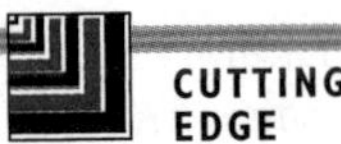

CUTTING EDGE

Preventing recurrent fetal loss

According to a recent report, the standard of care for preventing recurrent fetal loss due to antiphospholipid antibody syndrome should be low-molecular-weight heparin plus low-dose aspirin. Investigators have found that this combination is substantially more effective than I.V. immunoglobulin and recommend that it be considered a standard therapy.

embolic episode or a miscarriage. (See *Preventing recurrent fetal loss.*)

For women considering hormonal contraceptive use, counseling should be provided to explore other methods that are highly effective and don't carry the risk of thrombosis. For women considering hormone replacement therapy (HRT), the risks of thrombosis versus the benefits of HRT must be assessed.

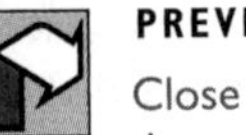

PREVENTION POINTER

Close surveillance for evidence of uteroplacental insufficiency and preeclampsia is indicated in pregnancies complicated by a antiphospholipid antibody syndrome. Early ultrasonography to confirm gestational age and serial scans to monitor fetal growth will prompt diagnosis of intrauterine growth retardation. Antepartum fetal surveillance consisting of nonstress tests, amniotic fluid volume assessment, biophysical profiles, contraction stress tests, or Doppler umbilical flow studies may be performed during the third trimester — or earlier, if indicated — for assessment of uteroplacental function.

Anxiety disorder, generalized

Anxiety is a feeling of apprehension that some describe as an exaggerated feeling of impending doom, dread, or uneasiness. Unlike fear — a reaction to danger from a specific external source — anxiety is a reaction to an internal threat, such as an unacceptable impulse or a repressed thought that's straining to reach a conscious level.

A rational response to a real threat, occasional anxiety is a normal part of life. Overwhelming anxiety, however, can result in generalized anxiety disorder — uncontrollable, unreasonable worry that persists for at least 6 months and narrows perceptions or interferes with normal functioning. Recent evidence indicates that the prevalence of generalized anxiety disorder is greater than previously thought and may be even greater than that of depression.

Generalized anxiety disorder can begin at any age but typically has an onset between ages 20 and 39. Anxiety disorder affects about 4 million Americans and about twice as many women than men.

Causes

Theorists share a common premise about generalized anxiety disorder:

Conflict, whether intrapsychic, sociopersonal, or interpersonal, promotes an anxiety state.

Signs and symptoms

Psychological or physiologic symptoms of anxiety states vary with the degree of anxiety. Mild anxiety mainly causes psychological symptoms, with unusual self-awareness and alertness to the environment. Moderate anxiety leads to selective inattention but with the ability to concentrate on a single task. Severe anxiety causes an inability to concentrate on more than scattered details of a task. A panic state with acute anxiety causes a complete loss of concentration, commonly with unintelligible speech.

Physical examination of the patient with generalized anxiety disorder may reveal signs or symptoms of motor tension, including trembling, muscle aches and spasms, headaches, and an inability to relax. Autonomic signs and symptoms include shortness of breath, tachycardia, sweating, and abdominal complaints.

In addition, the patient may startle easily and complain of feeling apprehensive, fearful, or angry. She may also experience difficulty concentrating, eating, and sleeping. Medical, psychiatric, and psychosocial histories of a patient with generalized anxiety disorder fail to identify a specific physical or environmental cause of the anxiety.

Diagnosis

Laboratory tests must rule out organic causes of the patient's signs and symptoms, such as hyperthyroidism, pheochromocytoma, coronary artery disease, supraventricular tachycardia, and Ménière's disease. For example, an electrocardiogram can rule out myocardial ischemia in a patient who complains of chest pain. Blood tests, including complete blood count, white blood cell count and differential, and serum lactate and calcium levels, can rule out hypocalcemia.

Because anxiety is the central feature of other mental disorders, psychiatric evaluation must rule out phobias, obsessive-compulsive disorders, depression, and acute schizophrenia. (See *Diagnosing generalized anxiety disorder*, page 206.)

Treatment

A combination of drug therapy and psychotherapy may help a patient with generalized anxiety disorder. Benzodiazepines, such as clonazepam and alprazolam, may relieve mild anxiety and improve the patient's ability to cope.

Antidepressants, such as venlafaxine or higher doses of short-acting benzodiazepines, may relieve the patient of severe anxiety and panic attacks. Antihistamines and sedatives may also be prescribed, which may pose less risk of physical and psychological dependence than benzodiazepines.

Psychotherapy for generalized anxiety disorder has two goals: helping the patient identify and deal with the cause of the anxiety, and eliminating environmental factors that precipitate an anxious reaction.

Diagnosing generalized anxiety disorder

When a patient's symptoms match criteria documented in *Diagnostic and Statistical Manual of Mental Disorders,* Fourth Edition, Text Revision, for generalized anxiety disorder, the diagnosis is confirmed. These criteria include:

- excessive anxiety and worry about a number of events or activities occur more days than not for at least 6 months
- difficulty controlling worry
- anxiety and worry associated with at least three of the following six symptoms:
  - restlessness or feeling keyed up or on edge
  - being easily fatigued
  - difficulty concentrating or mind going blank
  - irritability
  - muscle tension
  - sleep disturbances (difficulty falling or staying asleep, or restless, dissatisfying sleep).
- focus of anxiety and worry not confined to features of an axis I disorder
- anxiety, worry, or physical symptoms causing clinically significant distress or impairment in social, occupational, or other important areas of functioning
- disturbance not due to the direct physiologic effects of a substance or a general medical condition and not occurring exclusively during a mood disorder, a psychotic disorder, or a pervasive developmental disorder.

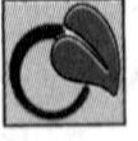

ALTERNATIVE THERAPIES

The patient can learn relaxation techniques, such as deep breathing, progressive muscle relaxation, focused relaxation, and visualization.

Special considerations

- Stay with the patient when she's anxious, and encourage her to discuss her feelings. Reduce environmental stimuli and remain calm. Additionally, tell the patient to avoid or reduce caffeine intake and other stimulants.
- Administer antianxiety drugs or antidepressants, and evaluate the patient's response. Teach the patient about prescribed medications, including the need for compliance with the medication regimen. Review adverse reactions.

PREVENTION POINTER

Teach the patient effective coping strategies and relaxation techniques. Help her identify stressful situations that trigger her anxiety, and provide positive reinforcement when she uses alternative coping strategies.

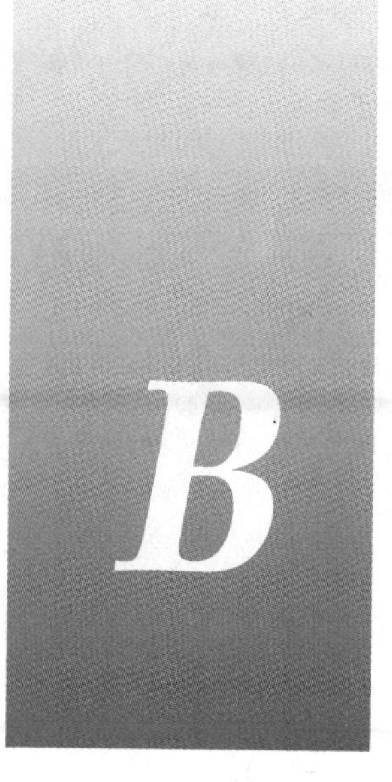

Bipolar disorder

Marked by severe mood swings from hyperactivity and euphoria to sadness and depression, bipolar disorder (also known as *manic depression*) involves various symptom combinations. Type I bipolar disorder is characterized by alternating episodes of mania and depression, whereas type II is characterized by recurrent depressive episodes and occasional manic episodes.

Women are more commonly diagnosed with type II bipolar disorder. In addition, women are more affected by rapid cycling bipolar disorder, a complex variant of the disorder, than men. (See *Rapid cycling*, page 208.) In some patients, bipolar disorder assumes a seasonal pattern, marked by a cyclic relation between the onset of the mood episode and a particular 60-day period each year.

The American Psychiatric Association estimates that over 2 million American adults suffer from bipolar disorder. Although this disorder affects men and women equally, recent studies suggest that gender differences exist in the prevalence, risks, symptoms, and clinical course of illness. For example, men tend to begin with a manic episode, while women tend to begin with a depressive episode. In addition, women with bipolar disorder

Rapid cycling

Rapid cycling in bipolar disorder is defined in the *Diagnostic and Statistical Manual of Mental Disorders,* Fourth Edition, Text Revision, as the occurrence of four or more episodes of illness per year. This rapid pattern is seen in approximately 10% to 20% of people with bipolar disorder, most of them women. This rapid cycling pattern usually develops later rather than earlier in the course of the illness. It occurs in all types of bipolar disorder, but is mainly seen in patients with bipolar I illness. The progression to rapid cycling commonly begins after an episode of depression rather than mania.

Causes

The cause of rapid cycling remains unknown; however, many factors triggering rapid cycling have been identified:

- antidepressants (especially the older tricyclic antidepressants)—women with bipolar disorder experience more depressive episodes than men, so they are more likely to receive antidepressant medications. This may explain why rapid cycling occurs in women more than men.
- L-dopa and other dopamine-stimulating drugs
- amphetamines
- certain estrogens
- cyproheptadine
- lithium (Lithotabs)
- hypothyroidism, which may explain why more women than men tend to develop rapid cycling because women have a much higher prevalence of hypothyroidism than men
- pregnancy
- hormonal changes
- stroke
- multiple sclerosis
- Graves' disease
- electroconvulsive therapy (ECT)

Treatment

Valproate and carbamazepine used alone or with lithium are the mood stabilizers of choice for people with rapid cycling bipolar disorder. Other treatments that have proven successful are thyroxine and clozapine.

Although no well-controlled studies exist, other treatments that may be useful include:

- calcium channel blockers
- ECT
- primidone (Mysoline)
- clonidine (Klonopin).

have a higher risk of alcoholism than men with bipolar disorder. Alcoholism is associated with a history of polysubstance use in women with bipolar disorder, while alcoholism is associated with a family history of alcoholism in men with bipolar disorder.

Bipolar disorder affects all ages, races, ethnic groups, and social classes. It usually manifests itself during late adolescence, but onset may start as early as childhood or much later in life. According to the American Academy of Child and Adolescent Psychiatry, up to one-third of the 3.4 million children and adolescents with depression in the United States actually may be experiencing the early onset of bipolar disorder.

Bipolar disorder recurs in 80% of patients; as they grow older, the episodes recur more frequently and last longer. This illness is associated with a significant mortality; 20% of patients commit suicide, many just as the depression lifts.

SPECIAL NEEDS

Older adults at highest risk for suicide are at least age 85, are depressed—but may appear to have high self-esteem—and need to control their own lives. Even a frail nursing home resident with these characteristics may have the strength to kill herself. Therefore, all persons, including elderly patients, must be considered at high risk for suicide.

Causes

The cause of bipolar disorder is unclear but hereditary, biological, and psychological factors may play a part. For example, the incidence of bipolar disorder among relatives of affected patients is higher than in the general population, and highest among maternal relatives. The closer the familial relationship, the greater the susceptibility. A child with one affected parent has a 25% chance of developing bipolar disorder; a child with two affected parents, a 50% chance. The incidence of this illness in siblings is 20% to 25%; in identical twins, the incidence is 66% to 96%. Recent studies have shown that postpartum women are also at particular risk for bipolar disorder through postpartum psychosis.

Although certain biochemical changes accompany mood swings, it isn't clear whether these changes cause the mood swings or result from them. In both mania and depression, intracellular sodium concentration increases during illness and returns to normal with recovery.

Patients with mood disorders have a defect in the way the brain handles certain neurotransmitters—chemical messengers that shuttle nerve impulses between neurons. Low levels of the chemicals dopamine and norepinephrine, for example, have been linked to depression, whereas excessively high levels of these chemicals are associated with mania. Changes in the concentration of acetylcholine and serotonin may also play a role. Although neurobiologists have yet to prove that these chemical shifts cause bipolar disorder, it's widely assumed that most antidepressant medications work by modifying these neurotransmitter systems. In addition, new data suggest that changes in the circadian rhythms that control hormone secretion, body temperature, and appetite may contribute to the development of bipolar disorder.

Emotional or physical trauma, such as bereavement, disruption of an important relationship, or a serious accidental injury, may precede the onset of bipolar disorder. However, bipolar disorder commonly appears without identifiable predisposing factors. Manic episodes may follow a stressful event, but they're also associated with antidepressant therapy and childbirth. Chronic physical illness, psychoactive drug dependence, psychosocial stressors, and childbirth may precipitate major depressive episodes. Other familial influences—especially the early loss of a parent, parental

Cyclothymic disorder

A chronic mood disturbance of at least 2 years' duration, cyclothymic disorder involves numerous episodes of hypomania or depression that aren't of sufficient severity or duration to qualify as a major depressive episode or a bipolar disorder.

Cyclothymic disorder commonly starts in adolescence or early adulthood. Beginning insidiously, this disorder leads to persistent social and occupational dysfunction.

Signs and symptoms

In the hypomanic phase of cyclothymic disorder, the patient may experience insomnia; hyperactivity; inflated self-esteem; increased productivity and creativity; overinvolvement in pleasurable activities, including an increased sexual drive; physical restlessness; and rapid speech. Depressive symptoms may include insomnia, feelings of inadequacy, decreased productivity, social withdrawal, lethargy, slow speech, crying, and loss of libido or interest in pleasurable activities.

Diagnosis

A number of medical disorders (for example, endocrinopathies such as Cushing's syndrome, stroke, brain tumors, and head trauma) and drug overdose can produce a similar pattern of mood alteration. These organic causes must be ruled out before making a diagnosis of cyclothymic disorder.

depression, incest, or abuse — may predispose a person to depressive illness. (See *Cyclothymic disorder.*)

Signs and symptoms

Signs and symptoms vary widely, depending on whether the patient is experiencing a manic or depressive episode. Before the onset of overt symptoms, however, many patients with bipolar disorder have an energetic and outgoing personality with a history of wide mood swings. Bipolar disorder may be associated with high levels of creativity or high levels of destruction.

During the assessment interview, the *manic* patient typically appears grandiose, euphoric, expansive, or irritable with little control over her activities and responses. She may describe hyperactive or excessive behavior, including elaborate plans for numerous social events, efforts to renew old acquaintances by telephoning friends at all hours of the night, buying sprees, or promiscuous sexual activity. She seldom hesitates to start projects for which she has little aptitude.

The patient's activities may have a bizarre quality, such as dressing in colorful or strange garments, wearing excessive makeup, or giving advice to passing strangers. She commonly expresses an inflated sense of self-esteem, ranging from uncritical self-confidence to marked grandiosity, which may be delusional.

Note the patient's speech patterns and concentration level. Accelerated and pressured speech, frequent topic changes, and flights of ideas are common features during the manic phase. The patient is easily distracted and responds rapidly to external stimuli, such as background noise or a ringing telephone.

Physical examination of the manic patient may reveal signs of malnutrition and poor personal hygiene. She may report sleeping and eating less as well as being more physically active than usual.

Hypomania, which is more common than acute mania, is similar to mania, but is less severe and delusions, hallucinations, and other symptoms of psychotic intensity aren't present. Three classic symptoms of hypomania may be recognized during the assessment interview: euphoric but unstable mood, pressured speech, and increased motor activity. The hypomanic patient may appear elated, hyperactive, easily distracted, talkative, irritable, impatient, impulsive, and full of energy but seldom exhibits flight of ideas.

The patient who experiences a *depressive episode* may report a loss of self-esteem, overwhelming inertia, social withdrawal, and feelings of hopelessness, apathy, or self-reproach. She may believe that she's wicked and deserves to be punished. Her growing sadness, guilt, negativity, and fatigue place extraordinary burdens on her family.

During the assessment interview, the depressed patient may speak and respond slowly. She may complain of difficulty concentrating or thinking clearly but usually isn't obviously disoriented or intellectually impaired.

Physical examination may reveal reduced psychomotor activity, lethargy, low muscle tonus, weight loss, slowed gait, and constipation. The patient may also report sleep disturbances (falling asleep, staying asleep, or early morning awakening), sexual dysfunction, headaches, chest pains, and heaviness in the limbs. Typically, symptoms are worse in the morning and gradually subside as the day goes on.

Concerns about her health may become hypochondriacal: She may worry excessively about having cancer or some other serious illness. In an elderly patient, physical symptoms may be the only clues to depression.

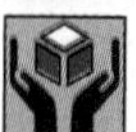

SPECIAL NEEDS

Symptoms of bipolar disorder may be especially difficult to discern in children because they may be mistaken for age-appropriate emotions and behaviors of children and adolescents. Also, their symptoms of bipolar disorder may vary somewhat from adults. For example, when manic, children and adolescents are more likely to be irritable and prone to destructive outbursts than to be elated or euphoric. When depressed, they may complain about headaches, stomach aches, tiredness, poor performance in school, poor communication, and extreme sensitivity to rejection or failure.

Suicide is an ever-present risk, no matter what age, especially as the depression begins to lift. At that point, a rising energy level may strengthen the patient's resolve to carry out suicidal plans. The suicidal patient may also harbor homicidal ideas — for example, thinking of killing her family either in anger or to spare them pain and disgrace.

Diagnosis

Most people are diagnosed between ages 20 and 35; many times, diagnosis in the adolescent or child is mistaken for attention deficit hyperactivity disorder, "teenage rebellion," or other age-appropriate behaviors. Physical examination and laboratory tests, such as endocrine function studies, rule out medical causes of mood disturbances, including intra-abdominal neoplasm, hypothyroidism, heart failure, cerebral arteriosclerosis, parkinsonism, psychoactive drug abuse, brain tumor, and uremia. Moreover, a review of the medications prescribed for other disorders may point to drug-induced depression or mania. (For characteristic findings in patients with bipolar disorder, see *Diagnosing bipolar disorders*.)

Treatment

Widely used to treat bipolar disorder, lithium (Lithotabs, Eskalith) has proven highly effective in relieving and preventing manic episodes. It curbs accelerated thought processes and hyperactive behavior without producing the sedating effect of antipsychotic drugs. In addition, it may prevent the recurrence of depressive episodes. Even so, it's ineffective in treating acute depression.

Because lithium has a narrow therapeutic range, treatment must be initiated cautiously and the dosage adjusted slowly. Therapeutic blood levels during the active manic period are 0.4 to 1.4 mEq/L. For safety, the level should never exceed 1.5 mEq/L. Therapeutic blood levels must be maintained for 7 to 10 days before the drug's beneficial effects appear; for this reason, antipsychotic drugs are commonly used in the interim to provide sedation and symptomatic relief. Because the kidneys excrete lithium, any renal impairment necessitates withdrawal of the drug.

Anticonvulsants, such as carbamazepine (Tegretol, Carbatrol), valproic acid (Depakene), and clonazepam (Klonopin), are used either alone or with lithium to treat mood disorders. Carbamazepine, a potent antimanic drug, is effective in many lithium-resistant patients.

Antidepressants are used to treat depressive symptoms, but they may trigger a manic episode.

Special considerations

For the *manic patient*:

- Remember the manic patient's physical needs. Encourage her to eat. Provide a diet high in calories, carbohydrates, and liquids.
- As the patient's symptoms subside, encourage her to assume responsibility for personal care.
- Provide emotional support, maintain a calm environment, and set realistic goals for behavior.
- Provide diversionary activities suited to a short attention span; firmly discourage the patient if she tries to overextend herself. Provide structured activities involving large motor movements to expend surplus energy. Re-

Diagnosing bipolar disorders

The diagnosis of a bipolar disorder is confirmed when the patient meets the criteria documented in the *Diagnostic and Statistical Manual of Mental Disorders*, Fourth Edition, Text Revision.

Manic episode

- A distinct period of abnormally and persistently elevated, expansive, or irritable mood must last at least 1 week (or any duration if hospitalization is needed)
- During the mood disturbance period, at least three of the following symptoms must have persisted (four, if the mood is only irritable) and have been present to a significant degree:
  - inflated self-esteem or grandiosity
  - decreased need for sleep
  - more talkative than usual or pressured to keep talking
  - flight of ideas or subjective experience that thoughts are racing
  - distractibility
  - increased goal-directed activity or psychomotor agitation
  - excessive involvement in pleasurable activities that have a high potential for painful consequences.
- The symptoms don't meet the criteria for a mixed episode.
- The mood disturbance is sufficiently severe to cause one of the following to occur:
  - marked impairment in occupational functioning or in usual social activities or relationships with others
  - hospitalization to prevent harm to self or others
  - evidence of psychotic features.
- The symptoms aren't due to the direct physiologic effects of a substance or a general medical condition.

Hypomanic episode

- A distinct period of abnormally and persistently elevated, expansive, or irritable mood must last at least 4 days and be clearly different from the usual nondepressed mood.
- During the mood disturbance period, at least three of the following symptoms must have persisted (four, if the mood is only irritable) and have been present to a significant degree:
  - inflated self-esteem or grandiosity
  - decreased need for sleep
  - more talkative than usual or pressured to keep talking
  - flight of ideas or subjective experience that thoughts are racing
  - distractibility
  - increased goal-directed activity or psychomotor agitation
  - excessive involvement in pleasurable activities that have a high potential for painful consequences.
- The episode is associated with an unequivocal change in functioning that's uncharacteristic of the person when not symptomatic.
- Others can recognize the disturbance in mood and the change in functioning.
- The episode isn't severe enough to markedly impair social or occupational functioning or to necessitate hospitalization to prevent harm to self or others. No psychotic features are evident.
- The symptoms aren't due to the direct physiologic effects of a substance or a general medical condition.

Bipolar I single manic episode

- Only one manic episode is present and no past major depressive episodes have occurred.
- The manic episode isn't better accounted for by schizoaffective disorder and isn't superimposed on schizophre-

(continued)

DIAGNOSING BIPOLAR DISORDERS *(continued)*

nia, schizophreniform disorder, delusional disorder, or psychotic disorder not otherwise specified.

Bipolar I disorder, most recent episode hypomanic

- The person is currently (or most recently) experiencing a hypomanic episode.
- The person previously had at least one manic episode or mixed episode.
- The mood symptoms cause clinically significant distress or impairment in social or occupational functioning or other important areas of functioning.
- The first two exacerbations of the mood episode (above) aren't better accounted for by schizoaffective disorder and aren't superimposed on schizophrenia, schizophreniform disorder, delusional disorder, or psychotic disorder not otherwise specified.

Bipolar I disorder, most recent episode manic

- The person is currently (or most recently) experiencing a manic episode.
- The person previously had at least one major depressive episode, manic episode, or mixed episode.
- The first two exacerbations of mood episode (above) aren't better accounted for by schizoaffective disorder and aren't superimposed on schizophrenia, schizophreniform disorder, delusional disorder, or psychotic disorder not otherwise specified.

Bipolar I disorder, most recent episode mixed

- The person is currently (or most recently) experiencing a mixed episode.
- The person previously had at least one major depressive episode, manic episode, or mixed episode.
- The first two exacerbations of mood episode (above) aren't better accounted for by schizoaffective disorder and aren't superimposed on schizophrenia, schizophreniform disorder, delusional disorder, or psychotic disorder not otherwise specified.

Bipolar I disorder, most recent episode depressed

- The person is currently (or most recently) experiencing a major depressive episode.
- The person previously had at least one manic episode or mixed episode.
- The first two exacerbations of mood episode (above) aren't better accounted for by schizoaffective disorder and aren't superimposed on schizophrenia, schizophreniform disorder, delusional disorder, or psychotic disorder not otherwise specified.

Bipolar I disorder, most recent episode unspecified

- All criteria, except for duration, are currently (or most recently) met for a manic, hypomanic, mixed, or major depressive episode.
- The person previously had at least one manic episode or mixed episode.
- The mood symptoms cause clinically significant distress or impairment in social or occupational functioning or other important areas of functioning.
- The first two exacerbations of mood episode (above) aren't better accounted for by schizoaffective disorder and aren't superimposed on schizophrenia, schizophreniform disorder, delusional disorder, or psychotic disorder not otherwise specified.
- The first two exacerbations of mood episode (above) aren't due to the direct physiologic effects of a substance or a general medical condition.

DIAGNOSING BIPOLAR DISORDERS *(continued)*

Bipolar II disorder

- The person is currently (or has a history of) experiencing one or more major depressive episodes
- The person is currently (or has a history of) at least one hypomanic episode.
- The patient has never had a manic episode or a mixed episode.
- The first two exacerbations of mood episode (above) aren't better accounted for by schizoaffective disorder and aren't superimposed on schizophrenia, schizophreniform disorder, delusional disorder, or psychotic disorder not otherwise specified.
- The symptoms cause clinically significant distress or impairment in social or occupational functioning or other important areas of functioning.

duce or eliminate group activities during acute manic episodes.

- When necessary, reorient the patient to reality. Tactfully divert conversations when they become intimately concerned with other patients or staff members.
- Set limits in a calm, clear, and self-confident manner for the manic patient's demanding, hyperactive, manipulative, and acting-out behaviors. Setting limits tells the patient that you'll provide security and protection by refusing inappropriate and possibly harmful requests. Avoid leaving an opening for the patient to test you or argue with you.
- Listen to requests attentively and with a neutral attitude. Avoid power struggles if a patient tries to put you on the spot for an immediate answer. Explain that you'll seriously consider the request and will respond later.
- Encourage solitary activities such as writing out one's thoughts.
- Collaborate with other staff members to provide consistent responses to the patient's manipulative or acting-out behaviors.
- Watch for early signs of frustration (when the patient's anger escalates from verbal threats to hitting an object). Tell the patient firmly that threats and hitting are unacceptable. Explain that these behaviors show that she needs help to control her behavior. Inform her that the staff will help her move to a quiet area to help her control her behavior so she won't hurt herself or others. Staff members who have practiced as a team can work effectively to prevent acting-out behavior or to remove and confine a patient.
- Alert the staff team promptly when acting-out behavior escalates. It's safer to have help available before you need it than to try controlling an anxious or frightened patient by yourself.
- Once the incident is over and the patient is calm and in control, discuss her feelings with her and offer suggestions on how to prevent a recurrence.

■ If the patient is taking lithium, tell her and her family to temporarily discontinue the drug and notify the physician if signs or symptoms of toxicity, such as diarrhea, abdominal cramps, vomiting, unsteadiness, drowsiness, muscle weakness, polyuria, and tremors, occur.

For the *depressed patient*:

■ The depressed patient needs continual positive reinforcement to improve her self-esteem. Provide a structured routine, including activities to boost her self-confidence and promote interaction with others (for instance, group therapy). Keep reassuring her that her depression will lift.

■ Encourage the patient to talk or to write down her feelings if she's having trouble expressing them. Listen attentively and respectfully; allow her time to formulate her thoughts if she seems sluggish. Record your observations and conversations.

PREVENTION POINTER

To prevent possible self-injury or suicide, remove harmful objects (such as glass, belts, rope, or bobby pins) from the patient's environment, observe her closely, and strictly supervise her medications. Institute suicide precautions as dictated by your facility's policy.

■ Don't forget the patient's physical needs. If she's too depressed to care for herself, help her with personal hygiene measures. Encourage her to eat, if necessary. If she's constipated, add high-fiber foods to her diet; offer small, frequent meals; and encourage physical activity.

PREVENTION POINTER

If the patient is taking an antidepressant, watch for signs of mania. Also, remember that the risk for suicide is highest when the patient's depression begins to lift.

Breast cancer

Breast cancer is the most common cancer affecting women and is the number two killer (after lung cancer) of women ages 35 to 54. One in nine women will develop breast cancer in her lifetime. It may develop any time after puberty but is most common after age 50 (about 20% of cases occur in women under age 30 and about 70% in women over age 50). In the United States, about 1,500 men are diagnosed with breast cancer each year.

The 5-year survival rate for localized breast cancer has improved from 72% in the 1940s to 96% today because of earlier diagnosis and the variety of treatments available. According to the most recent data, mortality rates continue to decline in White women and, for the first time, are also declining in younger Black women. Lymph node involvement is the most valuable prognostic predictor. With adjuvant therapy, 70% to 75% of women with negative nodes will survive 10 years or more compared with 20% to 25% of women with positive nodes. (See *Predicting breast cancer survival.*)

Causes

Although the cause of breast cancer isn't known, its high incidence in women implicates estrogen. In addition, certain predisposing factors are clear. For example, women at highest risk include those who have a family history of breast cancer, particularly first-degree relatives (mother, sister, or maternal aunt).

Other women at high risk include those who:

- have long menstrual cycles or began menses early or menopause late
- have never been pregnant
- were first pregnant after age 30
- have had unilateral breast cancer
- have had ovarian cancer, particularly at a young age
- were exposed to low-level ionizing radiation
- are obese
- who have taken or are on hormonal contraceptives or hormone replacement therapy (HRT).

Recently, scientists have discovered the BRCA 1 and BRCA 2 genes. Mutations in these genes are thought to cause less than 10% of breast cancer. However, these discoveries have made genetic predisposition testing an option for women at high risk.

Women at lower risk include those who:

- were pregnant before age 20
- have had multiple pregnancies
- are of Native American or Asian descent.

Breast cancer can affect various parts of the breast structures; however, it occurs more commonly in the left breast than the right and more commonly in the outer upper quadrant. Growth rates vary. Theoretically, slow-growing breast cancer may take up to 8 years to become palpable at 1 cm in size. It spreads by way of the lymphatic system and the bloodstream, through the right side of the heart to the lungs, and eventually to the other breast, the chest wall, liver, bone, and brain. (See *Where breast cancer starts*, page 218.) Many refer to the estimated growth rate of breast

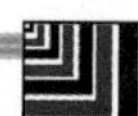

CUTTING EDGE

Predicting breast cancer survival

According to a recent study, a new test that measures the amount of cyclin E, a protein found in tumor tissue, may be a good predictor of breast cancer survival. Currently, the prognosis for women with breast cancer is determined by various factors, such as the size of the tumor and whether the cancer has metastasized to nearby lymph nodes.

According to the study, women with stages I, II, and III breast cancer who had high levels of cyclin E had died within a 6-year period, demonstrating poorer survival times. All women with stage I breast cancer who had low levels of cyclin E were still alive.

Although this study needs further trials to confirm its results before it becomes standard practice, researchers are hopeful that this test will be more sensitive in measuring prognosis and will become another tool in the fight against breast cancer.

Where breast cancer starts

Among American women, the most common breast cancer types are ductal carcinoma (79% of all types), lobular carcinoma (10%), and tubular carcinoma (6%). The remaining 5% of breast cancers are colloid, medullary, papillary, and inflammatory carcinomas.

Most ductal and lobular carcinomas originate in the upper, outer portion of the breast. Tubular carcinomas consist of small tubes or ducts within the fatty layers of the breast.

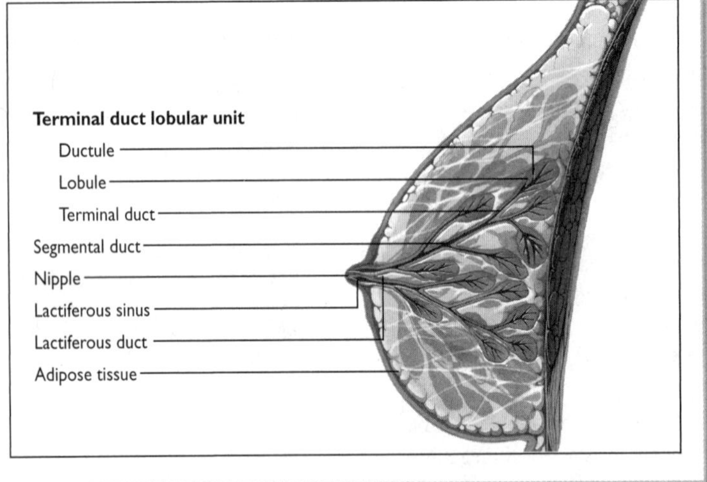

cancer as "doubling time," or the time it takes the malignant cells to double in number. Survival time for breast cancer is based on tumor size and spread. The number of involved nodes is the single most important factor in predicting survival time.

Breast cancer is classified by histologic appearance and location of the lesion:

- *adenocarcinoma* — arising from the epithelium
- *intraductal* — within the ducts (includes Paget's disease)
- *infiltrating* — occurring in parenchyma of the breast
- *inflammatory* (rare) — reflecting rapid tumor growth, in which the overlying skin becomes edematous, inflamed, and indurated
- *lobular carcinoma in situ* — reflecting tumor growth involving lobes of glandular tissue
- *medullary or circumscribed* — large tumor with rapid growth rate.

These histologic classifications should be coupled with a staging or nodal status classification system for a clearer understanding of the extent of the cancer. The most commonly used system for staging cancer before and after surgery is the tumor size, nodal involvement, metastatic progress (TNM) staging system.

Signs and symptoms

Warning signals of possible breast cancer include:

- lump or mass in the breast (firm, fixed, nontender, and irregular in shape)
- change in symmetry or size of the breast
- change in skin, such as thickening, scaly skin around the nipple, dimpling, peau d'orange, edema, or ulceration
- change in skin temperature, such as a warm, hot, or pink area (in a nonlactating woman past childbearing age)
- unusual drainage or discharge, such as greenish black, white or creamy (in a nonlactating woman), serous, or bloody (If a breast-fed infant rejects one breast, this may suggest possible breast cancer.)
- change in the nipple, such as itching, burning, erosion, or retraction
- pain (usually only when tumor is advanced)
- bone metastasis, pathologic bone fractures, and hypercalcemia
- edema of the arm.

Diagnosis

In 2003, the American Cancer Society published its most recent guidelines for early breast cancer screening.

Mammography is still the gold standard because it has been consistently proven to reduce deaths from breast cancer. One major change in the guidelines concerns breast self-examination (BSE). Although the American Cancer Society once considered BSE as the most reliable method of detecting breast cancer, evdience of its benefits is lacking.

The updated guidelines emphasize educating women, especially high-risk women, about mammography and other screening methods; offering more information to older women; and clarifying the role of clinical breast examinations. (See *Updated breast cancer screening guidelines*, pages 220 and 221.)

Mammography is indicated for any woman whose physical examination suggests breast cancer. It should be done as a baseline on women between ages 35 and 39; then annually for women age 40 and older. Women with a family history of breast cancer generally should begin breast cancer screening at an earlier age.

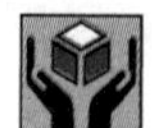

SPECIAL NEEDS

Unfortunately, many older women don't receive regular mammograms, even when recommended by health care professionals because they fear radiation, discovering cancer, or discomfort during the procedure; they can't afford the costs of the mammogram; or they're embarrassed about exposing their breasts.

The value of mammography remains questionable for women under age 35 (because of the density of the breasts), except those who are strongly suspected of having breast cancer. False-negative results can occur in as many as 30% of all tests. Consequently, with a suspicious mass, a negative

UPDATED BREAST CANCER SCREENING GUIDELINES

According to the American Cancer Society, these updated breast cancer screening guidelines place more emphasis on educating women, especially those at high-risk for breast cancer, on mammography and other screening methods, more information for

Population	Screening Tool	Former Guidelines (1997)
Women at average risk	Mammography	Annually starting at age 40
	CBE	Every three years for women ages 20 to 39; annually for women age 40 and older
	BSE	Monthly starting at age 20
Older women and women with serious health problems		Additional research is needed.
High-risk women		Women with a family history of breast cancer should discuss guidelines with their doctors.

mammogram should be disregarded, and a fine-needle aspiration or surgical biopsy should be done. Ultrasonography, such as the T-Scan 2000 that was approved by the Food and Drug Administration in 1999, can distinguish a fluid-filled cyst from a tumor as small as 1 cm and may be used instead of an invasive surgical biopsy. However, this scan is intended to be used alongside conventional diagnosing; not alone.

Bone scan, CT scan, measurement of alkaline phosphatase levels, liver function studies, and liver biopsy can detect distant metastases. A hormonal older women, and clarifies the role of clinical breast examinations (CBE) and breast self-examinations (BSE). The table below compares the updated guidelines with the previous guidelines.

Updated Guidelines (2003)	Explanation
No change from 1997 recommendation. There's a tremendous amount of additional, credible evidence of the benefit of mammography since 1997, especially regarding women in their 40s.	Women can feel confident about the benefits associated with regular screening mammography. However, mammography also has limitations: it will miss some cancers, and it sometimes leads to follow up of findings that are not cancer, including biopsies.
CBE should be part of a woman's periodic health examination, about every three years for women in their 20s and 30s and annually for women age 40 and older.	CBE is a complement to regular mammography screening and an opportunity for women and their health care providers to discuss changes in their breasts, risk factors, and early detection testing.
Women should report breast changes promptly to their healthcare provider. Beginning in their 20s, women should be told about the benefits and limitations of BSE. It's acceptable for women to choose not to do BSE or to do it occasionally.	Research has shown that BSE plays a small role in detecting breast cancer compared with self-awareness. However, doing BSE is one way for women to know how their breasts normally feel and to notice any changes.
Continue annual mammography, regardless of age, as long as a woman doesn't have serious, chronic health problems. For women with serious health problems or short life expectancy, evaluate ongoing early detection testing.	There's a need to balance the potential benefits of ongoing screening mammography in women with limited longevity against the limitations. The survival benefit of a current mammogram may not be seen for several years.
May benefit from earlier initiation of early detection testing or the addition of breast ultrasound or magnetic resonance imaging.	The evidence available is only sufficient to offer general guidance. This guidance will help women and their doctors make more informed decisions about screening.

receptor assay done on the tumor can determine if the tumor is estrogen or progesterone dependent. (This test guides decisions to use therapy that blocks the action of the estrogen hormone that supports tumor growth.)

Treatment

Much controversy exists over breast cancer treatments. In choosing therapy, the patient and doctor should take into consideration the stage of the disease, the woman's age and menopausal status, and the disfiguring effects of the surgery. Treatment of breast cancer may include one or any combination of the following:

- surgery
- chemotherapy
- peripheral stem cell therapy
- primary radiation therapy
- estrogen, progesterone, androgen, or antiandrogen aminoglutethimide therapy.

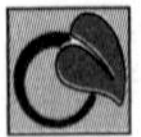

ALTERNATIVE THERAPIES

Soy-based diets are rich in genistein, an isoflavone thought to reduce the risk of breast cancer. Some studies suggest that soy may prevent breast cancer, especially in premenopausal women, while others suggest that soy may promote breast cancer, especially breast cancers that are estrogen-dependent. Data are insufficient to determine whether soy fights cancer or promotes cancer; however, soy products may remain as part of a healthy diet (in moderation) without any harmful effects.

Surgery involves either mastectomy or lumpectomy. A lumpectomy may be done on an outpatient basis and may be the only surgery needed, especially if the tumor is small and there is no evidence of axillary node involvement. In many cases, radiation therapy is combined with this surgery. A two-stage procedure in which the surgeon removes the lump and confirms that it's malignant and then discusses treatment options with the patient is desirable because it allows the patient to participate in her treatment plan. Sometimes, if the tumor is diagnosed as clinically malignant, such planning can be done before surgery. In lumpectomy and dissection of the axillary lymph nodes, the tumor and the axillary lymph nodes are removed, leaving the breast intact. Modified radical mastectomy removes the breast and the axillary lymph nodes. Radical mastectomy, the performance of which has declined, removes the breast, pectoralis major and minor, and the axillary lymph nodes. Postmastectomy reconstructive surgery can create a breast mound if the patient desires it and doesn't have evidence of advanced disease.

Chemotherapy, involving various cytotoxic drug combinations, is used as either adjuvant or primary therapy, depending on several factors, including TNM staging and estrogen receptor status. The most commonly used antineoplastic drugs are cyclophosphamide (Cytoxan), fluorouracil (5-FU, Adrucil), methotrexate (Trexall), doxorubicin (Adriamycin, Rubex), vincristine (Oncovin), paclitaxel (Taxol), and prednisone (Deltasone). A common drug combination used in both premenopausal and postmenopausal women is cyclophosphamide, methotrexate, and fluorouracil (CMF).

Tamoxifen, an estrogen antagonist, is the adjuvant treatment of choice for postmenopausal patients with positive estrogen receptor status. Tamoxifen has also been found to reduce the risk of breast cancer in women at high risk.

Peripheral stem cell therapy may be used for advanced breast cancer by replacing stem cells that were destroyed by high doses of chemotherapy. These healthy transplanted stem cells help to produce blood cells after chemotherapy.

Primary radiation therapy before or after tumor removal is effective for small tumors in early stages with no evidence of distant metastasis; it's also used to prevent or treat local recurrence. Presurgical radiation to the breast in inflammatory breast cancer helps make tumors more surgically manageable.

Estrogen, progesterone, androgen, or antiandrogen aminoglutethimide therapy may also be given to postmenopausal women with advanced breast cancer.

Special considerations

To provide good care for a breast cancer patient, begin with a history; assess the patient's feelings about her illness, and determine what she knows about it and what she expects. Preoperatively, make sure you know what kind of surgery is scheduled so you can prepare her properly. If a mastectomy is scheduled, in addition to the usual preoperative preparation (for example, skin preparations and not allowing the patient anything by mouth), provide the following information:

- Teach her how to deep breathe and cough to prevent pulmonary complications and how to rotate her ankles to help prevent thromboembolism.
- Tell her she can ease her pain by lying on the affected side or by placing a hand or pillow on the incision. Preoperatively, show her where the incision will be. Inform her that she'll receive pain medication and that she need not fear addiction. Remember, adequate pain relief encourages coughing and turning and promotes general well-being. Positioning a small pillow anteriorly under the patient's arm provides comfort.
- Encourage her to get out of bed as soon as possible (even as soon as the anesthesia wears off or the first evening after surgery).
- Explain that, after mastectomy, an incisional drain or suction device (Hemovac) will be used to remove accumulated serous or sanguineous fluid and to keep the tension off the suture line, promoting healing.

After the procedure:

- Inspect the dressing anteriorly and posteriorly, promptly reporting bleeding.
- Measure and record the amount and color of drainage. Expect drainage to be bloody during the first 4 hours and then to become serous.
- Check circulatory status (blood pressure, pulse, respirations, and bleeding).
- Monitor intake and output for at least 48 hours after general anesthesia.
- Prevent lymphedema of the arm, which may be an early complication of any breast cancer treatment that involves lymph node manipulation. Instruct her to exercise her hand and arm regularly and to avoid activities that might cause infection or impairment in this hand or arm, which increases the chance of developing lymphedema. (See *Postoperative arm and hand care,* page 224.)

Postoperative arm and hand care

Hand exercises for the patient who's prone to lymphedema can begin on the day of surgery. Plan arm exercises with the surgeon who can anticipate potential problems with the suture line:

- Have the patient open her hand and close it tightly six to eight times every 3 hours while she's awake.
- Elevate the arm on the affected side on a pillow above the heart level.
- Encourage the patient to wash her face and comb her hair—an effective exercise to prevent lymphedema.
- Measure and record the circumference of the patient's arm 2¼" (6 cm) from her elbow. Indicate the exact place you measured. By remeasuring a month after surgery and at intervals during and following radiation therapy, you'll be able to determine whether lymphedema is present. The patient may complain that her arm is heavy—an early symptom of lymphedema.
- When the patient is home, she can elevate her arm and hand by supporting it on the back of a chair or a couch.

- Tell the patient not to let anyone draw blood, start an I.V., give an injection, or take a blood pressure reading on the affected side because these activities will also increase the chances of developing lymphedema.
- Inspect the incision. Encourage the patient and her partner to look at her incision as soon as feasible, perhaps when the first dressing is removed.
- Advise the patient to ask her physician about reconstructive surgery or to call the local or state medical society for the names of plastic reconstructive surgeons who regularly perform surgery to create breast mounds. In many cases, reconstructive surgery may be planned prior to the mastectomy. Also, both surgeries may be performed at the same time.
- Instruct the patient about breast prostheses. The American Cancer Society's Reach to Recovery group can provide instruction, emotional support, counseling, and a list of area stores that sell prostheses.
- Give psychological and emotional support. Most patients fear cancer and possible disfigurement and worry about loss of sexual function. Explain that breast surgery doesn't interfere with sexual function and that the patient may resume sexual activity as soon as she desires after surgery.
- Also explain to the patient that she may experience "phantom breast syndrome" (a phenomenon in which a tingling or a pins-and-needles sensation is felt in the area of the amputated breast tissue) or depression following mastectomy. Listen to the patient's concerns, offer support, and refer her to an appropriate organization such as the American Cancer Society's Reach to Recovery, which offers caring and sharing groups to help breast cancer patients in the hospital and at home.
- Explain to the patient the importance of regular (monthly) breast self-examinations and routine follow-up.

Bulimia nervosa

The essential features of bulimia nervosa include eating binges followed by feelings of guilt, humiliation, and self-deprecation. These feelings cause the patient to engage in self-induced vomiting, abuse laxatives or diuretics, follow a strict diet, or fast to overcome the effects of the binges. Unless the patient spends an excessive amount of time bingeing and purging, bulimia nervosa is seldom incapacitating. However, electrolyte imbalances (metabolic alkalosis, hypochloremia, and hypokalemia) and dehydration can occur, increasing the risk for physical complications.

Bulimia nervosa usually begins in adolescence or early adulthood and can occur simultaneously with anorexia nervosa. It affects nine women for every man. Nearly 2% of adult women meet the diagnostic criteria for bulimia nervosa; 5% to 15% have some symptoms of the disorder. Eating disorders are most prevalent in affluent cultural groups and are essentially unknown in cultural groups where poverty and malnutrition are prevalent. In developing countries, almost no cases of eating disorders have been recognized.

Causes

The cause of bulimia nervosa is unknown, but psychosocial factors may contribute to its development. These factors include family disturbance or conflict, sexual abuse, maladaptive learned behavior, struggle for control or self-identity, cultural overemphasis on physical appearance, and parental obesity. Bulimia nervosa is commonly associated with depression, anxiety, phobias, and obsessive-compulsive disorder, all of which may interfere with recovery. Depression in a bulimic patient may lead to suicide attempts or a completed suicide.

Signs and symptoms

The history of a patient with bulimia nervosa is characterized by episodes of binge eating that may occur up to several times a day. The patient commonly reports a binge-eating episode during which she continues eating until abdominal pain, sleep, or the presence of another person interrupts it. The preferred food is usually sweet, soft, and high in calories and carbohydrates.

The bulimic patient may appear thin and emaciated. Typically, however, although her weight frequently fluctuates, it usually stays within normal limits — through the use of diuretics, laxatives, vomiting, and exercise. So, unlike the anorexic patient, the bulimic patient usually can hide her eating disorder.

Overt clues to this disorder include hyperactivity, peculiar eating habits or rituals, frequent weighing, and a distorted body image. (See *Characteristics of bulimia patients*, page 226.)

The patient may complain of abdominal and epigastric pain caused by acute gastric dilation. She may also have amenorrhea if she maintains a body weight too low to sustain a pregnancy. Repetitive vomiting may cause painless swelling of the salivary

Characteristics of bulimia patients

Recognizing the bulimia patient isn't always easy. Unlike anorexic patients, bulimic patients don't deny that their eating habits are abnormal, but they commonly conceal their behavior out of shame. If you suspect bulimia nervosa, be alert for the following features:

- difficulty with impulse control
- chronic depression
- exaggerated sense of guilt
- low tolerance for frustration
- recurrent anxiety
- feelings of alienation
- self-consciousness
- difficulty expressing feelings such as anger
- impaired social or occupational adjustment.

glands, hoarseness, throat irritation or lacerations, and dental erosion. The patient may also exhibit calluses on the knuckles or abrasions and scars on the dorsum of the hand, caused by tooth injury during self-induced vomiting, although many bulimic persons induce vomiting chemically, such as with ipecac.

Others may perceive a bulimic patient as the "perfect" student, mother, or career woman; an adolescent may be distinguished for participation in competitive activities such as sports. However, the patient's psychosocial history may reveal an exaggerated sense of guilt, symptoms of depression, childhood trauma (especially sexual abuse), parental obesity, or a history of unsatisfactory sexual relationships.

Diagnosis

Diagnosis of bulimia begins with a history and physical examination. The primary care provider may order tests to check the person's health status, including:

- blood tests such as a complete blood count
- electrocardiography to check for heart problems
- urinalysis to check for dehydration and infection
- chest X-ray to check for rib fractures, heart problems, or lung infection
- abdominal X-ray to look for digestive tract problems. (For characteristic findings in this condition, see *Diagnosing bulimia nervosa.*)

Additional diagnostic tools include the Beck Depression Inventory, which may identify coexisting depression, and laboratory tests to help determine the presence and severity of complications. Serum electrolyte studies may show elevated bicarbonate, decreased potassium, and decreased sodium levels.

Treatment

Treatment of bulimia nervosa may continue for several years. Interrelated physical and psychological symptoms must be treated simultaneously. Merely promoting weight gain isn't sufficient to guarantee long-term . A patient whose physical status is severely compromised by inadequate or chaotic eating patterns is difficult to engage in the psychotherapeutic process.

Psychotherapy concentrates on interrupting the binge-purge cycle and helping the patient regain control over her eating behavior. Inpatient or outpatient treatment includes behavior modification therapy, which may take place in highly structured psychoeducational group meetings. Individual psychotherapy and family therapy, which address the eating disorder as a symptom of unresolved conflict, may help the patient understand the basis of her behavior and teach her self-control strategies. Antidepressant drugs, particularly selective serotonin reuptake inhibitors (SSRIs), may be used as an adjunct to psychotherapy.

The patient may also benefit from participation in self-help groups such as Overeaters Anonymous or a drug rehabilitation program if she has a concurrent substance abuse problem.

Diagnosing bulimia nervosa

The diagnosis of bulimia is made when the patient meets criteria put forth in the *Diagnostic and Statistical Manual of Mental Disorders,* Fourth Edition, Text Revision. The behaviors listed below must occur at least twice a week for 3 months:

- recurrent episodes of binge eating (rapid consumption of a large amount of food in a discrete period of time and a feeling of lack of control over eating behavior during the eating binges)
- recurrent inappropriate compensatory behavior to prevent weight gain (self-induced vomiting; misuse of laxatives, diuretics, enemas, or other medications; fasting; excessive exercise).

Special considerations

- Supervise the patient during mealtimes and for a specified period after meals (usually 1 hour). Set a time limit for each meal. Provide a pleasant, relaxed environment for eating.
- Using behavior modification techniques, reward the patient for satisfactory weight gain.
- Establish an eating contract with the patient, specifying the amount and type of food to be eaten at each meal.
- Encourage her to recognize and express her feelings about her eating behavior. Maintain an accepting and nonjudgmental attitude, controlling your reactions to her behavior and feelings.
- Encourage the patient to talk about stressful issues, such as achievement, independence, socialization, sexuality, family problems, and control.
- Identify the patient's elimination patterns.
- Assess her suicide potential. If she is suicidal, place her on suicide precautions and establish a suicide contract with her.
- Refer the patient and her family to the American Anorexia/Bulimia Association and to Anorexia Nervosa and Related Eating Disorders for additional information and support.
- Teach the patient how to keep a food journal to monitor treatment progress.

- Outline the risks of laxative, emetic, and diuretic abuse for the patient.
- Provide assertiveness training to help the patient gain control over her behavior and achieve a realistic and positive self-image.
- If the patient is taking a prescribed tricyclic antidepressant, warn her to avoid consuming alcoholic beverages; exposing herself to sunlight, heat lamps, or tanning salons; and discontinuing the medication unless she has notified the physician.
- SSRIs may take up to 4 to 8 weeks to establish their therapeutic effectiveness. They interfere with sexual functioning, and patients should be questioned about their sexual activity. Some SSRIs must be tapered rather than discontinued abruptly.

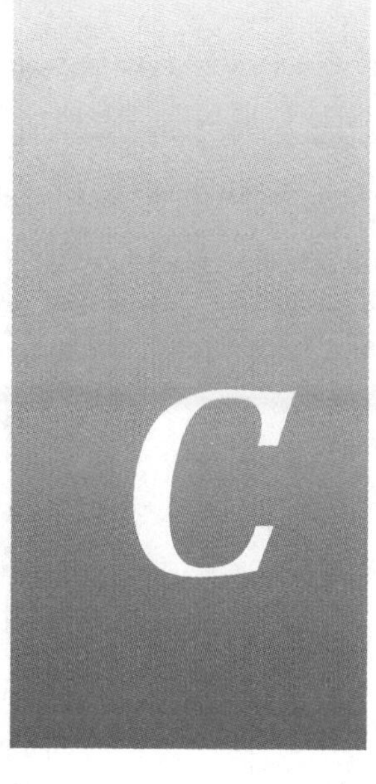

Carpal tunnel syndrome

Carpal tunnel syndrome, a form of repetitive stress injury, is the most common nerve entrapment syndrome. Carpal tunnel syndrome usually occurs in women between ages 30 and 60 (posing a serious occupational health problem). However, men who are employed as assembly-line workers and packers or who repeatedly use poorly designed tools, may also develop this disorder. Any strenuous use of the hands — sustained grasping, twisting, or flexing — aggravates this condition.

Causes

Carpal tunnel syndrome is mostly idiopathic, or it may result from:

- repetitive stress injury
- rheumatoid arthritis
- flexor tenosynovitis (commonly associated with rheumatic disease)
- nerve compression
- pregnancy
- multiple myeloma
- diabetes mellitus
- acromegaly
- hypothyroidism
- amyloidosis
- obesity
- benign tumor

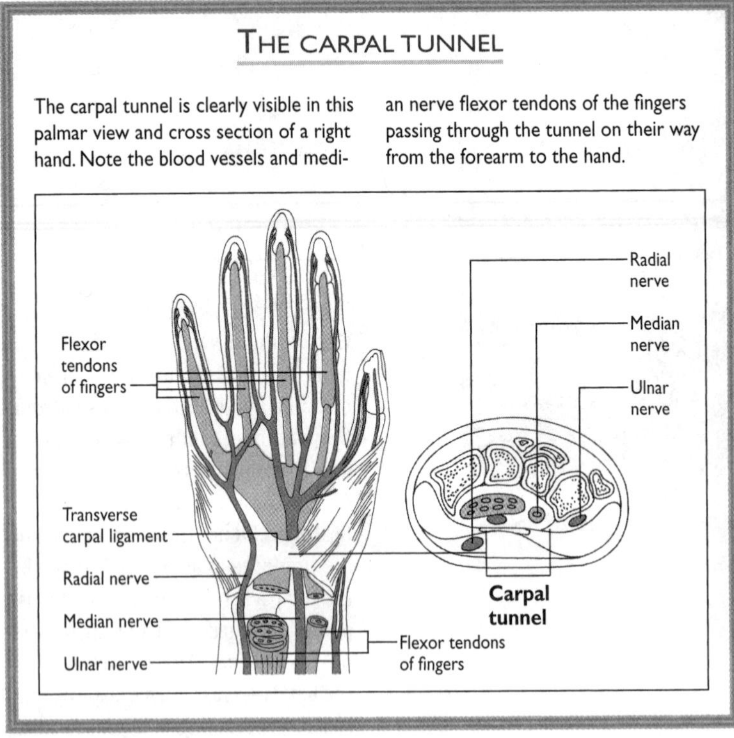

The carpal tunnel

The carpal tunnel is clearly visible in this palmar view and cross section of a right hand. Note the blood vessels and median nerve flexor tendons of the fingers passing through the tunnel on their way from the forearm to the hand.

- other conditions that increase fluid pressure in the wrist, including alterations in the endocrine or immune systems
- wrist dislocation or sprain, including Colles' fracture followed by edema.

The carpal bones and the transverse carpal ligament form the carpal tunnel. (See *The carpal tunnel.*) Inflammation or fibrosis of the tendon sheaths that pass through the carpal tunnel usually causes edema and compression of the median nerve. This compression neuropathy causes sensory and motor changes in the median distribution of the hands, initially impairing sensory transmission to the thumb, index finger, second finger, and inner aspect of the third finger.

Signs and symptoms

The patient with carpal tunnel syndrome usually complains of weakness, pain, burning, numbness, or tingling in one or both hands. This paresthesia affects the thumb, forefinger, middle finger, and half of the fourth finger. The patient is unable to clench her hand into a fist; the nails may be atrophic, and the skin may be dry and shiny.

Because of vasodilation and venous stasis, symptoms typically are worse at night and in the morning. The pain may spread to the forearm and, in severe cases, as far as the shoulder. The patient usually can relieve such pain by shaking or rubbing her hands vigorously or dangling her arms at her side.

- Continued use of the affected wrist may increase tendon inflammation, compression, and neural ischemia, causing a decrease in wrist function.
- Untreated, carpal tunnel syndrome can produce permanent nerve damage with loss of movement and sensation.

Diagnosis

Physical examination reveals decreased sensation to light touch or pinpricks in the affected fingers. Thenar muscle atrophy occurs in about half of all cases of carpal tunnel syndrome, but is usually a late sign.

The following tests provide rapid diagnosis of carpal tunnel syndrome:

- *Tinel's sign* — tingling over the median nerve on light percussion
- *Phalen's maneuver* — holding the forearms vertically and allowing both hands to drop into complete flexion at the wrists for 1 minute, which reproduces symptoms of carpal tunnel syndrome
- *compression test* — blood pressure cuff inflated above systolic pressure on the forearm for 1 to 2 minutes, which provokes pain and paresthesia along the distribution of the median nerve.

Other tests include electromyography to detect a median nerve motor conduction delay of more than 5 msec and laboratory tests to identify underlying disease.

Treatment

Conservative treatment should be tried first, including resting the hands by splinting the wrist in neutral extension for 1 to 2 weeks. Nonsteroidal anti-inflammatory drugs usually provide symptomatic relief. Injection of the carpal tunnel with hydrocortisone and lidocaine may provide significant but temporary relief. If a definite link has been established between the patient's occupation and the development of repetitive stress injury, she may have to seek other work. Effective treatment may also require correction of an underlying disorder. When conservative treatment fails, the only alternative is surgical decompression of the nerve by resecting the entire transverse carpal tunnel ligament or by using endoscopic surgical techniques. Neurolysis (freeing of the nerve fibers) may also be necessary.

Special considerations

Consider the following patient care for carpal tunnel syndrome:

- Administer mild analgesics as needed. Encourage the patient to use her hands as much as possible. If her dominant hand has been impaired, you may have to help her with eating and bathing.
- Teach the patient how to apply a splint. Tell her not to make it too tight. Show her how to remove the splint to perform gentle range-of-motion exercises, which should be done daily. Make sure the patient knows how to do these exercises before she's discharged.

- After surgery, monitor vital signs and regularly check the color, sensation, and motion of the affected hand.
- Advise the patient who is about to be discharged to exercise her hands occasionally in warm water. If the arm is in a sling, tell her to remove the sling several times per day to do exercises for her elbow and shoulder.
- Suggest occupational counseling for the patient who has to change jobs because of repetitive stress injury.

Cataract

A cataract is a gradually developing opacity of the lens or lens capsule of the eye. Light shining through the cornea is blocked by this opacity, and a blurred image is cast onto the retina. As a result, the brain interprets a hazy image. Cataracts commonly occur bilaterally, and each progresses independently. Exceptions are traumatic cataracts, which are usually unilateral, and congenital cataracts, which may remain stationary. Cataracts are most prevalent in people older than age 70 as part of the aging process. The prognosis is generally good; surgery improves vision in 95% of affected people. However, in recent studies, cataracts have been associated with a higher risk of mortality in older women.

Causes

Causes of cataracts include:

- aging (senile cataracts)
- congenital disorders
- genetic abnormalities
- maternal rubella during the first trimester of pregnancy
- traumatic cataracts
- foreign body injury
- complicated cataracts
- uveitis
- glaucoma
- retinitis pigmentosa
- retinal detachment
- diabetes mellitus
- hypoparathyroidism
- myotonic dystrophy
- atopic dermatitis
- exposure to ionizing radiation or infrared rays
- drugs that are toxic to the lens and that cause photosensitivity, such as prednisone (Deltasone), antihistamines, hormonal contraceptives, antidepressants, sulfa drugs, fluroquinone antibiotics, and tranquilizers.
- exposure to ultraviolet rays.

Some causes of cataract occur only in women — researchers suspect that these causes may be related to hormonal changes and adverse events in pregnancy and childbearing, which are linked to higher mortality. These and other factors are undergoing investigation.

Pathophysiology may vary with each form of cataract. Senile cataracts show evidence of protein aggregation, oxidative injury, and increased pigmentation in the center of the lens. In traumatic cataracts, phagocytosis of the lens or inflammation may occur when a lens ruptures. The mechanism of a complicated cataract varies with the disease process; for example, in diabetes, increased glucose in the lens causes it to absorb water.

Typically, cataract development goes through four stages:

- *immature.* The lens isn't completely opaque.
- *mature.* The lens is completely opaque and vision loss is significant.
- *tumescent.* The lens is filled with water, which may lead to glaucoma.
- *hypermature.* The lens proteins deteriorate, causing peptides to leak through the lens capsule. Glaucoma may develop if intraocular fluid outflow is obstructed.

Signs and symptoms

Possible signs and symptoms of cataracts include:

- gradual painless blurring and loss of vision due to lens opacity
- milky white pupil due to lens opacity
- blinding glare from headlights at night due to the inefficient reflection of light rays by the opacities
- poor reading vision caused by reduced clarity of images
- better vision in dim light than in bright light in patients with central opacity; as pupils dilate, patients can see around the opacity.

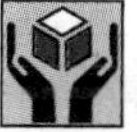

SPECIAL NEEDS

Elderly patients with reduced vision may become depressed and withdraw from social activities rather than complain about reduced vision.

Complications of cataracts include blindness and glaucoma. Surgical complications may include:

- loss of vitreous humor
- wound dehiscence from loosening of sutures and flat anterior chamber or iris prolapse into the wound
- hyphema, which is a hemorrhage into the eye's anterior chamber
- vitreous-block glaucoma
- retinal detachment
- infection.

Diagnosis

Diagnosis is based on the following tests:

- physical examination (shining a penlight on the pupil to show the white area behind the pupil, which remains unnoticeable until the cataract is advanced)
- indirect ophthalmoscopy and slit-lamp examination to show a dark area in the normally homogeneous red reflex
- visual acuity test to confirm vision loss.

Treatment

Treatment for cataract may include:

- extracapsular cataract extraction to remove the anterior lens capsule and cortex and intraocular lens (IOL) implant in the posterior chamber; typically performed by using phacoemulsification to fragment the lens with ultrasonic vibrations, then aspirating the pieces (see *Comparing methods of cataract removal*, page 234.)
- intracapsular cataract extraction to remove the entire lens within the intact capsule by cryoextraction (rare procedure in which the moist lens sticks to an extremely cold metal probe for easy and safe extraction) with subsequent placement of an IOL

Comparing methods of cataract removal

Cataracts can be removed by extracapsular or intracapsular techniques.

Extracapsular cataract extraction

The surgeon may use irrigation and aspiration or phacoemulsification for extracapsular cataract extraction. To irrigate and aspirate, he makes an incision at the limbus, opens the anterior lens capsule with a cystotome, and exerts pressure from below to express the lens. He then irrigates and suctions the remaining lens cortex.

In phacoemulsification, he uses an ultrasonic probe to break the lens into minute particles and aspirates the particles.

Irrigation and aspiration

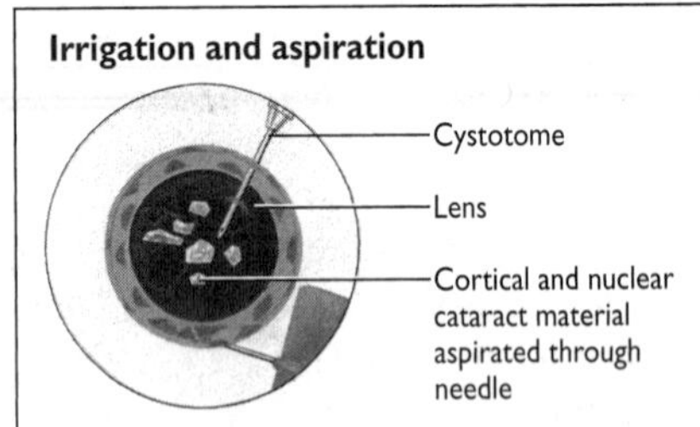

Phacoemulsification

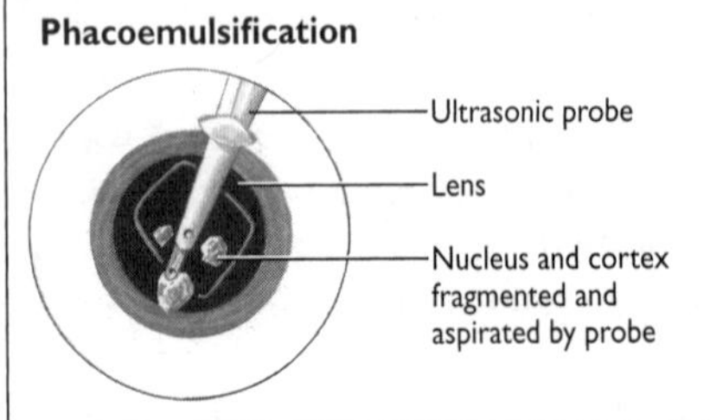

Intracapsular cataract extraction

The surgeon makes a partial incision at the superior limbus arc. He then removes the lens using specially designed forceps or a cryoprobe, which adheres to the frozen lens to facilitate its removal.

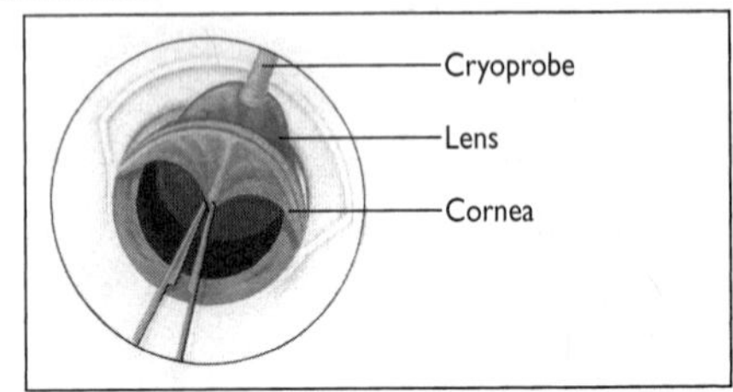

in the anterior or posterior chamber after lens removal; alternatively, use of contact lens or aphakic glasses to enhance vision

- laser surgery after an extracapsular cataract extraction to restore visual acuity when a secondary membrane forms in the posterior lens capsule that has been left intact
- discission (an incision) and aspiration in children with soft cataracts
- contact lenses or lens implantation after surgery to improve visual acuity, binocular vision, and depth perception.

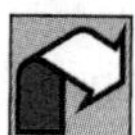

PREVENTION POINTER

A study showed that older women who took vitamin C consistently during their younger and middle-age years had a decreased risk of cataracts. However, the study isn't conclusive and advises women that large doses of vitamin C shouldn't be taken without the advice of their health care provider because it may cause renal calculi.

Special considerations

Consider these patient care measures after surgery to extract a cataract:

- Because the patient will be discharged after she recovers from anesthesia, remind her to return for a checkup the next day, and warn her to avoid activities that increase intraocular pressure such as straining.
- Urge the patient to protect the eye from accidental injury at night by wearing a plastic or metal shield with perforations; a shield or glasses should be worn for protection during the day.
- Before discharge, teach the patient to administer antibiotic ointment or drops to prevent infection and steroids to reduce inflammation; combination steroid-antibiotic eyedrops can also be used.
- Advise the patient to watch for the development of complications, such as a sharp pain in the eye uncontrolled by analgesics as a result of hyphema, or clouding in the anterior chamber (which may herald an infection), and to report them immediately.
- Caution the patient about activity restrictions, and advise her that she'll receive her corrective reading glasses or lenses in several weeks.

Cervical cancer

The third most common cancer of the female reproductive system, cervical cancer is classified as either preinvasive or invasive.

Preinvasive carcinoma ranges from minimal cervical dysplasia, in which the lower third of the epithelium contains abnormal cells, to carcinoma in situ, in which the full thickness of epithelium contains abnormally proliferating cells (also known as *cervical intraepithelial neoplasia* [CIN]). Preinvasive cancer is curable 75% to 90% of the time with early detection and proper treatment. If untreated (and depending on the form in which it appears), it may progress to invasive cervical cancer.

In invasive carcinoma, cancer cells penetrate the basement membrane and can spread directly to contiguous pelvic structures or disseminate to distant sites by lymphatic routes. In almost all cases of cervical cancer (95%), the histologic type is squamous cell carcinoma, which varies from well-differentiated cells to highly anaplastic spindle cells. Only 5% are adenocarcinomas. Usually, invasive carcinoma occurs between ages 30 and 50; rarely, under age 20.

Causes

Although the cause is unknown, several predisposing factors have been related to the development of cervical cancer:

- frequent intercourse at a young age (under age 16)
- multiple sexual partners
- multiple pregnancies
- exposure to sexually transmitted diseases (particularly genital warts caused by the human papillomavirus)
- smoking.

Signs and symptoms

Preinvasive cervical cancer produces no symptoms or other clinically apparent changes. Early invasive cervical cancer causes abnormal vaginal bleeding, persistent vaginal discharge, and postcoital pain and bleeding. In advanced stages, it causes pelvic pain, vaginal leakage of urine and feces from a fistula, anorexia, weight loss, and anemia.

Diagnosis

A cytologic examination (Papanicolaou [Pap] test) can detect cervical cancer before clinical evidence appears. (Systems of Pap test classification may vary from hospital to hospital.) Abnormal cervical cytology routinely calls for colposcopy, which can detect the presence and extent of preclinical lesions requiring biopsy and histologic examination. Staining with Lugol's solution (strong iodine) or Schiller's solution (iodine, potassium iodide, and purified water) may identify areas for biopsy when the smear shows abnormal cells, but there is no obvious lesion. Although the tests are nonspecific, they do distinguish between normal and abnormal tissues. Normal tissues absorb the iodine and turn brown; abnormal tissues are devoid of glycogen and won't change color. Additional studies, such as lymphangiography, cystography, and scans, can detect metastasis.

Treatment

Appropriate treatment depends on accurate clinical staging. Preinvasive lesions may be treated with total excisional biopsy, cryosurgery, laser destruction, conization (and frequent Pap test follow-up) or, rarely, hysterectomy. Therapy for invasive squamous cell carcinoma may include radical hysterectomy and radiation therapy (internal, external, or both).

Special considerations

Management of cervical cancer requires skilled preoperative and postoperative care, comprehensive patient teaching, and emotional and psychological support:

- If you assist with a biopsy, drape and prepare the patient as for routine Pap test and pelvic examination. Have a container of formaldehyde ready to preserve the specimen during transfer to the pathology laboratory. Explain to the patient that she may feel pressure, minor abdominal cramps, or a pinch from the punch forceps. Reassure her that pain will be minimal because the cervix has few nerve endings.
- If you assist with cryosurgery, drape and prepare the patient as if for a routine Pap test and pelvic examination. Explain that the procedure takes approximately 15 minutes, during which time the physician will use refrigerant to freeze the cervix. Warn

the patient that she may experience abdominal cramps, headache, and sweating, but reassure her that she'll feel little, if any, pain.

- If you assist with laser therapy, drape and prepare the patient as if for a routine Pap test and pelvic examination. Explain that the procedure takes approximately 30 minutes and may cause abdominal cramps.
- After excisional biopsy, cryosurgery, and laser therapy, tell the patient to expect discharge or spotting for about 1 week after these procedures, and advise her not to douche, use tampons, or engage in sexual intercourse during this time. Tell her to watch for and report signs of infection. Stress the need for a follow-up Pap test and a pelvic examination within 3 to 4 months after these procedures and periodically thereafter.
- Tell the patient what to expect postoperatively if she'll have a hysterectomy.
- After surgery, monitor vital signs every 4 hours.
- Watch for and immediately report signs or symptoms of complications, such as bleeding, abdominal distention, severe pain, breathing difficulties, and symptoms of deep vein thrombosis.
- Administer analgesics, prophylactic antibiotics, and subcutaneous heparin, as ordered.
- Encourage deep-breathing and coughing exercises.

For radiation therapy:

- Find out if the patient is to have internal or external therapy, or both. Usually, internal radiation therapy is the first procedure.
- Explain the internal radiation procedure, and answer the patient's questions. Internal radiation requires a 2 to 3-day hospital stay, bowel preparation, a povidone-iodine vaginal douche, a clear liquid diet, insertion of an indwelling urinary catheter, and nothing by mouth the night before the implantation.
- Explain to the patient that she'll have less contact with staff and visitors while the implant is in place.
- Tell the patient that the internal radiation applicator will be inserted in the operating room under general anesthesia and that the radioactive material (such as radium or cesium) will be loaded into it once she's back in her room.
- Remember that safety precautions — time, distance, and shielding — begin as soon as the radioactive source is in place. Inform the patient that she'll require a private room. (See *Internal radiation safety precautions*, page 238.)
- Encourage the patient to lie flat and limit movement while the implant is in place. If she prefers, elevate the head of the bed slightly.
- Check vital signs every 4 hours; watch for skin reaction, vaginal bleeding, abdominal discomfort, or evidence of dehydration. Make sure the patient can reach everything she needs without stretching or straining. Assist her in range-of-motion arm exercises (leg exercises and other body movements could dislodge the implant). If ordered, administer a tranquilizer to

Internal radiation safety precautions

There are three cardinal safety rules in internal radiation therapy:

- *Time*—Wear a radiosensitive badge. Remember, your exposure increases with time, and the effects are cumulative. Therefore, carefully plan your time with the patient to prevent overexposure. (However, don't rush procedures or ignore the patient's psychological needs.)
- *Distance*—Radiation loses its intensity with distance. Avoid standing at the foot of the patient's bed, where you're in line with the radiation.
- *Shield*—Lead shields reduce radiation exposure. Use them whenever possible.

In internal radiation therapy, remember that the patient is radioactive while the radiation source is in place, usually 48 to 72 hours:

- Pregnant women shouldn't be assigned to care for these patients.
- Check the position of the source applicator every 4 hours. If it appears dislodged, notify the physician immediately. If it's completely dislodged, remove the patient from the bed; pick up the applicator with long forceps, place it on a lead-shielded transport cart, and notify the physician immediately.
- *Never* pick up the source with your bare hands. Notify the doctor and radiation safety officer whenever there's an accident, and keep a lead-shielded transport cart on the unit as long as the patient has a source in place.

Positioning of internal radiation applicator for uterine cancer

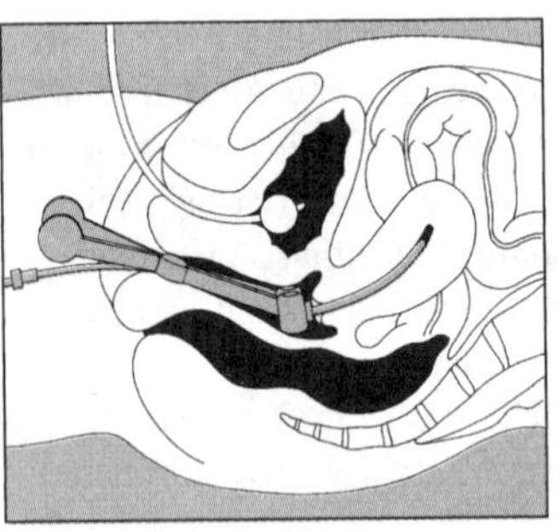

help the patient relax and remain still. Organize the time you spend with the patient to minimize your exposure to radiation.

- Inform visitors of safety precautions, and hang a sign listing these precautions on the patient's door.
- Explain that external outpatient radiation therapy, when necessary, continues for 4 to 6 weeks.
- Teach the patient to watch for and report uncomfortable adverse effects. Because radiation therapy may increase susceptibility to infection by lowering the white blood cell count, warn the patient to avoid persons with obvious infections during therapy.
- Teach the patient to use a vaginal dilator to prevent vaginal stenosis and to facilitate vaginal examinations and sexual intercourse.
- Reassure the patient that this disease and its treatment shouldn't radically alter her lifestyle or prohibit sexual intimacy.

Chlamydia

Chlamydia is one of the most common, yet curable sexually transmitted diseases (STDs) in the United States. It's most common in women and men under age 25. The Centers for Disease Control and Prevention estimates that more than 3 million people each year become infected with chlamydia. Chlamydial infections cost Americans more than $2 billion per year. Chlamydia, if not treated, can cause serious problems in men, women, and neonates of infected mothers. It's estimated that 20% to 50% of children born to infected women will be infected.

Causes

Chlamydial infections are caused by a bacterium called *Chlamydia trachomatis.* They are smaller than rickettsia and bacteria, but larger than viruses. They depend on host cells for replication and are susceptible to antibiotics. Chlamydiae are transmitted by direct contact, such as by vaginal and anal sexual intercourse. It can also spread from an infected woman to her fetus during childbirth. They're a common cause of various infections of the urethra, bladder, fallopian tubes, and prostate gland, including:

- *cervicitis* — cervical erosion, dyspareunia, mucopurulent discharge, pelvic pain
- *endometritis or salpingitis* — pain and tenderness of the lower abdomen, cervix, uterus, and lymph nodes; chills and fever; breakthrough bleeding, bleeding after intercourse, and vaginal discharge; dysuria
- *urethral syndrome* — dysuria, pyuria, urinary frequency
- *urethritis* — dysuria, erythema, and tenderness of the urethral meatus; urinary frequency; pruritus and urethral discharge (copious and purulent or scant and clear or mucoid)
- *epididymitis* — painful scrotal swelling, urethral discharge
- *prostatitis* — low back pain; urinary frequency, nocturia, and dysuria; painful ejaculation
- *proctitis* — diarrhea, tenesmus, pruritus, bloody or mucopurulent discharge, diffuse or discrete ulceration in the rectosigmoid colon.

Signs and symptoms

Usually, chlamydia has no symptoms. Up to 85% of women and 40% of men don't develop symptoms. Therefore, many people transmit the disease without even knowing they have a chlamydial infection until it's discovered by laboratory tests.

For those who do have symptoms, clinical expressions of infectious disease vary, depending on the pathogen involved and the organ system affected. Most of the signs and symptoms vary based on host responses. Symptoms may appear as early as 5 to 10 days after infection, but usually appear 1 to 3 weeks after being infected. During the prodromal stage, a person will complain of mild, common, and nonspecific signs and symptoms, such as fever, muscle aches, headache, and lethargy. In the acute stage, more specific signs and symptoms provide evidence of the microbe's target. Infection can also cause an inflamed, itching, or bleeding rectum. If it infects the eye, it may cause redness, itching, and a discharge (also known as *pink eye*). It may also infect the throat from oral sexual contact with an infected partner.

When women have symptoms, they may experience:

- abnormal discharge from the vagina
- bleeding between menstrual cycles
- vaginal bleeding or pain with sexual intercourse
- abdominal pain
- low-grade fever
- painful urination
- urinary urgency
- cervical inflammation
- mucopurulent cervicitis.

When men have symptoms, they may have:

- abnormal discharge from the penis
- pain or burning feeling with urination
- swollen or tender testicles.

If the infection isn't treated, complications may occur, including:

- pelvic inflammatory disease in women
- epididymitis in men
- Reiter's syndrome, usually in young men
- sterility in men and women.

In neonates, both the mother and neonate experience symptoms.

Neonates born of infected mothers are born with eye infections or pneumonia. Symptoms usually begin within 4 weeks of birth. Chlamydia is the leading cause of neonatal conjunctivitis, an eye infection that can lead to blindness.

Diagnosis

Diagnosis is confirmed through laboratory tests:

- A swab from the site of infection (vagina or penis) establishes a diagnosis of urethritis, cervicitis, salpingitis, endometritis, or proctitis.
- A culture of aspirated material establishes a diagnosis of epididymitis.
- Antigen-detection methods are the diagnostic tests of choice for identifying chlamydial infection.
- Polymerase chain reaction test is highly sensitive and specific.
- Urine tests don't require pelvic examinations or swabbing. Results from the urine tests are usually available within 24 hours.

Treatment

Usually, treatments for chlamydial infections include antibiotics, such as azithromycin, doxycycline, or erythromycin.

Special considerations

- Encourage the patient to take all of the medication as prescribed, even if her symptoms disappear.
- Tell the woman that she should have all of her sexual partners past, present, and future tested and treated for chlamydial infections.

PREVENTION POINTER

Teach her how to avoid future infections through such methods as abstinence, using condoms, avoiding intercourse until treatment is complete, and making sure that her sex partners are screened and treated at the same time.

Cholelithiasis and related disorders

Diseases of the gallbladder and biliary tract are common and, in many cases, painful conditions that may be life-threatening and usually require surgery. They are generally associated with deposition of calculi and inflammation. (See *Common sites of calculi formation.*)

Cholelithiasis is the fifth leading cause of hospitalization among adults and accounts for 90% of all gallbladder and duct diseases. Women have two to three times the incidence as men of developing cholelithiasis. The disease may also be more prevalent in persons who are obese, who have high cholesterol, or who are on cholesterol-lowering drugs. The prognosis is usually good with treatment unless infection occurs, in which case prognosis depends on its severity and response to antibiotics.

In most cases, gallbladder and bile duct diseases occur during middle age. Between ages 20 and 50, they're six times more common in women, but incidence in men and women becomes equal after age 50. Incidence rises with each succeeding decade.

Common sites of calculi formation

The illustration below shows sites where calculi typically collect. Stones vary in size; small stones may travel.

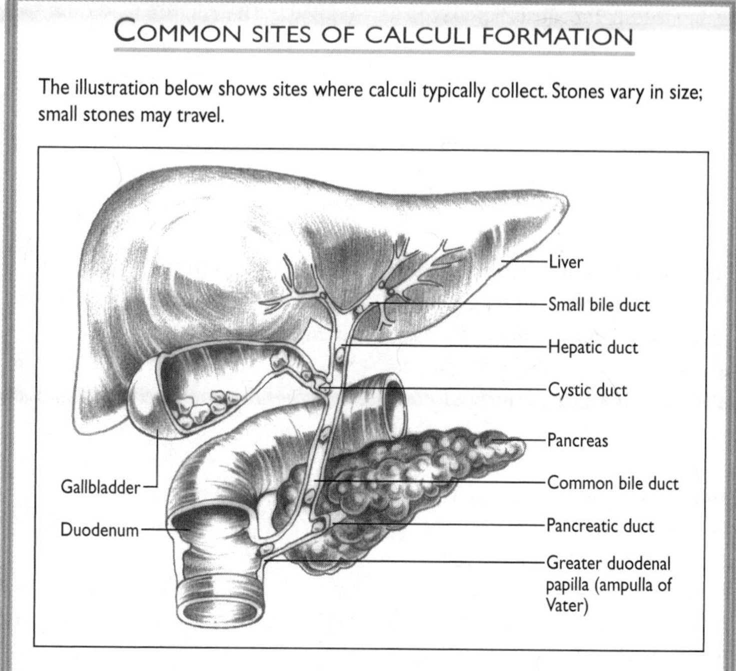

Causes

Cholelithiasis, stones or calculi (gallstones) in the gallbladder, results from changes in bile components. Gallstones are made of cholesterol, calcium bilirubinate, or a mixture of cholesterol and bilirubin pigment. They arise during periods of sluggishness in the gallbladder due to pregnancy, hormonal contraceptives, diabetes mellitus, celiac disease, cirrhosis of the liver, and pancreatitis.

One out of every 10 patients with gallstones develops *choledocholithiasis*, or gallstones in the common bile duct (sometimes called *common duct stones*). This condition occurs when stones pass out of the gallbladder and lodge in the hepatic and common bile ducts, obstructing the flow of bile into the duodenum. Prognosis is good unless infection occurs.

Cholangitis, infection of the bile duct, is commonly associated with choledocholithiasis and may follow percutaneous transhepatic cholangiography or occlusion of endoscopic stents. Predisposing factors may include bacterial or metabolic alteration of bile acids. Widespread inflammation may cause fibrosis and stenosis of the common bile duct. The prognosis for this rare condition is poor without stenting or surgery.

Cholecystitis, acute or chronic inflammation of the gallbladder, is usually associated with a gallstone impacted in the cystic duct, causing painful distention of the gallbladder. Cholecystitis accounts for 10% to 25% of all patients requiring gallbladder surgery. The acute form is most common during middle age; the chronic form occurs most commonly among the elderly. The prognosis is good with treatment.

Cholesterolosis, polyps or crystal deposits of cholesterol in the gallbladder's submucosa, may result from bile secretions containing high concentrations of cholesterol and insufficient bile salts. The polyps may be localized or speckle the entire gallbladder. Cholesterolosis, the most common pseudotumor, isn't related to widespread inflammation of the mucosa or lining of the gallbladder. The prognosis is good with surgery.

Biliary cirrhosis, ascending infection of the biliary system, sometimes follows viral destruction of liver and duct cells, but the primary cause is unknown. This condition usually leads to obstructive jaundice and involves the portal and periportal spaces of the liver. It's nine times more common among women ages 40 to 60 than among men. The prognosis is poor without liver transplantation.

Gallstone ileus results from a gallstone lodging at the terminal ileum; it's more common in the elderly. The prognosis is good with surgery.

Postcholecystectomy syndrome commonly results from residual gallstones or stricture of the common bile duct. It occurs in 1% to 5% of all patients whose gallbladders have been surgically removed and may produce right upper quadrant abdominal pain, biliary colic, fatty food intolerance, dyspepsia, and indigestion. The prognosis is good with selected radiologic procedures, endoscopic procedures, or surgery.

Acalculous cholecystitis is more common in critically ill patients, accounting for about 5% of cholecystitis cases. It may result from primary infection with such organisms as *Salmonella typhi*, *Escherichia coli*, or *Clostridium* or from obstruction of the cystic duct due to lymphadenopathy or a tumor. It appears that ischemia, usually related to a low cardiac output, also has a role in the pathophysiology of this disease. Signs and symptoms of acalculous cholecystitis include unexplained sepsis, right upper quadrant pain, fever, leukocytosis, and a palpable gallbladder.

Signs and symptoms

Although gallbladder disease may produce no symptoms, acute cholelithiasis, acute cholecystitis, choledocholithiasis, and cholesterolosis produce the symptoms of a classic gallbladder attack. Attacks commonly follow meals rich in fats or may occur at night, suddenly awakening the patient. They begin with acute abdominal pain in the right upper quadrant that may radiate to the back, between the shoulders, or to the front of the chest; the pain may be so severe that the patient seeks emergency department care. Other features may include recurring fat intolerance, biliary colic, belching, flatulence, indigestion, diaphoresis, nausea, vomiting, chills, low-grade fever, jaundice (if a stone obstructs the common bile duct), and clay-colored stools (with choledocholithiasis).

Clinical features of cholangitis include a rise in eosinophils, jaundice, abdominal pain, high fever, and chills; biliary cirrhosis may produce jaundice, related itching, weakness, fatigue, slight weight loss, and abdominal pain. Gallstone ileus produces signs and symptoms of small bowel obstruction — nausea, vomiting, abdominal distention, and absent bowel sounds if the bowel is completely obstructed. Its most telling symptom is intermittent recurrence of colicky pain over several days. Each of these disorders produces its own set of complications. (See *Complications of cholelithiasis and related disorders*, page 244.)

Diagnosis

Differential diagnosis is essential in gallbladder and biliary tract disease because gallbladder disease can mimic other diseases (myocardial infarction, angina, pancreatitis, pancreatic head cancer, pneumonia, peptic ulcer, hiatal hernia, esophagitis, and gastritis). Serum amylase distinguishes gallbladder disease from pancreatitis. With suspected heart disease, serial cardiac enzyme tests and electrocardiogram should precede gallbladder and upper GI diagnostic tests. Tests used to diagnose gallbladder and biliary tract disease include:

- *Ultrasound* reflects stones in the gallbladder with 96% accuracy. It's also considered the primary tool for diagnosing cholelithiasis.
- *Percutaneous transhepatic cholangiography*, done under fluoroscopic control, distinguishes between gall-

Complications of cholelithiasis and related disorders

Cholelithiasis may lead to any of the disorders associated with gallstone formation: cholangitis, cholecystitis, choledocholithiasis, and gallstone ileus. Cholecystitis can progress to gallbladder complications, such as empyema, hydrops or mucocele, or gangrene. Gangrene may lead to perforation, resulting in peritonitis, fistula formation, pancreatitis, limy bile, and porcelain gallbladder. Other complications include chronic cholecystitis and cholangitis.

Choledocholithiasis may lead to cholangitis, obstructive jaundice, pancreatitis, and secondary biliary cirrhosis. Cholangitis, especially in the suppurative form, may progress to septic shock and death. Gallstone ileus may cause bowel obstruction, which can lead to intestinal perforation, peritonitis, septicemia, secondary infection, and septic shock.

bladder or bile duct disease and cancer of the pancreatic head in patients with jaundice.

- *Endoscopic retrograde cholangiopancreatography (ERCP)* visualizes the biliary tree after insertion of an endoscope down the esophagus into the duodenum, cannulation of the common bile and pancreatic ducts, and injection of contrast medium.
- *HIDA scan* of the gallbladder detects obstruction of the cystic duct.
- *Computed tomography scan*, although not used routinely, helps distinguish between obstructive and nonobstructive jaundice.
- *Flat plate of the abdomen* identifies calcified, but not cholesterol, stones with 15% accuracy.
- *Oral cholecystography*, which is rarely used, shows stones in the gallbladder and biliary duct obstruction.

Elevated icteric index, total bilirubin, urine bilirubin, and alkaline phosphatase support the diagnosis. White blood cell count is slightly elevated during a cholecystitis attack.

Treatment

Surgery, usually elective, is the treatment of choice for gallbladder and biliary tract diseases and may include open or laparoscopic cholecystectomy, cholecystectomy with operative cholangiography and, possibly, exploration of the common bile duct. Other treatments include a low-fat diet to prevent attacks and vitamin K for itching, jaundice, and bleeding tendencies due to vitamin K deficiency. Treatment during an acute attack may include insertion of a nasogastric tube and an I.V. line and, possibly, antibiotic and analgesic administration.

A nonsurgical treatment for choledocholithiasis involves placement of a catheter through the percutaneous transhepatic cholangiographic route. Guided by fluoroscopy, the catheter is directed toward the stone. A basket is threaded through the catheter, opened, twirled to entrap the stone, closed, and withdrawn. This procedure can be performed endoscopically.

Ursodiol (Actigall), which dissolves radiolucent stones, provides an alternative for patients who are poor surgical risks or who refuse surgery.

However, use of urdodiol is limited by the need for prolonged treatment, the high incidence of adverse effects, and the frequency of stone formation after treatment ends.

Extracorporeal shock wave lithotripsy (ESWL) has also been adapted for the treatment of gallstones. ESWL is a nonsurgical procedure used to crush stones inside the gallbladder. A lithotripsy machine focuses sound waves against the gallstones to break them into smaller pieces that can pass out of the gallbladder through the cystic duct and common bile duct into the small intestine.

SPECIAL NEEDS

Lithotripsy is contraindicated in pregnant women and those who have a pacemaker or serious heart problems.

Special considerations

Patient care for gallbladder and biliary tract diseases focuses on supportive care and close postoperative observation:

- Before surgery, teach the patient to deep-breathe, cough, expectorate, and perform leg exercises that are necessary after surgery. Also teach splinting, repositioning, and ambulation techniques. Explain the procedures that will be performed before, during, and after surgery to help ease the patient's anxiety and help ensure cooperation.
- After surgery, monitor vital signs for signs of bleeding, infection, or atelectasis.
- Evaluate the incision site for bleeding. Serosanguineous drainage is common during the first 24 to 48 hours if the patient has a wound drain. If, after a choledochostomy, a T-tube drain is placed in the duct and attached to a drainage bag, make sure that the drainage tube has no kinks. Also check that the connecting tubing from the T tube is well secured to the patient to prevent dislodgment.
- Measure and record T-tube drainage daily. (200 to 300 ml is normal.)
- Teach patients who will be discharged with a T tube how to perform dressing changes and routine skin care.
- Monitor intake and output. Allow the patient nothing by mouth for 24 to 48 hours or until bowel sounds return and nausea and vomiting cease. (Postoperative nausea may indicate a full bladder.)
- If the patient doesn't void within 8 hours (or if the amount voided is inadequate based on I.V. fluid intake), percuss over the symphysis pubis for bladder distention (especially in patients receiving anticholinergics). Patients who have had a laparoscopic cholecystectomy may be discharged the same day or within 24 hours after surgery. These patients should have minimal pain, be able to tolerate a regular diet within 24 hours after surgery, and be able to return to normal activity within a few days to 1 week.
- Encourage deep-breathing and leg exercises every hour. The patient should ambulate after surgery. Provide antiembolism stockings to support leg muscles and promote venous

blood flow, thus preventing stasis and clot formation.

- Evaluate the location, duration, and character of any pain. Administer adequate medication to relieve pain, especially before such activities as deep breathing and ambulation, which increase pain.
- At discharge, advise the patient against heavy lifting or straining for 6 weeks. Urge her to walk daily. Tell her that food restrictions are unnecessary unless she has an intolerance to a specific food or some underlying condition (such as diabetes, atherosclerosis, or obesity) that requires such restriction.
- Instruct the patient to notify the surgeon if she has pain for more than 24 hours, notices jaundice, anorexia, nausea or vomiting, fever, or tenderness in the abdominal area because these may indicate a biliary tract injury from cholecystectomy that requires immediate attention.

Chronic fatigue and immune dysfunction syndrome

Chronic fatigue and immune dysfunction syndrome (CFIDS), sometimes called *chronic fatigue syndrome, chronic Epstein-Barr virus (EBV)*, or *myalgic encephalomyelitis*, is typically marked by debilitating fatigue, neurologic abnormalities, and persistent symptoms that suggest chronic mononucleosis. It commonly occurs in adults under age 45 and primarily in women.

Causes

The cause of chronic fatigue and immune dysfunction syndrome is unknown, but researchers suspect that it may be found in HHV-6 or in other herpesviruses, enteroviruses, or retroviruses. Rising levels of antibodies to EBV, once thought to implicate EBV infection as the cause of CFIDS, are now considered a result of this disease. CFIDS may be associated with a reaction to viral illness that's complicated by dysfunctional immune response and by other factors that may include gender, age, genetic disposition, prior illness, stress, and environment.

Signs and symptoms

The characteristic symptom of CFIDS is prolonged, often overwhelming fatigue that is commonly associated with a varying complex of other symptoms, including but not limited to myalgia, arthralgia with arthritis, low-grade fever, pain, cervical adenopathy, sore throat, headache, memory deficits, and sleep disturbances. To aid identification of the disease, the Centers for Disease Control and Prevention (CDC) uses a "working case definition" to group symptoms and severity.

Diagnosis

Because the cause and nature of CFIDS are still unknown, no single test unequivocally confirms its presence. Therefore, physicians base this diagnosis on the patient's history and the CDC's criteria. (See *CDC criteria for diagnosing CFIDS.*) Because the

CDC CRITERIA FOR DIAGNOSING CFIDS

To meet the Centers for Disease Control and Prevention (CDC) case definition of chronic fatigue immune dysfunction syndrome (CFIDS), a patient must fulfill 2 major criteria and either 8 of 11 symptom criteria; or, 6 of the symptom criteria and 2 of 3 physical criteria.

Major criteria

- New onset of persistent or relapsing debilitating fatigue in a person without a history of similar symptoms; fatigue doesn't resolve with bed rest and is severe enough to reduce or impair average daily activity by 50% for 6 months.
- Exclusion of other disorders after evaluation through history, physical examination, and laboratory findings.

Symptom criteria

The symptom criteria include the initial development of the main symptom complex over a few hours or days and 10 other symptoms:

- profound or prolonged fatigue, especially after exercise levels that would have been easily tolerated previously
- low-grade fever
- painful lymph nodes
- muscle weakness
- muscle discomfort or myalgia
- sleep disturbances (insomnia or hypersomnia)
- headaches of a new type, severity, or pattern
- migratory arthralgia without joint swelling or redness
- photophobia, forgetfulness, irritability, confusion, depression, transient visual scotomata, difficulty thinking, and inability to concentrate.

Physical criteria

Physical criteria must be recorded on at least two occasions, at least 1 month apart:

- low-grade fever
- nonexudative pharyngitis
- palpable or tender nodes.

CDC criteria are admittedly a working concept that may not include all forms of this disease and are based on symptoms that can result from other diseases, diagnosis is difficult and uncertain.

Treatment

No treatment is known to cure CFIDS. Rather, treatment is symptomatic and may include tricyclic antidepressants (such as doxepin [Sinequan]), histamine-2 blocking agents (such as cimetidine [Tagamet]), and antianxiety agents (such as alprazolam [Xanax]). In some patients, avoidance of environmental irritants and certain foods may help to relieve symptoms.

Experimental treatments include the antiviral agent acyclovir and selected immunomodulating agents, such as I.V. gamma globulin, Ampligen, transfer factor, and others.

Special considerations

Because patients with CFIDS may benefit from supportive contact with others who share this disease, refer the patient to the CFIDS Association for information and to local support groups. Patients may also benefit from psychological counseling.

Colorectal cancer

Colorectal cancer is the second most common visceral malignant neoplasm in the United States and Europe. It's the third most common cancer in women and the second leading cause of cancer death. Incidence is equally distributed between men and women; however, it's estimated that, in 2003, over 100,000 new cases of colon cancer were diagnosed and almost 54% in women. Colorectal malignant tumors are usually adenocarcinomas. About half of these are sessile lesions of the rectosigmoid area; the rest are polypoid lesions.

Colorectal cancer tends to progress slowly and remains localized for a long time. Consequently, it's potentially curable in about 90% of patients if early diagnosis allows resection before nodal involvement. With improved diagnosis, the overall 5-year survival rate is about 60% for adjacent organ or nodal spread, and greater than 90% for early, localized disease.

Causes

The exact cause of colorectal cancer is unknown, but studies showing higher concentrations in areas of greater economic development suggest a relationship to diet (excess saturated animal fat). Other factors that magnify the risk of developing colorectal cancer include:

- other diseases of the digestive tract
- age (over 40)
- history of ulcerative colitis (average of 11 to 17 years between onset of ulcerative colitis and onset of cancer)
- familial polyposis (cancer onset almost always by age 50).

Most colorectal cancers arise from adenomatous polyps (adenomas), which are inner growths of the colon and the rectum. Although these seemingly benign polyps are common in men and women over age 50, 5% to 10% become malignant. Fortunately, this may take many years, so there is a good chance of identifying and removing them before they progress to cancer. (See *Staging colorectal cancer.*)

Signs and symptoms

Signs and symptoms of colorectal cancer result from local obstruction and, in later stages, from direct extension to adjacent organs (bladder, prostate, ureters, vagina, sacrum) and distant metastasis (usually liver). In the early stages, signs and symptoms are typically vague and depend on the anatomic location and function of the bowel segment containing the tumor. Later signs or symptoms usually include pallor, cachexia, ascites, hepatomegaly, or lymphangiectasis.

SPECIAL NEEDS

Older patients may ignore bowel symptoms, believing that they result from constipation, poor diet, or hemorrhoids. Evaluate your older patient's responses to your questions carefully.

On the right side of the colon (which absorbs water and electrolytes), early tumor growth causes no signs of obstruction because the tumor tends to grow along the bowel rather than surround the lumen, and

Staging colorectal cancer

Named for pathologist Cuthbert Dukes, the Dukes' cancer classification system assigns tumors to four stages. These stages (with substages) reflect the extent of bowel-mucosa and bowel-wall infiltration, lymph node involvement, and metastasis.

Stage A

Malignant cells are confined to the bowel mucosa, and the lymph nodes contain no cancer cells. Treated promptly, about 90% of these patients remain disease-free 5 years later.

Stage B

Malignant cells extend through the bowel mucosa, but remain within the bowel wall. The lymph nodes are normal. In substage B_2, all bowel wall layers and immediately adjacent structures contain malignant cells but the lymph nodes remain normal. About 63% of patients with substage B_2 survive for 5 or more years.

Stage C

Malignant cells extend into the bowel wall and the lymph nodes. In substage C_2, malignant cells extend through the entire thickness of the bowel wall and into the lymph nodes. The 5-year survival rate for patients with stage C disease is about 25%.

Stage D

Metastasizing to distant organs by way of the lymph nodes and mesenteric vessels, malignant cells typically lodge in the lungs and liver. Only 7% of patients with stage D cancer survive 5 or more years.

the fecal content in this area is normally liquid. It may, however, cause black, tarry stools; anemia; and abdominal aching, pressure, or dull cramps. As the disease progresses, the patient develops weakness, fatigue, exertional dyspnea, vertigo and, eventually, diarrhea, obstipation, anorexia, weight loss, vomiting, and other signs or symptoms of intestinal obstruction. In addition, a tumor on the right side may be palpable.

On the left side, a tumor causes signs of an obstruction even in early stages because stool consistency in this area is formed. A tumor on the left side commonly causes rectal bleeding (in many cases ascribed to hemorrhoids), intermittent abdominal fullness or cramping, and rectal pressure. As the disease progresses, the patient develops obstipation, diarrhea, or "ribbon" or pencil-shaped stools. Typically, he notices that passage of a stool or flatus relieves the pain. At this stage, bleeding from the colon becomes obvious, with dark or bright red blood in the feces and mucus in or on the stools.

With a rectal tumor, the first symptom is a change in bowel habits, in many cases beginning with an urgent need to defecate on rising (morning diarrhea) or obstipation alternating with diarrhea. Other signs are blood or mucus in stool and a sense of incomplete evacuation. Late in the disease, pain begins as a feeling of rectal fullness that later becomes a dull, and sometimes constant, ache confined to the rectum or sacral region.

Diagnosis

Only a tumor biopsy can verify colorectal cancer, but other tests help detect it:

- Digital rectal examination can detect almost 15% of colorectal cancers.
- Hemoccult test (guaiac), also known as *fecal occult blood test (FOBT)*, can detect blood in stools. This test is recommended yearly after age 50 for colorectal cancer screening and prevention.
- Proctoscopy or sigmoidoscopy can detect up to 66% of colorectal cancers. This test is recommended every 5 years after age 50 for colorectal cancer screening and prevention.
- Colonoscopy permits visual inspection (and photographs) of the colon up to the ileocecal valve, and gives access for polypectomies and biopsies of suspected lesions. This test is the single most accurate test for detecting cancer or polyps. This test is recommended every 10 years after age 50 for colorectal cancer screening.
- CT scan helps to detect areas affected by metastasis.
- Barium X-ray, using a dual contrast with air, can locate lesions that are undetectable manually or visually. Barium examination should follow endoscopy or excretory urography because the barium sulfate interferes with these tests. This test is recommended every 5 to 10 years for colorectal cancer screening beginning at age 50.
- Carcinoembryonic antigen, though not specific or sensitive enough for early diagnosis, is helpful in monitoring patients before and after treatment to detect metastasis or recurrence.

Treatment

The best treatment for colorectal cancer is prevention. Colorectal screening decreases the incidence of the disease by 75% to 90%. Other treatments recommended to prevent colorectal cancer include a diet:

- high in fruits and vegetables
- low in red and processed meats
- low in fat
- high in calcium and folic acid.

A recent study found that women who took aspirin twice a week or more had a 44% reduction in risk after 20 years. The risk was also reduced in women who took a multivitamin with folic acid for more than 15 years. However, it may take more than a decade for aspirin use to benefit and may cause gastric ulcers and hemorrhagic strokes. Thus, these aren't substitutes for regular colorectal cancer screening.

The most effective treatment once colorectal cancer is diagnosed is surgery to remove the malignant tumor and adjacent tissues and any lymph nodes that may contain cancer cells. The type of surgery depends on the location of the tumor:

- *cecum and ascending colon* — right hemicolectomy (for advanced disease), which may include resection of the terminal segment of the ileum, cecum, ascending colon, and right half of the transverse colon with corresponding mesentery

- *proximal and middle transverse colon* — right colectomy, which includes transverse colon and mesentery corresponding to midcolic vessels, or segmental resection of transverse colon and associated midcolic vessels
- *sigmoid colon* — surgery usually limited to sigmoid colon and mesentery
- *upper rectum* — anterior or low anterior resection, employing a newer method that uses a stapler and allows for resections much lower than were previously possible
- *lower rectum* — abdominoperineal resection and permanent sigmoid colostomy.

Chemotherapy is indicated for patients with metastasis, residual disease, or a recurrent inoperable tumor. Drugs used in such treatment commonly include fluorouracil with levamisole, leucovorin, methotrexate, or streptozocin. Patients whose tumors have extended to regional lymph nodes may receive fluorouracil and levamisole for 1 year postoperatively.

Radiation therapy induces tumor regression and may be used before or after surgery or combined with chemotherapy, especially fluorouracil.

Special considerations

Before surgery:

- Monitor the patient's diet modifications, laxatives, enemas, and antibiotics — all used to clean the bowel and to decrease abdominal and perineal cavity contamination during surgery.
- If the patient is having a colostomy, teach the patient and her family about the procedure.
- Emphasize that the stoma will be red, moist, and swollen and that postoperative swelling will eventually subside.
- Show them a diagram of the intestine before and after surgery, stressing how much of the bowel will remain intact. Supplement your teaching with instructional aids. Arrange a postsurgical visit from a recovered ostomate.
- Prepare the patient for postoperative I.V. infusions, nasogastric tube, and indwelling urinary catheter.
- Discuss the importance of cooperating during deep-breathing and coughing exercises.

After surgery:

- Explain to the patient's family the importance of their positive reactions to the patient's adjustment. Consult with an enterostomal therapist, if available, to help set up a regimen for the patient.
- Encourage the patient to look at the stoma and participate in its care as soon as possible. Teach good hygiene and skin care. Allow her to shower or bathe as soon as the incision heals. If appropriate, instruct the patient with a sigmoid colostomy to irrigate it as soon as possible after surgery. Schedule irrigation for the time of day when the person normally evacuated before surgery. Many patients find that irrigating every 1 to 3 days is necessary for regularity. If flatus, diarrhea, or constipation occurs, eliminate suspected causative foods from

the patient's diet. Those foods may be reintroduced in the patient's diet later.

- After several months, many ostomates establish control with irrigation and no longer need to wear a pouch. A stoma cap or gauze sponge placed over the stoma protects it and absorbs mucoid secretions.
- Before achieving such control, the patient can resume physical activities, including sports, provided that there's no threat of injury to the stoma or surrounding abdominal muscles. However, caution the patient to avoid heavy lifting because herniation or prolapse may occur through weakened muscles in the abdominal wall. A structured and gradually progressive exercise program to strengthen abdominal muscles may be instituted under medical supervision.
- If appropriate, refer the patient to a home health agency for follow-up care and counseling. Suggest sexual counseling, especially after an abdominoperineal resection.
- Anyone who has had colorectal cancer is at increased risk for recurrence and should have yearly screening and testing.

Cytomegalovirus infection

Cytomegalovirus (CMV) infection is caused by the cytomegalovirus, a deoxyribonucleic acid, ether-sensitive virus belonging to the herpes family. CMV infection occurs worldwide and is transmitted by human contact. About four out of five people over age 35 have been infected with CMV, usually during childhood or early adulthood. In most of these people, the disease is so mild that it's overlooked. However, CMV infection during pregnancy can be hazardous to the fetus, possibly leading to stillbirth, brain damage, and other birth defects or to severe neonatal illness. About 1% of all neonates have CMV. It's the most common cause of congenital infection in the United States. It's also common in those with human immunodeficiency virus infection or in those who are otherwise immunocompromised.

Causes

CMV has been found in saliva, urine, semen, breast milk, feces, blood, and vaginal and cervical secretions of infected people. The virus is usually transmitted through contact with these infected secretions, which harbor the virus for months or even years. It may be transmitted by sexual contact and can travel across the placenta, causing a congenital infection. Immunosuppressed patients, especially those who have received transplanted organs, have a 90% chance of contracting CMV infection. Recipients of blood transfusions from donors with positive CMV antibodies are at some risk.

Signs and symptoms

CMV is thought to spread through the body in lymphocytes or mononuclear cells to the lungs, liver, GI tract, eyes, and central nervous system, where it commonly produces inflammatory reactions.

Most patients with CMV infection have mild, nonspecific complaints or none at all, even though antibody titers indicate infection. In these patients, the disease usually runs a self-limiting course. However, immunodeficient patients and those receiving immunosuppressants may develop pneumonia or other secondary infections. In patients with acquired immunodeficiency syndrome, disseminated CMV infection may cause chorioretinitis (resulting in blindness), colitis, encephalitis, abdominal pain, diarrhea, or weight loss. Infected infants ages 3 to 6 months usually appear asymptomatic, but may develop hepatic dysfunction, hepatosplenomegaly, spider angiomas, pneumonitis, and lymphadenopathy.

Congenital CMV infection is seldom apparent at birth, although the neonate's urine contains the virus. CMV can cause brain damage that may not show up for months after birth. It can also produce a rapidly fatal neonatal illness characterized by jaundice, petechial rash, hepatosplenomegaly, thrombocytopenia, hemolytic anemia, microcephaly, psychomotor retardation, mental deficiency, and hearing loss. Infants with congenital CMV infection may also present with abnormal muscle tone, lethargy, and chorioretinitis. Occasionally, this form is rapidly fatal.

In some adults, CMV may cause cytomegalovirus mononucleosis, with 3 weeks or more of irregular, high fever. Other findings may include a normal or elevated white blood cell (WBC) count, lymphocytosis, and increased atypical lymphocytes.

Diagnosis

Although virus isolation in urine is the most sensitive laboratory method, diagnosis can also rest on virus isolation from saliva, throat, cervix, WBC, and biopsy specimens.

Other laboratory tests support the diagnosis of CMV, including complement fixation studies, hemagglutination inhibition antibody tests and, for congenital infections, indirect immunofluorescent tests for CMV immunoglobulin M antibody.

Treatment

There is no current treatment for maternal CMV infection or for the congenital disease in the neonate. Rather, treatment aims to relieve symptoms and prevent complications. In the immunosuppressed patient, CMV is treated with acyclovir, ganciclovir and, possibly, foscarnet. (*Note:* Ganciclovir is the only drug approved by the Food and Drug Administration for prevention and maintenance treatment of CMV and CMV retinitis.) Most important, parents of children with severe congenital CMV infection need support and counseling to help them cope with the possibility that their child will suffer serious and chronic medical problems or even death.

Special considerations

To help prevent CMV infection:

- For patients taking ganciclovir, monitor complete blood count because the drug causes bone marrow suppression. Administer G-CSF (Neupogen) or erythropoietin (Procrit), as ordered.

- Encourage vaccination for hepatitis and the flu to prevent further complications and opportunistic infections.
- Monitor the patient for thrush and encourage antifungal prophylaxis.

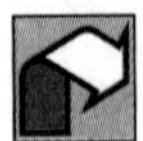

PREVENTION POINTER

Be sure to observe standard precautions when handling body secretions.

- Warn immunosuppressed patients and pregnant women to avoid exposure to confirmed or suspected CMV infection. (Maternal CMV infection can cause fetal abnormalities, such as hydrocephaly, microphthalmia, seizures, encephalitis, hepatosplenomegaly, hematologic changes, microcephaly, and blindness.
- Urge patients with CMV infection to wash their hands thoroughly to prevent spreading it. Stress this also with young children.

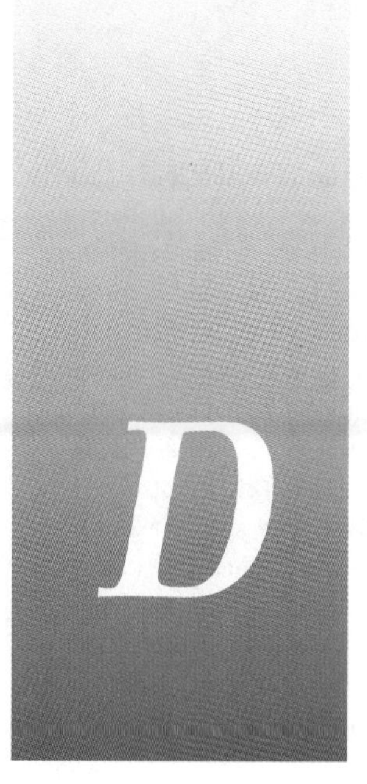

Deep vein thrombophlebitis

Deep vein thrombophlebitis, or thrombosis, (DVT) is an acute condition characterized by inflammation and thrombus formation, occurring in deep (intermuscular or intramuscular) or superficial (subcutaneous) veins. DVT usually occurs in the lower leg and affects small veins, such as the soleal venous sinuses, or large veins, such as the vena cava and the femoral, iliac, and subclavian veins, causing venous insufficiency. (See *Chronic venous insufficiency*, page 256.) Although this disorder isn't fatal, it's typically progressive and can lead to a pulmonary embolism (PE), a potentially lethal complication. Superficial thrombophlebitis is usually self-limiting and seldom leads to pulmonary embolism. Thrombophlebitis usually begins with localized inflammation alone (phlebitis), but such inflammation rapidly provokes thrombus formation. Rarely, venous thrombosis develops without associated inflammation of the vein (phlebothrombosis).

About two million people experience DVT each year. Although DVT is more common in elderly people, pregnant women are also at high risk for

Chronic venous insufficiency

Chronic venous insufficiency results from the valvular destruction by deep vein thrombophlebitis (DVT), usually in the iliac and femoral veins and occasionally in the saphenous veins. It's commonly accompanied by incompetence of the communicating veins at the ankle, causing increased venous pressure and fluid migration into the interstitial tissue. Clinical effects include chronic swelling of the affected leg from edema, leading to tissue fibrosis and induration, skin discoloration from extravasation of blood in subcutaneous tissue, and stasis ulcers around the ankle.

Treatment of small ulcers includes bed rest, elevation of the legs, warm soaks, and antimicrobial therapy for infection. Treatment to counteract increased venous pressure, the result of reflux from the deep venous system to surface veins, may include compression dressings, such as a sponge rubber pressure dressing or a zinc gelatin boot (Unna's boot). This therapy begins after massive swelling subsides with leg elevation and bed rest.

Large stasis ulcers unresponsive to conservative treatment may require excision and skin grafting. Patient care includes daily inspection to assess healing. Other care measures are the same as for varicose veins.

DVT and, subsequently, PE. Further, women develop PE more commonly than men, especially those who are obese, smoke, or who take hormonal contraceptives.

Causes

DVT may be idiopathic, but it usually results from endothelial damage, accelerated blood clotting, and reduced blood flow. Predisposing factors are prolonged bed rest, immobilization, physical trauma, major surgical procedures, childbirth, and use of hormonal contraceptives. There are many known causes of clot formation. Prolonged inactivity, such as a long plane ride, can cause reduced circulation in the legs, which provides the opportunity for clot formation. In fact, the Department of Health published advisories to pregnant women and women taking hormonal contraceptives that they're at an increased risk of developing DVT during long plane rides and should consult with their physician before flying.

A thrombus occurs when an alteration in the epithelial lining causes platelet aggregation and consequent fibrin entrapment of red and white blood cells and additional platelets. Thrombus formation is more rapid in areas where blood flow is slower, due to greater contact between platelet and thrombin accumulation. The rapidly expanding thrombus initiates a chemical inflammatory process in the vessel epithelium, which leads to fibrosis. The enlarging clot may occlude the vessel lumen partially or totally, or it may detach and embolize to lodge elsewhere in the systemic circulation.

Causes of superficial thrombophlebitis include trauma, infection, I.V. drug abuse, and chemical irritation due to extensive use of the I.V.

route for medications and diagnostic tests.

Signs and symptoms

In both types of thrombophlebitis, clinical features vary with the site and length of the affected vein. Although DVT may produce no symptoms, it may cause severe pain, fever, chills, malaise and, possibly, swelling and cyanosis of the affected arm or leg — walking may also be painful. Superficial thrombophlebitis produces visible and palpable signs, such as heat, pain, swelling, redness, tenderness, and induration along the length of the affected vein. Varicose veins may also be present. Extensive vein involvement may cause lymphadenitis.

Diagnosis

Contrast venography is the standard for the diagnosis of DVT, although this test is invasive and may precipitate adverse and life-threatening reactions. It's also contraindicated in patients with kidney failure. As a result, venography is mostly used for confirmation when the diagnosis can't be established by other means.

Diagnosis of superficial thrombophlebitis is based on physical examination (redness and warmth over affected area, palpable vein, and pain during palpation or compression). Differential diagnosis must rule out arterial occlusive disease, lymphangitis, cellulitis, and myositis.

Other noninvasive tests tools for diagnosing DVT in the leg veins include ultrasound; magnetic resonance imaging; phlebography, which shows filling defects and diverted blood flow and usually confirms the diagnosis; and physical examination, which in some patients may reveal signs of inflammation and, possibly, a positive Homans' sign (pain on dorsiflexion of the foot). Other patients may be asymptomatic.

Essential laboratory tests include the following:

- *D-dimer test* is a blood test that has recently been found to confirm the presence of coagulation by measuring the D-dimer levels. This test is highly sensitive and has a negative predictive value, which is useful in excluding the presence of DVT or PE in patients with low susceptibility. However, it can't confirm the presence of DVT. This test also has a low specificity in patients taking oral anticoagulants and in patients older than age 70.
- *Duplex Doppler ultrasonography* and *impedance plethysmography* allow noninvasive examination of the major veins (but not calf veins).
- *Plethysmography* shows decreased circulation distal to the affected area. This test is more sensitive than ultrasound in detecting DVT.

Treatment

The goals of treatment are to control thrombus development, prevent complications, relieve pain, and prevent recurrence of the disorder. Symptomatic measures include bed rest with elevation of the affected arm or leg, analgesics, and warm, moist soaks to the affected area. After the acute episode of DVT subsides, the patient may resume activity while wearing antiembolism stockings applied before getting out of bed.

Initially, the patient is given heparin, an anticoagulant, to prevent the formation of new clots. Additionally, if the patient isn't pregnant, treatment with warfarin (Coumadin) is started. It takes about 5 days for the warfarin to become fully effective, during which time the patient continues to get heparin to prevent new clots from forming. Low-molecular-weight (LMW) heparin has proven effective in treating DVT. Although LMW heparin is more expensive, it doesn't require monitoring for its anticoagulant effect. Full anticoagulant doses must be discontinued during any operative period because of the risk of hemorrhage. After some types of surgery, especially major abdominal or pelvic operations, prophylactic doses of anticoagulants may reduce the risk of DVT and PE. For lysis of acute, extensive DVT, treatment should include streptokinase. Rarely, DVT may cause complete venous occlusion, which necessitates venous interruption through simple ligation to vein plication, or clipping. Embolectomy and insertion of a vena caval umbrella or filter may also be done.

Therapy for severe superficial thrombophlebitis may include an anti-inflammatory drug such as indomethacin, antiembolism stockings, warm soaks, and elevation of the leg.

Special considerations

Patient teaching, identification of high-risk patients, and measures to prevent venostasis can prevent DVT. Close monitoring of anticoagulant therapy can prevent serious complications such as internal hemorrhage:

- Enforce bed rest, as ordered, and elevate the patient's affected arm or leg. If you plan to use pillows for elevating the leg, place them so they support the entire length of the affected extremity to prevent possible compression of the popliteal space.
- Apply warm soaks to increase circulation to the affected area and to relieve pain and inflammation. Give analgesics to relieve pain.
- Measure and record the circumference of the affected arm or leg daily, and compare this measurement to the other arm or leg. To ensure accuracy and consistency of serial measurements, mark the skin over the area, and measure at the same spot daily.
- Administer heparin I.V. with an infusion monitor or pump to control the flow rate, if necessary.
- Measure partial thromboplastin time regularly for the patient on heparin therapy; prothrombin time (PT) and International Normalized Ratio (INR) for the patient on warfarin (therapeutic anticoagulation values are one and a half to two times control values for prothrombin time and an INR of 2 to 3). Watch for signs and symptoms of bleeding, such as dark, tarry stools, coffee-ground vomitus, and ecchymoses. Encourage the patient to use an electric razor and to avoid medications that contain aspirin.
- Be alert for signs of pulmonary emboli (crackles, dyspnea, hemoptysis, sudden changes in mental status, restlessness, and hypotension).

To prepare the patient with DVT for discharge:

- Emphasize the importance of follow-up blood studies to monitor anticoagulant therapy.
- If the patient is being discharged on heparin therapy, teach her and her family how to give subcutaneous injections. If she requires further assistance, arrange for a home health nurse.
- If the patient is being discharged on warfarin therapy, stress the importance of regular blood tests to monitor the patient's INR and PT levels, monitoring for signs and symptoms of bleeding, and avoiding cuts by using an electric razor and a soft toothbrush.
- Tell the patient to avoid prolonged sitting or standing to help prevent recurrence.
- Teach the patient how to properly apply and use antiembolism stockings. Tell her to report any complications such as cold, blue toes.

PREVENTION POINTER

To prevent DVT, perform range-of-motion exercises while the patient is on bed rest, use intermittent pneumatic calf massage during lengthy surgical or diagnostic procedures, apply antiembolism stockings postoperatively, and encourage early ambulation.

Depression, major

Also known as *unipolar disorder,* major depression is a syndrome of persistently sad, dysphoric mood, accompanied by disturbances in sleep and appetite, lethargy, and an inability to experience pleasure (anhedonia). Major depression occurs in up to 17% of adults, affecting all racial, ethnic, and socioeconomic groups. It affects both sexes, but is more common in women.

About 50% of all depressed patients experience a single episode and recover completely; the rest have at least one recurrence. Major depression can profoundly alter social, family, and occupational functioning. However, suicide is the most serious consequence of major depression; the patient's feelings of worthlessness, guilt, and hopelessness are so overwhelming that she no longer considers life worth living. Nearly twice as many women as men attempt suicide, but men are far more likely to succeed.

Causes

The multiple causes of depression aren't completely understood. Current research suggests possible genetic, familial, biochemical, physical, psychological, and social causes. Psychological causes (the focus of many nursing interventions) may include feelings of helplessness and vulnerability, anger, hopelessness and pessimism, and low self-esteem. They may be related to abnormal character and behavior patterns and troubled personal relationships. In many patients, the history identifies a specific personal loss or severe stressor that probably interacts with the person's predisposition to provoke major depression.

Depression may be secondary to a specific medical condition, for example:

Dysthymic disorder

Dysthymic disorder is a chronic disturbance of mood (irritable mood in children), characterized by mild depression or loss of interest in usual activities. Dysthymic disorder persists for at least 2 years in adults and 1 year in children and adolescents. The disorder typically begins in childhood, adolescence, or early adulthood and causes only mild social or occupational impairment. In adults, it's more common in women; in children and adolescents, it's equally common in both sexes.

Signs and symptoms

During periods of depression, the patient may also experience poor appetite or overeating, insomnia or hypersomnia, low energy or fatigue, low self-esteem, poor concentration or difficulty making decisions, and feelings of hopelessness.

Diagnosis

Dysthymic disorder is confirmed when the patient exhibits at least two of the signs or symptoms nearly every day, with intervening normal moods lasting no more than 2 months during a 2-year period.

- metabolic disturbances, such as hypoxia and hypercalcemia
- endocrine disorders, such as diabetes and Cushing's syndrome
- neurologic diseases, such as Parkinson's disease and Alzheimer's disease
- cancer (especially of the pancreas)
- viral and bacterial infections, such as influenza and pneumonia
- cardiovascular disorders such as heart failure
- pulmonary disorders such as chronic obstructive pulmonary disease
- musculoskeletal disorders such as degenerative arthritis
- GI disorders such as irritable bowel syndrome
- genitourinary problems such as incontinence
- collagen vascular diseases such as lupus
- anemias.

Drugs prescribed for medical and psychiatric conditions as well as many commonly abused substances can also cause depression. Examples include antihypertensives, psychotropics, narcotic and nonnarcotic analgesics, antiparkinsonian drugs, numerous cardiovascular medications, oral antidiabetics, antimicrobials, steroids, chemotherapeutic agents, cimetidine, and alcohol.

Signs and symptoms

The primary features of major depression are a predominantly sad mood and a loss of interest or pleasure in daily activities. The patient may complain of feeling "down in the dumps," express doubts about his self-worth or ability to cope, or simply appear unhappy and apathetic. She may also report feeling angry or anxious. Symptoms tend to be more severe than those caused by dysthymic disorder, which is a milder, chronic form of depression. (See *Dysthymic disorder.*) Other common signs include difficulty concentrating or thinking clearly, distractibility, and indecisiveness. All physiologic and psychologic processes are slowed. Anergia and fatigue are common as well as anhedonia and insomnia. Take special note if the patient reveals suicidal thoughts, a preoccupation with death, or previous suicide attempts.

The psychosocial history may reveal life problems or losses that can account for the depression. Alternatively, the patient's medical history may implicate a physical disorder or the use of prescription, nonprescription, or illegal drugs that might cause depression.

The patient may report an increase or a decrease in appetite, sleep disturbances (such as insomnia or early awakening), a lack of interest in sexual activity, constipation, or diarrhea. Other signs include agitation (such as hand wringing or restlessness) and reduced psychomotor activity (such as slowed speech).

SPECIAL NEEDS

Members of different cultures may experience depression differently. For instance, in some Asian cultures, there are more somatic manifestations of depression than overt psychological signs or symptoms.

Diagnosis

The diagnosis of depression is supported by psychological tests such as the Beck Depression Inventory, which may help determine the onset, severity, duration, and progression of depressive symptoms. A toxicology screening may suggest drug-induced depression. (For characteristic findings in patients with depression, see *Diagnosing major depression*, page 262.)

Treatment

Depression is difficult to treat, especially in children, adolescents, elderly patients, and those with a history of chronic disease. The primary treatment methods are drug therapy, electroconvulsive therapy (ECT), and psychotherapy.

Drug therapy for depression includes:

- tricyclic antidepressants (TCAs) such as amitriptyline. TCAs are the most widely used class of antidepressant drugs. They prevent the reuptake of norepinephrine or serotonin (or both) into the presynaptic nerve endings, resulting in increased synaptic concentrations of these neurotransmitters. They also cause a gradual loss in the number of beta-adrenergic receptors.
- monoamine oxidase (MAO) inhibitors such as isocarboxazid (Marplan). MAO inhibitors block the enzymatic degradation of norepinephrine and serotonin. However, they're commonly prescribed for patients with atypical depression (for example, depression marked by an increased appetite and need for sleep, rather than anorexia and insomnia) and for some patients who fail to respond to TCAs. MAO inhibitors are associated with a high risk of toxicity; patients treated with one of these drugs must be able to comply with the necessary dietary restrictions.
- selective serotonin reuptake inhibitors (SSRIs), such as fluoxetine

Diagnosing major depression

A patient is diagnosed with major depression when she fulfills the following criteria for a single major depressive episode put forth in the *Diagnostic and Statistical Manual of Mental Disorders,* Fourth Edition, Text Revision:

- At least five of the following symptoms must have been present during the same 2-week period and must represent a change from previous functioning; one of these must either be depressed mood or loss of interest in previously pleasurable activities:
  - depressed mood (irritable mood in children and adolescents) most of the day, nearly every day, as indicated by either subjective account or observation by others
  - markedly diminished interest or pleasure in all, or almost all, activities most of the day, nearly every day
  - significant weight loss or weight gain when not dieting or decrease or increase in appetite nearly every day (in children, consider failure to make expected weight gains)
  - insomnia or hypersomnia nearly every day
  - psychomotor agitation or retardation nearly every day
  - fatigue or loss of energy nearly every day
  - feelings of worthlessness or excessive or inappropriate guilt nearly every day
  - diminished ability to think or concentrate, or indecisiveness, nearly every day
  - recurrent thoughts of death, recurrent suicidal ideation without a specific plan, a suicide attempt, or a specific plan for committing suicide.
- The symptoms don't meet criteria for a mixed episode.
- The symptoms cause clinically significant distress or impairment in social or occupational function or other important areas of functioning.
- The symptoms aren't due to the direct physiologic effects of a substance or a general medical condition.
- The symptoms aren't better accounted for by bereavement; they persist for longer than 2 months; or are characterized by marked functional impairment, morbid preoccupation with worthlessness, suicidal ideation, psychotic symptoms, or psychomotor retardation.

(Prozac), paroxetine (Paxil), and sertraline (Zoloft). SSRIs are becoming the drugs of choice for treating depression. They're effective and produce fewer adverse effects than TCAs. Even so, they're associated with sleep and GI problems and alterations in sexual desire and function.

- maprotiline, trazodone (Desyrel), and bupropion (Wellbutrin) aren't chemically related to the other antidepressants listed above; however, they're effective in treating depression by blocking the reuptake of norepinephrine, serotonin, and epinephrine, respectively. However, the reason they aren't used as commonly as the other compounds is because of increased adverse effects.

Alternative treatments for depression include:

- electroconvulsive therapy (ECT). When a depressed patient is incapacitated, suicidal, or psychotically depressed or when antidepressants are contraindicated or ineffective, ECT commonly is the treatment of choice for depression. Usually, 6 to 12 treatments are needed, although in many cases improvement is evident after only a few treatments. Even so, ECT has been associated with later short-term memory loss, arrhythmias, and seizure activity. Researchers hypothesize that ECT affects the same receptor sites as antidepressants.

- short-term psychotherapy. Many psychiatrists believe that the best results are achieved with a combination of individual, family, or group psychotherapy and medication. After resolution of the acute episode, patients with a history of recurrent depression may be maintained on low doses of antidepressants as a preventive measure.

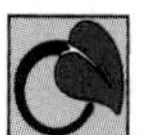

ALTERNATIVE THERAPIES

Complementary and alternative therapies may be used with such conventional therapies as medication, ECT, or psychotherapy to treat depression. Although scientific evidence of their effectiveness remains inconclusive, examples of possible alternative therapies include acupuncture, guided imagery, hypnosis, biofeedback, and many others. Experimental therapies for treatment of depression include vagal nerve stimulation and transcranial magnetic stimulation. The safety and effectiveness of these therapies are still being studied. Also, for less severe forms of depression, herbal remedies, such as St. John's wort or SAMe, have been found to be effective. However, these shouldn't be taken with other prescription medications.

Special considerations

- Share your observations of the patient's behavior with her. For instance, you might say, "You're sitting all by yourself, looking very sad. Is that how you feel?" Because the patient may think and react sluggishly, speak slowly and allow ample time for her to respond. Avoid feigned cheerfulness. However, don't hesitate to laugh with the patient and point out the value of humor.
- Show the patient she's important by listening attentively and respectfully, preventing interruptions, and avoiding judgmental responses.
- Provide a structured routine, including noncompetitive activities, to build the patient's self-confidence and encourage interaction with others. Urge her to join group activities and to socialize.
- Inform the patient that she can help ease depression by expressing her feelings, participating in pleasurable activities, and improving grooming and hygiene.

PREVENTION POINTER

Ask the patient if she thinks of death or suicide. Such thoughts signal an immediate need for consultation and assessment. Failure to detect suicidal thoughts early may encourage the patient to attempt suicide. The risk of suicide increases as depression lifts. (See *Suicide prevention guidelines*, page 264.)

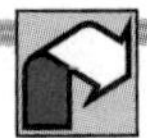

PREVENTION POINTER

Suicide prevention guidelines

When your patient is diagnosed with major depression, keep in mind the following guidelines.

Assess for suicide clues

Be alert for the patient's suicidal thoughts, threats, and messages; describing a suicide plan; hoarding medication; talking about death and feelings of futility; giving away prized possessions; and changing behavior, especially as depression begins to lift.

Provide a safe environment

Check patient areas and correct dangerous conditions, such as exposed pipes, windows without safety glass, and access to the roof or balconies.

Remove dangerous objects

Take away potentially dangerous objects, such as belts, razors, suspenders, light cords, glass, knives, nail files and clippers, and metal and hard plastic objects.

Consult with staff

Recognize and document both verbal and nonverbal suicidal behaviors; keep the physician informed; share data with all staff members; clarify the patient's specific restrictions; assess risk and plan for observation; clarify day and night staff responsibilities and the frequency of consultations.

Observe the suicidal patient

Be alert when the patient is using a sharp object (such as a razor), taking medication, or using the bathroom (to prevent hanging or other injury). Assign the patient to a room near the nurses' station and with another patient. Continuously observe the acutely suicidal patient.

Maintain personal contact

Help the suicidal patient feel that she isn't alone or without resources or hope. Encourage continuity of care and consistency of primary nurses. Building emotional ties to others is the ultimate technique for preventing suicide.

PREVENTION POINTER

Tell the patient to inform her primary care provider or any other health care professional if she's taking TCAs or MAO inhibitors to prevent possible drug-drug interactions.

- While tending to the patient's psychological needs, don't forget her physical needs. If she's too depressed to take care of herself, help her with personal hygiene. Encourage her to eat. If she's constipated, add high-fiber foods to her diet; offer small, frequent meals; and encourage physical activity and fluid intake.
- Inform the patient that certain antidepressants may take several weeks to produce an effect.
- Teach the patient about depression. Emphasize that effective methods are available to relieve her symptoms. Help her to recognize distorted perceptions that may contribute to her depression. Once the patient learns to

recognize depressive thought patterns, she can consciously begin to substitute self-affirming thoughts.

- Instruct the patient about prescribed medications. Stress the need for compliance and review adverse effects. For drugs that produce strong anticholinergic effects, such as amitriptyline (Endep, Emitrip) and amoxapine, suggest sugarless gum or hard candy to relieve dry mouth. Many antidepressants are sedating (for example, amitriptyline and trazodone [Desyrel]); warn the patient to avoid activities that require alertness, including driving and operating mechanical equipment until the central nervous system (CNS) effects of the drug are known.
- Caution the patient taking a TCA to avoid drinking alcoholic beverages or taking other CNS depressants during therapy.

PREVENTION POINTER

If the patient is taking an MAO inhibitor, emphasize that she must avoid foods that contain tyramine, caffeine, or tryptophan. The ingestion of tyramine can cause a hypertensive crisis. Examples of foods that contain these substances are cheese, sour cream, beer, Chianti, sherry, pickled herring, liver, canned figs, raisins, bananas, avocados, chocolate, soy sauce, fava beans, yeast extracts, meat tenderizers, coffee, and colas.

Diabetes mellitus

Diabetes mellitus is a serious, chronic disease of absolute or relative insulin deficiency or resistance that's characterized by disturbances in carbohydrate, protein, and fat metabolism. A leading cause of death by disease in the United States, this syndrome is a contributing factor in about 50% of myocardial infarctions and about 75% of strokes as well as in renal failure and peripheral vascular disease. It's also the leading cause of new blindness. Diabetes mellitus affects an estimated 6.2% of the population of the United States (17 million people); more than 50% are women.

SPECIAL NEEDS

The prevalence of diabetes mellitus is at least 2 to 4 times higher in women of certain races and ethnic groups—especially Blacks, Hispanics, Native Americans, and Asian Pacific Islanders—than in White women.

As women are living longer and more minority women are entering the United States, the number of women at high risk for diabetes and its complications will increase.

Diabetes mellitus occurs in four forms classified by etiology: type 1, type 2, other specific types, and gestational diabetes mellitus (GDM). Type 1 is further subdivided into immune-mediated diabetes and idiopathic diabetes. Children and adolescents with type 1 immune-mediated diabetes rapidly develop ketoacidosis, but most adults with this type experience only modest fasting hyperglycemia unless they develop an infection or experience another stressor. Patients with type 1 idiopathic diabetes are prone to ketoacidosis.

About 90% to 95% of women with diabetes have type 2. Those who were previously in the type 2 or non–insulin-dependent diabetes (NIDDM) diabetes group also fall into this category. The "other specific types" category includes people who have diabetes because of a genetic defect, endocrinopathies, or exposure to certain drugs or chemicals.

GDM only occurs during pregnancy. It usually ends after the baby is born, but women with GDM have up to a 45% risk of recurrence in the next pregnancy and up to a 63% risk of developing type 2 diabetes later in life.

SPECIAL NEEDS

Native American women have higher rates of GDM than the national average and are, therefore, at greater risk for complications during pregnancy, such as preeclampsia, or the need for cesarean delivery.

Causes

In type 1 diabetes, pancreatic beta-cell destruction or a primary defect in beta-cell function results in failure to release insulin and ineffective glucose transport. Type 1 immune-mediated diabetes is caused by cell-mediated destruction of pancreatic beta cells. The rate of beta-cell destruction is usually higher in children than in adults. The idiopathic form of type 1 diabetes has no known cause. Patients with this form have no evidence of autoimmunity and don't produce insulin.

In type 2 diabetes, beta cells release insulin, but receptors are insulin-resistant and glucose transport is variable and ineffective. Risk factors for type 2 diabetes include:

- obesity (even just an increased percentage of body fat primarily in the abdominal region); risk decreases with weight loss and drug therapy
- lack of physical activity
- history of GDM
- hypertension or dyslipidemia
- Black, Latino, or Native American origin
- strong family history of diabetes
- increasing age (usually develops in women over age 40).

As the body ages, the cells become more resistant to insulin, thus reducing the older adult's ability to metabolize glucose. In addition, the release of insulin from the pancreatic beta cells is reduced and delayed. These combined processes result in hyperglycemia. In the older patient, sudden concentrations of glucose cause increased and more prolonged hyperglycemia.

SPECIAL NEEDS

Because, on average, women live 7 years longer than men, there are nearly twice as many older women over age 65 than older men over age 65. Thus, there are more elderly women with diabetes than elderly men with diabetes in the United States. About 25% of these women don't know they have diabetes; however, diabetes is one of the leading underlying causes of death among women age 65 and older.

Other types of diabetes mellitus result from various conditions (such as a genetic defect of the beta cells or endocrinopathies). They may also result from use of or exposure to certain drugs or chemicals.

GDM is considered present whenever a woman has any degree of abnormal glucose during pregnancy. This form may result from weight gain and increased levels of estrogen and placental hormones, which antagonize insulin. During pregnancy, the fetus relies on maternal glucose as a primary fuel source. Pregnancy triggers protective mechanisms that have anti-insulin effects: increased hormone production (placental lactogen, estrogen, and progesterone), which antagonizes the effects of insulin; degradation of insulin by the placenta; and prolonged elevation of stress hormones (cortisol, epinephrine, and glucagon), which raise blood glucose levels.

In a normal pregnancy, an increase in anti-insulin factors is counterbalanced by an increase in insulin production to maintain normal blood glucose levels. However, females who are prediabetic or diabetic are unable to produce sufficient insulin to overcome the insulin antagonist mechanisms of pregnancy, or their tissues are insulin-resistant. As insulin requirements rise toward term, the patient who is prediabetic may develop GDM, necessitating dietary management and, possibly, exogenous insulin to achieve glycemic control, whereas the patient who is insulin-dependent may need increased insulin dosage. In GDM, glucose tolerance levels usually return to normal after delivery. However, children who are exposed to diabetes in the womb have a greater likelihood of becoming obese during childhood and adolescence and developing type 2 diabetes later in life. (See *Pregnancy and diabetes*, pages 268 and 269.)

Signs and symptoms

Diabetes may begin dramatically with ketoacidosis or insidiously. Its most common symptom is fatigue from energy deficiency and a catabolic state. Insulin deficiency causes hyperglycemia, which pulls fluid from body tissues, causing osmotic diuresis, polyuria, dehydration, polydipsia, dry mucous membranes, poor skin turgor and, in most patients, unexplained weight loss.

SPECIAL NEEDS

Because the thirst mechanism functions less effectively in an older adult, she may not report polydipsia, a hallmark of diabetes in a younger adult.

In ketoacidosis and hyperosmolar hyperglycemic nonketotic syndrome, dehydration may cause hypovolemia and shock. Wasting of glucose in the urine usually produces weight loss and hunger in type 1 diabetes, even if the patient eats voraciously.

Long-term complications of diabetes may include retinopathy, nephropathy, atherosclerosis, and peripheral and autonomic neuropathy. Peripheral neuropathy usually affects the hands and feet and may cause numbness or pain. Autonomic neu-

Pregnancy and diabetes

Pregnancy places special demands on carbohydrate metabolism and causes insulin requirements to increase, even in a healthy female. Consequently, pregnancy may lead to a prediabetic state, to the conversion of an asymptomatic subclinical diabetic state to a clinical one (also known as gestational diabetes, which occurs in about 2% to 5% of all pregnancies), or to complications in a previously stable diabetic state.

Gestational diabetes is usually diagnosed (with a routine screening test) between the 24th and 28th week of pregnancy. The risk of developing gestational diabetes increases with advanced age, African or Hispanic descent, obesity, previous birth of a neonate larger than 9 lbs, recurrent infections, and unexplained death of a previous neonate. And, although gestational diabetes disappears after birth, these women are at risk for developing type 2 diabetes later in life.

Importance of control

Uncontrolled diabetes in a pregnant female can cause stillbirth, fetal anomalies, premature delivery, and birth of a neonate who is large or small for gestational age. Such neonates are predisposed to severe episodes of hypoglycemia shortly after birth. These neonates may also develop hypocalcemia, hyperbilirubinemia (with jaundice), and respiratory distress syndrome. Maternal and fetal prognoses can be equivalent to those in nondiabetic females if maternal blood glucose is well controlled and ketosis and other complications are prevented. Neonate morbidity and mortality depend on recognizing and successfully controlling hypoglycemia, which may develop within hours after delivery. Preconceptual counseling is helpful in optimizing pregnancy outcomes.

Signs and symptoms

Women with gestational diabetes are usually asymptomatic; however, those with symptoms may complain of:

- increased thirst
- increased urination
- weight loss despite increased hunger
- fatigue
- nausea and vomiting
- blurred vision
- recurrent monilial infections.

Treatment

For pregnant patients with diabetes, therapy includes:

- bimonthly visits to the obstetrician and the internist during the first 6 months of pregnancy, with weekly visits possibly necessary during the 3rd trimester
- maintenance of fasting blood glucose levels at or below 100 mg/dl and 2-hour postprandial blood glucose levels at or below 120 mg/dl during the pregnancy
- frequent monitoring for glycosuria and ketonuria (because ketosis presents a grave threat to the fetal central nervous system)
- weight control (gain not to exceed 3 to 3¼ lb [1.4 to 1.5 kg] per month during the last 6 months of pregnancy)
- high-protein diet of 2 g/day/kg of body weight, or a minimum of 80 g/day during the second half of pregnancy; daily calorie intake of 30 to 40 calories/kg of body weight; daily carbohydrate intake of 200 g; and enough fat to provide 36% of total calories (although, vigorous calorie restriction can cause starvation ketosis)
- exogenous insulin if diet doesn't control blood glucose levels. (Be alert for changes in insulin requirements from

Pregnancy and diabetes *(continued)*

one trimester to the next and immediately postpartum. Oral antidiabetic drugs are contraindicated during pregnancy because they may cause fetal hypoglycemia and congenital anomalies.)

Generally, the optimal time for delivery is between 37 and 39 weeks' gestation, although with reassuring antenatal testing and no evidence of macrosomia, 40 weeks is also feasible. Depending on fetal status and maternal history, the obstetrician may induce labor or perform a cesarean delivery. During labor and delivery, the patient with diabetes should receive continuous I.V. infusion of dextrose with regular insulin in water. Maternal and fetal status must be monitored closely throughout labor. The patient may benefit from half her prepregnancy dosage of insulin before a cesarean delivery. Her insulin requirement will fall markedly after delivery.

ropathy may manifest itself in several ways, including gastroparesis (leading to delayed gastric emptying and a feeling of nausea and fullness after meals), nocturnal diarrhea, impotence, and orthostatic hypotension.

Heart disease is the most common complication of diabetes. Although more men with diabetes suffer from heart disease, it's more serious among women because they have lower survival rates and suffer a poorer quality of life than men. In addition, women with diabetes have a shorter life expectancy than women without diabetes (almost threefold). They are also at greater risk for blindness from diabetes than men with the disorder. Because hyperglycemia impairs the patient's resistance to infection, diabetes may also result in skin and urinary tract infections and vaginitis. Glucose content of the epidermis and urine encourages bacterial growth.

Diagnosis

The gold standard for diagnosis of diabetes used to be the 2-hour plasma glucose test; however, the fasting plasma glucose (FPG) is also recommended because it's easier (no waiting and better tolerated), has better reproducibility and reliability, and has lower costs. Also, there's inadequate evidence to show that either test is superior.

According to the American Diabetes Association's (ADA) latest guidelines, diabetes mellitus can be diagnosed if any of the following exist:

- symptoms of diabetes (polyuria, polydipsia, unexplained weight loss) plus a casual plasma glucose value (obtained without regard to the time of the patient's last food intake) greater than or equal to 200 mg/dl
- fasting plasma glucose level (no caloric intake for at least 8 hours) greater than or equal to 126 mg/dl
- plasma glucose value in the 2-hour sample of the oral glucose tolerance test greater than or equal to 200 mg/dl. This test should be performed after

a glucose load dose of 75 g of anhydrous glucose.

To confirm suspected GDM, a screening 50-gram, 1-hour glucose tolerance test is normally performed at 24 to 28 weeks' gestation. In addition, women with a history of fetal macrosomia or who may have nongestational diabetes should be formally tested for diabetes with a 3-hour glucose tolerance test. A 100-gram, 3-hour glucose tolerance test confirms diabetes mellitus when two or more values are above normal.

If any results are questionable, the diagnosis should be confirmed by a repeat test on a different day. The ADA also recommends the following testing guidelines:

- In patients with newly diagnosed diabetes, a confirmatory test is recommended after the initial test.
- Test people age 45 or older without symptoms every 3 years.
- Test people with the classic symptoms immediately.
- Those with an abnormal FPG should have a 2-hour plasma glucose test.

SPECIAL NEEDS

Certain high-risk groups should be tested frequently:

- Blacks, Latinos, and Native Americans
- those who are obese (more than 20% over ideal body weight)
- those who have a close relative with diabetes
- those with high blood pressure (140/90 mm Hg or higher)
- those with high levels of high-density lipoprotein cholesterol (35 mg/dl or higher) or triglycerides (250 mg/dl or higher)
- women who have delivered a baby weighing more than 9 lb (4.1 kg) or who have a history of GDM
- those previously diagnosed with impaired glucose tolerance (IGT) or impaired fasting glucose (IFG).

Note: Individuals with IGT usually have normal blood levels unless challenged by a glucose load, such as a piece of pie or glass of orange juice. Two hours after a glucose load, the glucose level ranges from 140 to 199 mg/dl. Individuals with IFG have an abnormal fasting glucose level between 110 and 125 mg/dl. Because the fasting plasma glucose test is sufficient to make the diagnosis of diabetes, it replaces the oral glucose tolerance test. (See *Classifying blood glucose levels.*)

An ophthalmologic examination may show diabetic retinopathy. Other diagnostic and monitoring tests include urinalysis for acetone and blood testing for glycosylated hemoglobin (hemoglobin A), which reflects recent glucose cortisol.

Treatment

Effective treatment normalizes blood glucose and decreases complications. In diabetes type 1, this goal is achieved with insulin replacement, diet, and exercise. Current forms of insulin replacement include single-dose, mixed-dose, split-mixed dose, and multiple-dose regimens. The multiple-dose regimens may use an insulin pump. Insulin may be very rapid-acting (Humalog, Novo Log), rapid-acting (Velosulin, Regular), intermediate-acting (NPH), long-acting (Ultralente), or a combination of rapid-acting and intermediate-acting (Mixtard); standard or purified; and derived from beef, pork, or human sources. Purified human insulin is most commonly used.

Pancreas transplantation is experimental and requires chronic immunosuppression. Islet cell transplantation is another experimental treatment option that is less complicated than whole pancreas transplantation, but also requires chronic immunosuppression.

Treatment of all types of diabetes also requires a strict diet planned to meet nutritional needs, to control blood glucose levels, and to reach and maintain appropriate body weight. For the obese patient with type 2 diabetes, weight reduction is a goal. In type 1 diabetes, the calorie allotment may be high, depending on growth stage and activity level. For success, the diet must be followed consistently and meals eaten at regular times.

Type 2 diabetes may require oral antidiabetic drugs to stimulate endogenous insulin production, increase insulin sensitivity at the cellular level, and suppress hepatic gluconeogenesis.

Five types of drugs have been used to treat diabetes. Sulfonylureas (such as tolbutamide [Orinase]) stimulate pancreatic insulin release, increase tissue sensitivity to insulin, and require insulin's presence to work.

Classifying Blood Glucose Levels

The American Diabetes Association 2003 Clinical Practice guidelines classifies blood glucose diagnoses following a glucose tolerance test as follows:

- normal—when the 2-hour glucose test level is less than or equal to 110 mg/dl.
- impaired fasting glucose—when the glucose level is 100 to 125 mg/dl.
- diabetes—when the 2-hour glucose test level is 200 mg/dl or more (confirmed by a second test), and the patient has symptoms of diabetes; or, fasting blood glucose is 126 mg/dl or more on two separate occasions.
- gestational diabetes—when the patient has two or more of the following: fasting glucose level of more than 105 mg/dl, 1-hour glucose level of more than 190 mg/dl, 2-hour glucose level of more than 165 mg/dl, 3-hour glucose level of more than 145 mg/dl.

Repaglinide (Prandin) and nateglinide (Starlix) cause immediate, brief release of insulin and are taken immediately before meals. Biguanides (such as metformin [Glucophage]) decrease hepatic glucose production and increase tissue sensitivity to insulin. Alpha-glucosidase inhibitors (such as acarbose [Precose]) slow the breakdown of glucose and decrease postprandial glucose peaks. The thiazolidinediones (such as roglitazone [Avandia]) enhance the action of insulin; however, insulin must be present for them to work. These drugs also reduce insulin resistance by decreasing hepatic glucose production and increasing glucose uptake. They have also been shown to lower blood pressure in diabetic hypertensive patients. Cholesterol and triglyceride levels may also be reduced.

Treatment of long-term diabetic complications may include transplantation or dialysis for renal failure, photocoagulation for retinopathy, and vascular surgery for large-vessel disease. Meticulous blood glucose control is essential.

Any patient with a wound that has lasted more than 8 weeks and who has tried standard wound care and revascularization without improvement should consider hyperbaric oxygen therapy. This treatment may speed healing by allowing more oxygen to get to the wound and may therefore result in fewer amputations.

The Diabetes Control and Complications Trial has shown that, in type 1 diabetes, intensive drug therapy that focuses on keeping glucose at near-normal levels for 5 years or more reduces both the onset and progression of retinopathy (up to 63%), nephropathy (up to 54%), and neuropathy (up to 60%). The United Kingdom Diabetes Study Group demonstrated that in type 2 diabetes, blood pressure control as well as smoking cessation reduced the onset and progression of complications, including cardiovascular disease.

Special considerations

- Stress the importance of complying with the prescribed treatment program. Tailor your teaching to the patient's needs, abilities, and developmental stage. Include diet; purpose, administration, and possible adverse effects of medication; exercise; monitoring; hygiene; and the prevention and recognition of hypoglycemia and hyperglycemia. Stress the effect of blood glucose control on long-term health.
- Watch for acute complications of diabetic therapy, especially hypoglycemia (vagueness, slow cerebration, dizziness, weakness, pallor, tachycardia, diaphoresis, seizures, and coma); immediately give carbohydrates, ideally in the form of fruit juice, hard candy, honey, or glucose tablets or gels, if available. If the patient is unconscious, administer glucagon or dextrose I.V. Also, be alert for signs of ketoacidosis (acetone breath, dehydration, weak and rapid pulse, Kussmaul's respirations) and hyperosmolar coma (polyuria, thirst, neurologic abnormalities, stupor). These hyperglycemic crises require I.V. fluids, insulin and, usually, potassium replacement.
- Monitor diabetes control by obtaining blood glucose, glycohemoglobulin, lipid levels, and blood pressure measurements regularly.
- Watch for diabetic effects on the cardiovascular system, such as cerebrovascular, coronary artery, and peripheral vascular impairment, and on the peripheral and autonomic nervous systems. Treat all injuries, cuts, and

blisters (particularly on the legs or feet) meticulously. Be alert for signs of urinary tract infection and renal disease.

- Urge regular ophthalmologic examinations to detect diabetic retinopathy.
- Assess for signs of diabetic neuropathy (numbness or pain in hands and feet, footdrop, neurogenic bladder). Stress the need for personal safety precautions because decreased sensation can mask injuries. Minimize complications by maintaining strict blood glucose control.
- Teach the patient to care for her feet by washing them daily, drying carefully between toes, and inspecting for corns, calluses, redness, swelling, bruises, and breaks in the skin. Urge her to report any changes to the physician. Advise her to avoid wearing constricting shoes or walking barefoot. Instruct her to use over-the-counter athlete's foot remedies and seek professional care should athlete's foot not improve.
- Teach the patient how to manage her diabetes when she has a minor illness, such as a cold, the flu, or an upset stomach.
- To delay the clinical onset of diabetes, teach people at high risk to avoid risk factors. Advise genetic counseling for young adults with diabetes who are planning families.
- Further information may be obtained from the Juvenile Diabetes Foundation, the ADA, and the American Association of Diabetes Educators.

Dysfunctional uterine bleeding

Dysfunctional uterine bleeding (DUB) refers to any abnormal endometrial bleeding without recognizable organic lesions. It's a diagnosis of exclusion and, therefore, is used broadly. DUB is most common during postmenarchal and perimenopausal periods in a woman's reproductive life. The prognosis varies with the cause. DUB is the indication for almost 25% of gynecologic surgical procedures.

Causes

DUB usually results from an imbalance in the hormonal-endometrial relationship, where persistent and unopposed stimulation of the endometrium by estrogen occurs. Disorders that cause sustained high estrogen levels are polycystic ovary syndrome (see "Polycystic ovary syndrome," page 395), obesity, immaturity of the hypothalamic-pituitary-ovarian mechanism (in postpubertal teenagers), and anovulation (in women in their late 30s or early 40s). (See *Causes of abnormal premenopausal bleeding*, page 274.)

In most cases of DUB, the endometrium shows no pathologic changes. However, in chronic unopposed estrogen stimulation (as from a hormone-producing ovarian tumor), the endometrium may show hyperplastic or malignant changes.

Signs and symptoms

DUB usually occurs as metrorrhagia (irregular episodes of vaginal bleeding between menses); it may also occur as

Causes of abnormal premenopausal bleeding

In addition to complications of pregnancy, which may be as mild as spotting or as severe as hypermenorrhea, causes of abnormal premenopausal bleeding vary with the type of bleeding:

- Oligomenorrhea (infrequent menses) and polymenorrhea (menses occurring too frequently) usually result from anovulation due to an endocrine or systemic disorder.
- Hypomenorrhea (decreased amount of menstrual fluid) results from local, endocrine, or systemic disorders or blockage caused by partial obstruction by the hymen or cervical obstruction.
- Hypermenorrhea (excessive bleeding occurring at regular intervals) usually results from local lesions, such as uterine leiomyomas, endometrial polyps, and endometrial hyperplasia. It may also result from endometritis, salpingitis, and anovulation.
- Cryptomenorrhea (no external bleeding, although menstrual symptoms are experienced) may result from an imperforate hymen or cervical stenosis.
- Metrorrhagia (bleeding occurring at irregular intervals) usually results from slight physiologic bleeding from the endometrium during ovulation, but may also result from local disorders, such as uterine malignancy, cervical erosions, polyps (which tend to bleed after intercourse), or inappropriate estrogen therapy.

hypermenorrhea (heavy or prolonged menses, longer than 8 days) or chronic polymenorrhea (menstrual cycle of less than 18 days). Such bleeding is unpredictable and can cause anemia.

Diagnosis

Diagnostic studies must rule out other causes of excessive vaginal bleeding, such as organic, systemic, psychogenic, and endocrine causes, including certain cancers, polyps, incomplete abortion, pregnancy, and infection. Dilatation and curettage (D&C) and biopsy results confirm the diagnosis by revealing endometrial hyperplasia.

Less invasive diagnostic tools such as sonographic uterine imaging may help evaluate the cause. Hemoglobin levels and hematocrit determine the need for blood or iron replacement.

Differential diagnosis must rule out:

- pregnancy
- hematologic abnormalities, such as idiopathic thrombocytopenic purpura (ITP), von Willebrand's disease, and leukemia
- exogenous hormones such as hormonal contraceptives
- infections, such as sexually transmitted diseases and pelvic inflammatory disease
- underlying medical conditions such as thyroid disease
- genital tract neoplasia.

Treatment

High-dose estrogen-progestogen combination therapy (hormonal contraceptives), the primary treatment, is designed to control endometrial growth and reestablish a normal cyclic pattern of menstruation. These drugs are usually administered four times daily for 5 to 7 days, although bleeding usually stops in 12 to 24 hours. The patient's age and the cause of bleeding help determine the drug choice and dosage. In patients over age 35, endometrial biopsy is necessary before the start of estrogen therapy to rule out endometrial adenocarcinoma. Progestogen therapy is a necessary alternative in some women such as those susceptible to the adverse effects of estrogen (thrombophlebitis, for example). Progestins may be delivered locally via intrauterine devices without systemic adverse effects.

If drug therapy is ineffective, a D&C serves as a supplementary treatment through removal of a large portion of the bleeding endometrium. D&C can also help determine the original cause of hormonal imbalance and aid in planning further therapy. If fertility isn't an issue, endometrial ablation may be a treatment option. Regardless of the primary treatment, the patient may need iron replacement or transfusions of packed cells or whole blood, as indicated, because of anemia caused by recurrent bleeding.

Special considerations

- Explain the importance of adhering to the prescribed hormonal therapy. If a D&C or endometrial ablation is ordered, explain this procedure and its purpose.
- Stress the need for regular checkups to assess the effectiveness of treatment.

Dysmenorrhea

Dysmenorrhea is painful menstruation associated with ovulation that isn't related to pelvic disease. It's the most common gynecologic complaint and a leading cause of absenteeism from school (affecting 10% of high school girls each month) and work (an estimate of 140 million work hours lost annually). The incidence peaks in women in their early 20s and then slowly decreases.

Dysmenorrhea can occur as a primary disorder or secondary to an underlying disease. Because primary dysmenorrhea is self-limiting, the prognosis is generally good. The prognosis for secondary dysmenorrhea depends on the underlying disease.

Causes

Although primary dysmenorrhea is unrelated to an identifiable cause, possible contributing factors include:

- hormonal imbalance
- psychogenic factors.

Dysmenorrhea may also be secondary to such gynecologic disorders as:

- endometriosis
- cervical stenosis
- uterine leiomyomas (benign fibroid tumors)
- pelvic inflammatory disease
- pelvic tumors.

The pain of dysmenorrhea probably results from increased prostaglandin secretion in menstrual blood, which intensifies normal uterine contractions. Prostaglandins intensify myometrial smooth muscle contraction and uterine blood vessel constriction, thereby worsening the uterine hypoxia normally associated with menstruation. This combination of intense muscle contractions and hypoxia causes the intense pain of dysmenorrhea. Prostaglandins and their metabolites can also cause GI disturbances, headache, and syncope.

Because dysmenorrhea usually follows an ovulatory cycle, both the primary and secondary forms are rare during the anovulatory cycle of menses. After age 20, dysmenorrhea is generally secondary.

Signs and symptoms

Possible signs and symptoms of dysmenorrhea include sharp, intermittent, cramping, lower abdominal pain, usually radiating to the back, thighs, groin, and vulva. Such pain typically starts with or immediately before menstrual flow and peaks within 24 hours.

Dysmenorrhea may also be associated with signs and symptoms that suggest premenstrual syndrome, including:

- urinary frequency
- nausea
- vomiting
- diarrhea
- headache
- backache
- chills
- abdominal bloating
- painful breasts
- depression
- irritability.

A possible but rare complication of dysmenorrhea is dehydration due to nausea, vomiting, and diarrhea.

Diagnosis

Differential diagnosis must rule out other causes of pelvic pain, including pregnancy, impending abortion, or various other disorders. (See *Causes of pelvic pain.*)

Methods used to diagnose dysmenorrhea may include:

- pelvic examination and a detailed patient history to help suggest the cause
- ruling out secondary causes for menses painful since menarche (primary dysmenorrhea)
- tests, such as laparoscopy, hysteroscopy, and pelvic ultrasound, to diagnose underlying disorders in secondary dysmenorrhea.

Treatment

Initial treatment aims to relieve pain and may include:

- analgesics, such as nonsteroidal anti-inflammatory drugs, for mild to moderate pain (most effective when taken 24 to 48 hours before onset of menses) — especially effective due to inhibition of prostaglandin synthesis through inhibition of the enzyme cyclooxygenase
- cyclooxygenase (COX)-2-specific inhibitors, which recently have been

used to relieve the pain of dysmenorrhea
- opioids for severe pain (rarely used)
- prostaglandin inhibitors (such as mefenamic acid [Ponstel]and ibuprofen [Advil, Motrin]) to relieve pain by decreasing the severity of uterine contractions
- heat applied locally to the lower abdomen (may relieve discomfort in mature women), used cautiously in young adolescents because appendicitis may mimic dysmenorrhea.

For primary dysmenorrhea:
- sex steroids (effective alternative to treatment with antiprostaglandins or analgesics), such as hormonal contraceptives, to relieve pain by suppressing ovulation and inhibiting endometrial prostaglandin synthesis (patients attempting pregnancy should rely on antiprostaglandin therapy)
- psychological evaluation and appropriate counseling due to possible psychogenic cause of persistently severe dysmenorrhea.

Treatment of secondary dysmenorrhea is designed to identify and correct the underlying cause and may include surgical treatment of underlying disorders, such as endometriosis or uterine leiomyomas (after conservative therapy fails).

Special considerations

Effective management of the patient with dysmenorrhea focuses on relief of symptoms, emotional support, and appropriate patient teaching, especially for the adolescent.

- Obtain a complete history focusing on the patient's gynecologic complaints, including detailed information on symptoms of pelvic disease, such as excessive bleeding, changes in bleeding pattern, vaginal discharge, and dyspareunia (painful intercourse).
- Provide thorough patient teaching, including explanation of normal female anatomy and physiology as well as the nature of dysmenorrhea (depending on circumstances, providing the adolescent patient with information on pregnancy and contraception).

Causes of pelvic pain

The characteristic pelvic pain of dysmenorrhea must be distinguished from the acute pain caused by many other disorders, such as:
- *GI disorders*—appendicitis, acute diverticulitis, acute or chronic cholecystitis, chronic cholelithiasis, acute pancreatitis, peptic ulcer perforation, intestinal obstruction
- *urinary tract disorders*—cystitis, renal calculi
- *reproductive disorders*—acute salpingitis, chronic inflammation, degenerating fibroid, ovarian cyst torsion
- *pregnancy disorders*—impending abortion (pain and bleeding early in pregnancy), ectopic pregnancy, abruptio placentae, uterine rupture, leiomyoma degeneration, toxemia
- *emotional conflicts*—psychogenic (functional) pain
- *other*—ovulation and normal uterine contractions experienced in pregnancy.

- Encourage the patient to keep a detailed record of her menstrual cycle and symptoms and to seek medical care if symptoms persist.

Dysuria

Dysuria is defined as pain, burning, difficulty, or discomfort related to urination. It's a common problem; even so, its importance shouldn't be minimized because it could be an indication of a serious problem. Generally, dysuria occurs more frequently in women than men. Approximately 25% of women complain of acute dysuria each year. Its prevalence is greatest in women between ages 25 and 54 and in those who are sexually active.

Causes

The most common cause of dysuria is infection. Bacteria can easily gain access through local contamination and ascend to the affected region. *Escherichia coli* is the most common offending organism. Dysuria may also be a symptom of genital herpes. Infection occurs differently depending on the part of the genitourinary tract that's affected. The various forms include:

- cystitis
- prostatitis
- pyelonephritis
- urethritis
- vulvitis
- vaginitis
- cervicitis.

Noninfectious causes can also cause dysuria:

- Postmenopausal women can suffer from dysfunction of the lower urinary tract due to a decrease in estrogen; atrophy and dryness may give rise to dysuria and other symptoms, such as frequency and urgency.
- Patients with renal calculi or cancer of the bladder and renal tract may present with dysuria as one of the symptoms.
- Urethral trauma can occur during sexual intercourse.
- Patients may be sensitive to scented creams, sprays, soaps, or toilet paper.
- Physical activities, such as bicycle riding and horseback riding, can cause urethral trauma.
- Dysuria may be a feature of some psychogenic conditions, such as depression and somatization disorder.
- Medications, such as those used for chemotherapy, can inflame the bladder.

Signs and symptoms

A thorough history is essential for evaluating the timing, frequency, and location of dysuria — important areas for investigation to ascertain possible causes for the dysuria. Vaginal infection may be suspected if the pain occurs as urine passes over the labia. Pain inside the body suggests urethritis or cystitis. If the pain occurs at the onset of urination, it's usually caused by inflammation of the urethra; however, if it occurs after urination, bladder infection may be the cause. Also, acute dysuria suggests bacterial infection, whereas gradual onset may be seen with *Chlamydia trachomatis* infection.

Other signs and symptoms that may accompany dysuria also help the clinician determine the underlying cause. Associated findings may include:

- hematuria, or blood in the urine
- urinary frequency
- urinary hesitation
- urinary slowness
- urinary urgency
- urethral discharge
- vaginal discharge
- dyspareunia, or pain during sexual intercourse
- abnormal vaginal bleeding.

Acute pyelonephritis is manifested by systemic symptoms, such as:

- fever
- chills
- fatigue
- back pain
- flank pain
- nausea
- vomiting
- costovertebral tenderness.

Diagnosis

Urinalysis is an easy, inexpensive test to identify a urinary tract infection (UTI) by evaluating the urine for the presence of blood, bacteria, and pus. However, a negative test doesn't rule out a UTI, and further testing is necessary. Urine culture and gram stain can identify the presence of a UTI and the specific offending organism.

If the patient has urethral or vaginal discharge or is sexually active, urethral and vaginal specimens should be evaluated using wet mount and gram staining. Vaginal pH testing, potassium hydroxide evaluation by microscopy, and yeast cultures are additional valuable diagnostic tools. Cultures for *Chlamydia trachomatis* and *Neisseriae gonorrhoeae* should also be done. These organisms can also be detected using ligase chain reaction and polymerase chain reaction tests.

More invasive testing is indicated when the diagnosis isn't clear, if a patient is severely ill, or a patient doesn't respond adequately to antibiotic treatment. These tests include:

- urine cytology to screen for bladder cancer
- radiographic examination of the kidneys, ureter, and bladder
- excretory urography
- voiding cystourethrography
- computed tomography (CT) scan
- magnetic resonance imaging (MRI)
- cystoscopy.

Treatment

Treatment of dysuria should focus on treating the underlying cause. Infections must be treated with the appropriate antibiotics for the offending organism. (For more details, see "Urinary tract infection," page 467.) Urinary analgesics, such as phenazopyridine (Pyridium, Urogesic), may alleviate acute pain associated with UTI and can be used before a culture is done and antibiotic therapy is begun.

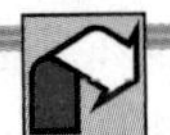

PREVENTION POINTER

Dysuria: Prevention tips

Patient education to prevent future episodes of dysuria should include the following:

- Avoid feminine douching.
- Avoid tight clothes.
- Wear cotton underwear because it's breathable.
- Use condoms, and have only one sexual partner.
- Urinate after sexual intercourse.
- Drink large amounts of fluids, especially water and cranberry juice.
- After urination, wipe from front to back.
- Use a lubricant as needed during sexual intercourse.
- Avoid intercourse until infection is gone.
- Discourage bubble baths.
- Avoid topical irritants, such as scented creams, sprays, soaps, or toilet paper.
- Change sanitary napkins or tampons every 4 hours.

Special considerations

Education regarding the underlying cause of dysuria is essential. If dysuria is the result of infection, a focus on preventive measures would be beneficial to the patient. (See *Dysuria: Prevention tips.*)

It's also important to reinforce the need for medical evaluation should dysuria occur again. Attempts at self-treatment should be discouraged due to the variety of possible causes.

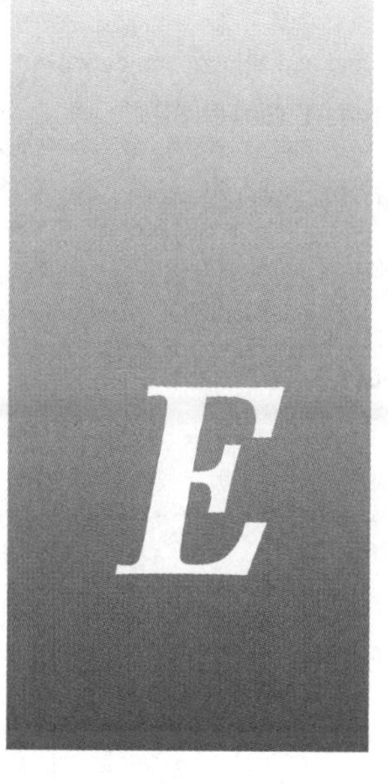

Ectopic pregnancy

Ectopic pregnancy is the implantation of a fertilized ovum outside the uterine cavity. The most common site is the fallopian tube, with more than 90% of ectopic implantations occurring in the fimbria, ampulla, or isthmus. Other possible sites include the interstitium, tubo-ovarian ligament, ovary, abdominal viscera, and internal cervical os. (See *Ectopic pregnancy implantation sites*, page 282.) In whites, ectopic pregnancy occurs in 1 in 200 pregnancies; in nonwhites, in 1 in 120. The prognosis is good with prompt diagnosis, appropriate surgical intervention, and control of bleeding; rarely, in cases of abdominal implantation, the fetus may survive to term. Usually, a subsequent and successful intrauterine pregnancy is achieved.

Causes

Conditions that prevent or retard the passage of the fertilized ovum through the fallopian tube and into the uterine cavity include:

- *diverticula* — the formation of blind pouches that cause tubal abnormalities
- *endometriosis* — the presence of endometrial tissue outside the lining of the uterine cavity

Ectopic pregnancy implantation sites

In 90% of patients with ectopic pregnancy, the ovum implants in the fallopian tube, either in the fimbria, ampulla, or isthmus. Other possible sites include the interstitium, tubo-ovarian ligament, ovary, abdominal viscera, and internal cervical os.

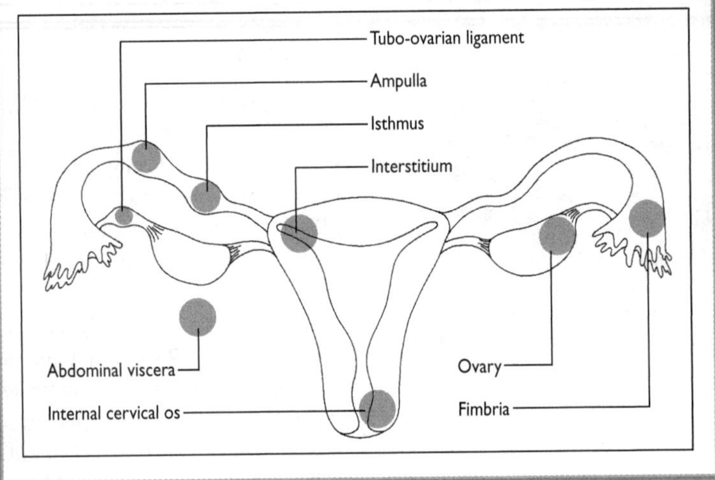

- *endosalpingitis* — an inflammatory reaction that causes folds of the tubal mucosa to agglutinate, narrowing the tube
- *pelvic inflammatory disease* — an infection of the oviducts and ovaries with adjacent tissue involvement
- *previous surgery* — tubal ligation or resection or adhesions from previous abdominal or pelvic surgery
- *tumors* pressing against the tube.

Ectopic pregnancy may result from congenital defects in the reproductive tract or ectopic endometrial implants in the tubal mucosa. The increased prevalence of sexually transmitted tubal infection may also be a factor.

Signs and symptoms

Ectopic pregnancy sometimes produces symptoms of normal pregnancy or sometimes no symptoms other than mild abdominal pain, thus, making diagnosis difficult. Characteristic clinical effects after fallopian tube implantation include amenorrhea or abnormal menses, followed by slight vaginal bleeding, and unilateral pelvic pain over the mass.

Rupture of the fallopian tube, however, causes life-threatening complications, including hemorrhage, shock, and peritonitis. The woman usually experiences sharp and severe lower abdominal pain, possibly radiating to the shoulders and neck, commonly precipitated by activities that increase abdominal pressure such as a bowel movement. She may also feel extreme pain upon motion of the cervix and palpation of the adnexa during a pelvic examination.

Diagnosis

Clinical features, patient history, and the results of a pelvic examination suggest ectopic pregnancy. The following tests may be used to confirm it:

- *Serum pregnancy test* shows presence of human chorionic gonadotropin.
- *Real-time ultrasonography* determines extrauterine pregnancy (performed if serum pregnancy test is positive).
- In *culdocentesis*, fluid is aspirated from the pouch of Douglas through the posterior vaginal fornix to detect free or nonclotting blood in the peritoneum (sometimes performed if ultrasonography fails to detect a gestational sac in the uterus).
- *Laparoscopy* or *laparotomy* is used to diagnose and treat an ectopic pregnancy by either removal of the tube (salpingectomy) or removal of the pregnancy with preservation of the tube (salpingostomy).

Decreased hemoglobin level and hematocrit due to blood loss support the diagnosis. Differential diagnosis must rule out uterine abortion, appendicitis, ruptured corpus luteum cyst, salpingitis, and torsion of the ovary.

Treatment

If culdocentesis is positive or the patient has peritoneal signs consistent with a surgical abdomen, laparoscopy and laparotomy are indicated. (*Note:* If the fallopian tube hasn't ruptured, laparoscopy is performed; if the tube has ruptured, laparotomy is performed.) The ovary is preserved as a rule; however, ovarian pregnancy may necessitate oophorectomy. Interstitial pregnancy rarely may require hysterectomy; abdominal pregnancy requires a laparotomy to remove the fetus, except in rare cases, when the fetus survives to term or calcifies undetected in the abdominal cavity.

Supportive treatment includes transfusion with whole blood or packed red cells to replace excessive blood loss, administration of broad-spectrum antibiotics I.V. for septic infection, and administration of supplemental iron by mouth or I.M. (using the Z-track method of injection). Methotrexate (Trexall) I.M. is also a therapeutic option in stable patients, which helps avoid surgery in most cases.

Special considerations

Patient care measures include careful monitoring and assessment of vital signs and vaginal bleeding, preparing the patient with excessive blood loss for emergency surgery as well as providing her with blood and fluid replacement, and offering the patient and the family emotional support and reassurance.

- Record the location and character of the pain and administer analgesics. (Remember, however, that analgesics may mask the symptoms of intraperitoneal rupture of the ectopic pregnancy.)

- Check the amount, color, and odor of vaginal bleeding. Ask the patient the date and characteristics of her last menstrual period.
- Observe for signs of pregnancy (enlarged breasts, soft cervix).
- Provide a quiet, relaxing environment, and encourage the patient to freely express her feelings of fear, loss, and grief.

To prevent ectopic pregnancy:

- Advise prompt treatment of pelvic infections to prevent diseases of the fallopian tube.
- Inform patients who have undergone surgery involving the fallopian tubes or those with confirmed pelvic inflammatory disease that they're at increased risk for ectopic pregnancy.

PREVENTION POINTER

Tell the patient who's vulnerable to ectopic pregnancy to delay using an intrauterine device until after she's finished bearing children.

Endometriosis

Endometriosis is the presence of endometrial tissue outside the lining of the uterine cavity. Ectopic endometrial tissue responds to normal stimulation in the same way as the endometrium, but much less predictably. The endometrial cells respond to estrogen and progesterone with proliferation and secretion. During menstruation, the ectopic tissue bleeds, which causes inflammation of the surrounding tissues. This inflammation causes fibrosis, leading to adhesions that produce pain and infertility. Ectopic tissue is generally confined to the pelvic area, usually around the ovaries, uterovesical peritoneum, uterosacral ligaments, and cul-de-sac, but it can appear anywhere in the body.

Active endometriosis may occur at any age, including adolescence. As many as 50% of infertile women may have endometriosis; however, the true incidence in both fertile and infertile women remains unknown.

Severe symptoms of endometriosis may have an abrupt onset or may develop over many years. Infertility occurs in 30% to 40% of women with endometriosis. Endometriosis usually manifests during the menstrual years; after menopause, it tends to subside.

Causes

The cause of endometriosis remains unknown. The main theories that attempt to explain this disorder (one or more are perhaps true for certain populations of women) include:

- retrograde menstruation with implantation at ectopic sites (although retrograde menstruation alone may not be sufficient for endometriosis to occur because it occurs in women with no clinical evidence of endometriosis)
- genetic predisposition and depressed immune system (may predispose one to endometriosis)
- coelomic metaplasia (repeated inflammation inducing metaplasia of mesothelial cells to the endometrial epithelium)

- lymphatic or hematogenous spread (extraperitoneal disease).

Signs and symptoms

Signs and symptoms of endometriosis include:

- dysmenorrhea, abnormal uterine bleeding, and infertility (classic symptoms)
- pain that begins 5 to 7 days before menses and peaks and lasts for 2 to 3 days (varies among patients), although severity of pain isn't indicative of extent of disease.

Other signs and symptoms depend on the location of the ectopic tissue and may include:

- infertility and profuse menses (ovaries and oviducts)
- deep-thrust dyspareunia (ovaries or cul-de-sac)
- suprapubic pain, dysuria, and hematuria (bladder)
- abdominal cramps, pain on defecation, constipation; bloody stools due to bleeding of ectopic endometrium in the rectosigmoid musculature (large bowel and appendix)
- bleeding from endometrial deposits in these areas during menses; pain on sexual intercourse (cervix, vagina, and perineum).

Complications of endometriosis include:

- infertility due to fibrosis, scarring, and adhesions (major complication)
- chronic pelvic pain
- ovarian carcinoma (rare).

Diagnosis

The only definitive way to diagnose endometriosis is through laparoscopy or laparotomy. Pelvic examination may suggest endometriosis or may be unremarkable. Findings that suggest endometriosis include:

- multiple tender nodules on uterosacral ligaments or in the rectovaginal septum (in approximately one-third of patients)
- ovarian enlargement in the presence of endometrial cysts on the ovaries.

Although laparoscopy is recommended to diagnose and determine the extent of disease, some clinicians recommend:

- empiric trial of gonadotropin-releasing hormone (GnRH) agonist therapy to confirm or refute the impression of endometriosis before resorting to laparoscopy (controversial but possibly cost-effective)
- biopsy at the time of laparoscopy (helpful to confirm the diagnosis), although diagnosis is confirmed by visual inspection in some instances.

Treatment

Treatment of endometriosis varies according to the stage of the disease and the patient's age and desire to have children. Hormonal treatments of endometriosis (continuous use of hormonal contraceptives, danazol [Danocrine], and GnRH agonists) are potentially effective in relieving discomfort (hormones stop ovulation, thereby decreasing inflammation and any menstrual tissue that may be distributed throughout the body), although treatment for advanced stages of endometriosis usually isn't as successful because of impaired follicular development. However, nonsurgical treatment of endometriosis generally remains inadequate. Surgery appears more effective to enhance fertility, although definitive class I evidence currently doesn't exist. Pharmacologic and surgical treatment of endometriosis may be beneficial for managing chronic pelvic pain. Conservative therapy for young women who want to have children includes:

- androgens such as danazol
- progestins and continuous combined hormonal contraceptives (pseudopregnancy regimen) to relieve symptoms by causing a regression of endometrial tissue
- GnRH agonists to induce pseudomenopause (medical oophorectomy), causing remission of the disease (commonly used).

No pharmacologic treatment has been shown to cure the disease or be effective in all women. Some disadvantages of nonsurgical therapy include:

- adverse reaction to drug-induced menopause (including osteoporosis if used for more than 6 months), high expense if used for an extended time, and possible recurrence of endometriosis after discontinuation of GnRH agonists
- high expense and weight gain when using danazol (Danocrine)
- lowest fertility rates of any medical treatment for endometriosis when using continuous hormonal contraceptive pills
- weight gain and depressive symptoms when using progestin (but as effective as GnRH agonists).

When ovarian masses are present, surgery must rule out cancer. Conservative surgery includes:

- laparoscopic removal of endometrial implants with conventional or laser techniques (no benefit shown for laser laparoscopy over electrocautery or suture methods)
- presacral neurectomy for central pelvic pain; effective in about 50% or less of appropriate candidates
- laparoscopic uterosacral nerve ablation (LUNA) also for central pelvic pain, although definitive studies supporting the efficacy of LUNA are lacking
- total abdominal hysterectomy with or without bilateral salpingo-oophorectomy. (Although success rates vary, it's unclear whether ovarian conservation is appropriate. This is a treatment of last resort for women who don't want to have children or for extensive disease.)

Special considerations

- Minor gynecologic procedures are contraindicated immediately before and during menstruation.
- Advise adolescents to use sanitary napkins instead of tampons; this can help prevent retrograde flow in girls with a narrow vagina or small introitus.
- Because infertility is a possible complication, advise the patient who wants children not to postpone childbearing.
- Recommend an annual pelvic examination and Papanicolaou test to all patients.

Fibromyalgia syndrome

Fibromyalgia syndrome (FMS), previously called *fibrositis,* is a diffuse pain syndrome and one of the most common causes of chronic musculoskeletal pain. It's characterized by diffuse daily fatigue; widespread pain in the muscles, tendons, and ligaments; and nonrestorative sleep, along with multiple tender points on examination (in specific areas). It affects an estimated 3 to 8 million people in the United States. Approximately 80% to 90% of those affected are women. Although FMS may occur at almost any age, it occurs most commonly in women of childbearing age (between ages 20 and 60) and sometimes may occur in elderly persons and men. FMS has also been reported in children, who have more diffuse pain and sleep disturbances than adult patients. They may have fewer tender points and commonly improve over 2 to 3 years of treatment. (See *Tender points of fibromyalgia*, page 288.)

Causes

The cause of FMS isn't certain. It may be a primary disorder or associated with an underlying disease, such as systemic lupus erythematosus,

Tender points of fibromyalgia

These illustrations show common areas of tenderness (tender points) in patients with fibromyalgia.

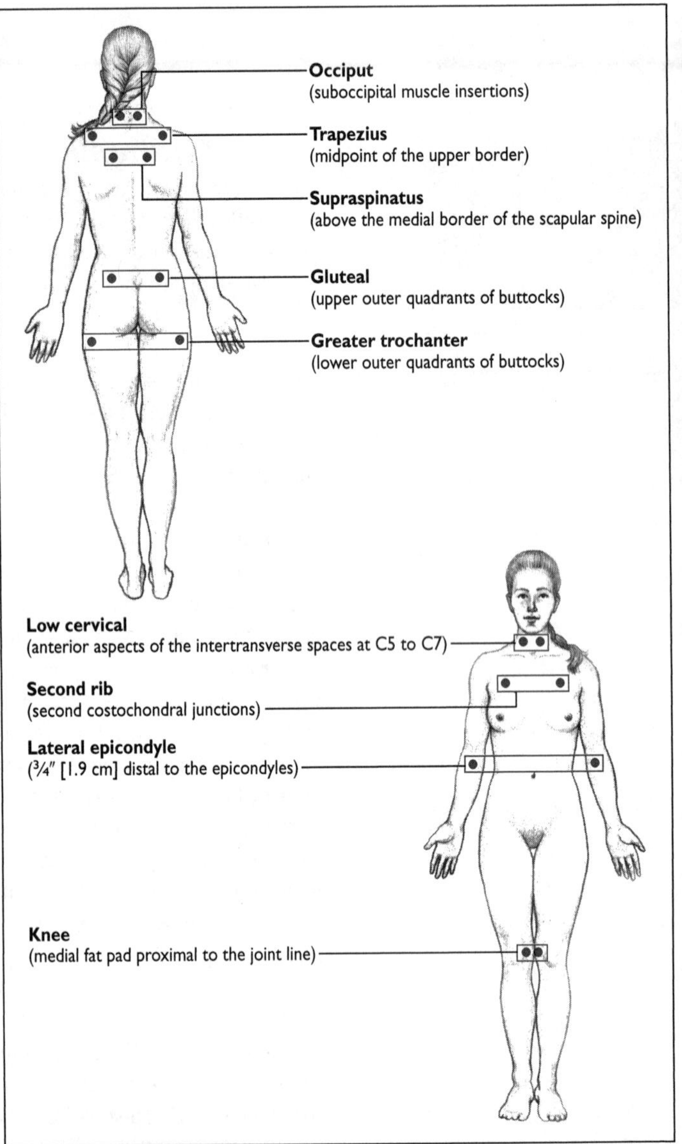

rheumatoid arthritis, osteoarthritis, and sleep apnea syndromes.

Many theories regarding the pathophysiology of FMS have been explored. The pain is located mainly in muscle areas; however, no distinct abnormalities have been documented on microscopic evaluation of tender point biopsies when compared with normal muscle. One theory suggests that blood flow to the muscle is decreased (due to poor muscle aerobic conditioning, rather than other physiologic abnormalities); another suggests that blood flow in the thalamus and caudate nucleus is decreased, leading to a lowered pain threshold. Still other theories suggest that the cause lies in endocrine dysfunction, such as abnormal pituitary-adrenal axis responses, or in abnormal levels of the neurotransmitter serotonin in brain centers, which affect pain and sleep. Abnormal functioning of other pain-processing pathways may also be involved. Considerable overlap of symptoms with other pain syndromes, such as chronic fatigue syndrome, raises the question of an association with infection, such as parvovirus B19 and others.

The development of FMS may be multifactorial and influenced by stress (physical and mental), physical conditioning, nonrestorative sleep, neuroendocrine factors, psychiatric factors and, possibly, hormonal factors (due to the predominance in women). Other associated features that can occur with FMS include irritable bowel syndrome, migraine or tension headaches, primary dysmenorrhea, temporomandibular joint pain, myofascial pain syndrome, puffy hands (hand swelling, especially in the morning), and paresthesia. All of these conditions, which commonly overlap, have been grouped under the umbrella term *central sensitivity syndrome*, which is now under research.

Signs and symptoms

The primary symptom of FMS is diffuse, dull, aching pain that's typically concentrated across the neck and shoulders and in the lower back and proximal limbs. It can involve all body quadrants (bilateral upper trunk and arms and bilateral lower trunk and legs) and is typically worse in the morning, when it's sometimes associated with stiffness. The pain can vary from day to day and be exacerbated by stress, lack of sleep, weather changes, and inactivity.

Sleep disturbance in FMS is another suggested factor in the development of symptoms. Many patients with this syndrome describe a habit of being a light sleeper, with frequent arousal and fragmented sleep (possibly secondary to pain in patients with underlying illnesses, such as osteoarthritis and rheumatoid arthritis). Other patients awaken frequently throughout the night but are unaware of the arousals. The patient awakens feeling fatigued and remains so throughout the day, hence the term *nonrestorative sleep*. Fatigue is commonly present from a half-hour to several hours after rising in the morning and can last for the rest of the day.

Women with fibromyalgia typically have pelvic pain, painful menorrhea, and pain during sexual intercourse. Some people have urinary symptoms, including a strong urge to urinate and bladder pain.

Diagnosis

Diagnosis of fibromyalgia is difficult because many of the symptoms mimic those of other disorders. Also, diagnostic testing in FMS that isn't associated with an underlying disease is generally negative for any significant abnormalities. Examination of joints doesn't reveal synovitis or significant swelling; the neurologic examination is normal; and no laboratory or radiologic abnormalities are common in patients with FMS.

Tender points are elicited by applying a moderate amount of pressure to a specific location. This examination can be fairly subjective, but many patients with true tender points wince or withdraw when pressure is applied to an appropriate intensity. Nontender control points, such as midforehead, distal forearm, and midanterior thigh, can also be tested to assess for conversion reactions (psychogenic rheumatism), in which patients hurt everywhere or exhibit other psychosomatic illnesses.

Overall, the diagnosis of FMS is made clinically in a patient with characteristic symptoms, such as widespread pain for more than 3 months, tenderness in at least 11 of the 18 specific tender point sites, and exclusion of other illnesses that can cause similar features. A workup for rheumatoid arthritis, primary sleep disorders, endocrinopathies (such as hypothyroidism), infections (such as Lyme disease and human immunodeficiency virus infection), neuropathies, and psychiatric illness (such as major depression) should be ruled out.

Treatment

The most important aspect in FMS management is patient education. Patients must understand that although FMS pain can be severe and is commonly chronic, it's treatable and doesn't lead to deforming or life-threatening complications.

Treatment of fibromyalgia usually requires a comprehensive approach, combining exercise, medication, physical therapy, and relaxation. A regular, low-impact aerobic exercise program, such as swimming, walking, or biking, has been shown to be effective in improving muscle conditioning, energy levels, and the patient's overall sense of well-being. The patient with FMS should be taught stretching before and after exercise to minimize injury and told to begin at a low intensity with slow and gradual increases.

Medications are typically used to improve sleep and control pain. A bedtime dose of amitriptyline, nortriptyline (Pamelor), trazodone (Desyrel), or doxepin (Sinequan) may be useful to improve sleep; however, they can be associated with anticholinergic adverse effects and daytime drowsiness. The combination of a tricyclic antidepressant at bedtime and a daytime dose of a serotonin uptake inhibitor, such as fluoxetine (Prozac), sertraline (Zoloft), or paroxetine (Paxil) have been found effective. Muscle relaxants such as cyclobenzaprine at bedtime may decrease muscle pain and spasms. Benzodiazepines are usually avoided because they haven't shown any long-term benefits and have the potential for drug dependence.

Nonsteroidal anti-inflammatory drugs (NSAIDs) and corticosteroids typically haven't been effective in relieving FMS pain, although NSAIDs may be used for coexisting tendinitis or arthritis. However, the combination of oral corticosteroids and an NSAID can put a patient at increased risk for peptic ulcer disease. For patients who require steroids for treatment and don't tolerate the discontinuation of their regular NSAID (for underlying arthritis, for example), the addition of a GI protective agent, such as misoprostol (Cytotec), should be considered. Some patients may get relief from a cyclooxygenase-2 inhibitor, which doesn't have the adverse GI effects associated with most NSAIDs. Tramadol (Ultram) has also been effective for patients who aren't sensitive to codeine preparations. Narcotics to control the chronic pain of FMS should be used only with extreme caution, preferably under the guidance of a pain clinic, because of their potential for dependence and addiction.

ALTERNATIVE THERAPIES

Many complementary and alternative therapies for pain and stress have been used for centuries. Although they're becoming more popular and more widely used among patients, many of these therapies haven't been studied adequately. Because members of the medical community are still at odds about the efficacy of these therapies, they remain controversial. Despite that fact, many patients are using these therapies because they have found several to be effective in treating their FMS symptoms. Some of the more common therapies include massage therapy, acupuncture, acupressure, chiropractic care, meditation, trigger point therapy, and botox. (See *Is botox the answer?* page 292.) Additionally, in some double-blind studies, bioelectromagnetic therapy has proven to be effective in relieving symptoms of FMS in some patients.

Special considerations

- Reassurance and social and emotional support are extremely important for the patient with FMS. She commonly goes through extensive diagnostic workups and multiple consultations with no significant abnormal findings. The patient may think that no one believes that the pain is present and that it's "all in her head." Reassure the patient that FMS is common and, although chronic, can be treated.

PREVENTION POINTER

Joints that aren't put through regular range of motion (ROM) (because of stiffness or pain) can "freeze" because of tendon and ligament shortening or adhesive capsulitis. A daily stretching program can help preserve ROM in the neck, shoulders, and hips. A physical therapist may assist in selecting appropri-

CUTTING EDGE

Is botox the answer?

There has been little research on the effects of botox (botulinum toxin type A) in treating the symptoms of fibromyalgia syndrome (FMS). Thus far, one double-blind study at Ohio State University using botox in patients with FMS had to be terminated because of adverse effects, including confusion, increased pain, and flulike symptoms. Another study, limited to 16 patients, reported that some patients who had multiple injections of botox had intensified pain in areas not injected with botox while others reported improvements.

Although the Food and Drug Administration (FDA) has approved botox for various other conditions, it hasn't approved botox for the treatment of FMS. Thus, it shouldn't be used as such until more clinical trials have shown that it's safe and effective.

The FDA has approved botox for:

- eye muscle spasms
- strabismus
- involuntary neck muscle contractions
- muscle spasticity
- migraines
- facial wrinkles
- sweating
- tremors.

ate exercises for the patient's tolerance level. Teach the patient how to do stretches safely and effectively and encourage her to perform them regularly.

- The deconditioned FMS patient may experience increased muscle pain with the initiation of a new exercise program. Reassure her that this may occur and, if it does, she may reduce the duration or intensity of her exercise.
- Encourage the patient not to stop exercising altogether (unless specifically told to do so) because even a limited amount of exercise each day may be beneficial.
- A bedtime dose of a tricyclic antidepressant can cause morning drowsiness in some patients. Taking the dose 1 to 2 hours before bedtime can sometimes improve sleep benefits while reducing this morning-after effect.

PREVENTION POINTER

Stress and poor sleep may exacerbate the symptoms of fibromyalgia. Encourage the patient to reduce stress and develop good sleeping habits in addition to eating a balanced diet, exercising regularly, and following her physician's treatment regimen.

G

Genital herpes

Genital herpes is an inflammatory disease of the genitalia for which there's no cure. This chronic infection can be classified by its cause, either herpes simplex virus-1 (HSV-1) or HSV-2. The prognosis varies, depending on the patient's age, the strength of her immune defenses, and the infection site. HSV-2 is usually self-limiting but is more likely to cause painful and severe outbreaks; therefore, individuals are more likely to seek medical attention than those with HSV-1. (See *Understanding the genital herpes cycle*, page 294.) In neonates and immunocompromised patients, such as those with acquired immunodeficiency syndrome, genital herpes is commonly severe, resulting in complications and a high mortality.

Genital herpes is very common in the United States, affecting people ages 12 and older. HSV-2 is more common in women than men, probably because male-to-female transmission is more efficient than female-to-male transmission. Also, it's more common in Blacks (45.9%) than in Whites (17.6%). However, as the number of infected people increases, the largest increase in the past 20 years is currently seen in White teenagers.

Understanding the genital herpes cycle

After a patient is infected with genital herpes, a latency period follows. The virus takes up permanent residence in the nerve cells surrounding the lesions, and intermittent viral shedding may take place. Repeated outbreaks may develop at any time, again followed by a latent stage during which the lesions heal completely. Outbreaks may recur as often as three to eight times yearly. Although the cycle continues indefinitely, some people remain symptom-free for years.

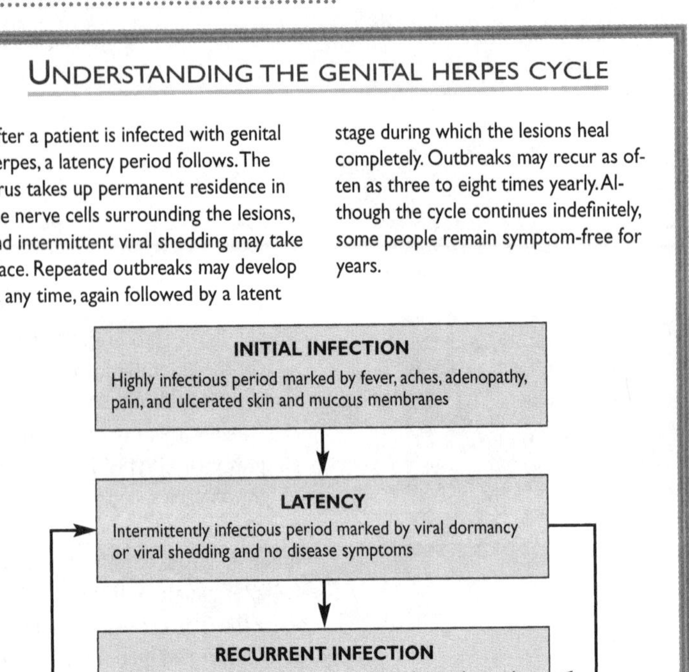

Causes

Genital herpes is usually caused by infection with HSV-2; however, HSV-1, which more commonly affects the lips and causes cold sores or fever blisters, can also cause genital herpes. Genital herpes is typically transmitted through sexual intercourse, oral-genital sexual activity, kissing, and hand-to-body contact with someone who's experiencing an outbreak (when HSV is active). Pregnant women may transmit the infection to neonates during vaginal delivery if an active infection is present. Such transmitted infection may be localized (for instance, in the eyes) or disseminated and may be associated with central nervous system involvement.

Signs and symptoms

Typically, when a person is first infected with HSV, symptoms may appear after a 2- to 10-day incubation period and may last 2 to 3 weeks. Early symptoms may include itching or burning in the genital or anal area; pain in the legs, buttocks, or genital area; vaginal discharge; and abdominal pressure. Then, after a few days, sores will begin to appear. For women, fluid-filled vesicles appear, usually on the cervix (the primary infection site) and, possibly, on the labia, perianal skin, vulva, or vagina. For men, these vesicles appear on the glans penis, foreskin, or penile shaft. In both males and females, extragenital lesions may appear on the mouth or anus. The vesicles, usually painless at first, rupture and develop into extensive, shallow, painful ulcers, with characteristic yellow, oozing centers. Redness, marked edema, tender inguinal lymph nodes, and cervical lymphadenopathy also develop. Over several days, the sores will begin to crust over and then heal without leaving a scar.

Other features of initial mucocutaneous infection include fever, malaise, dysuria and, in females, leukorrhea. Rare complications (generally from extragenital lesions) include herpetic keratitis, which may lead to blindness, and potentially fatal herpetic encephalitis.

Diagnosis

Diagnosis may be based on physical examination and patient history. However, approximately 20% of patients with HSV infections are asymptomatic and 60% of patients with HSV infections have only mild symptoms. In these patients, diagnosis using physical examination and patient history may be difficult. Helpful diagnostic tools include laboratory data showing increased antibody titers, smears of genital lesions showing atypical cells, and cytologic preparations (Tzanck test) revealing giant cells. Diagnosis can be confirmed by demonstration of HSV in vesicular fluid, using tissue culture techniques, or by antigen tests that identify specific antigens.

Treatment

There's no known cure for genital herpes. Rather, treatment is symptomatic and geared toward preventing outbreaks. Acyclovir (Zovirax) is an effective treatment for the symptoms of genital herpes. I.V. administration may be required for patients who are hospitalized with severe genital herpes or for those who are immunocompromised and have a potentially life-threatening herpes infection. Oral acyclovir may be prescribed for patients with first-time infections or recurrent outbreaks. Newer drug therapies include famciclovir (Famvir) and valacyclovir (Valtrex). Daily prophylaxis with acyclovir reduces the frequency of recurrences by at least 50% but is only appropriate for patients with frequent outbreaks and may not decrease transmission rate of the disease. (See *Genital herpes vaccination,* page 296.)

Special considerations

- Practice standard precautions.
- Encourage the patient to get adequate rest and nutrition and to keep the lesions dry.

PREVENTION POINTER

Teach the patient steps to avoid spreading the infection to other places on her body or to other people:

- Keep the infected area clean and dry.
- Avoid touching the sores.

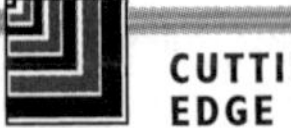

CUTTING EDGE

Genital herpes vaccination

In November of 2002, GlaxoSmithKline along with the National Institute of Allergy and Infectious Diseases launched its HERPEVAC Trial for Women with a new prophylactic genital herpes vaccination. The double-blind randomized trial conducted throughout the world will determine whether the vaccine protects women against genital herpes infection. Two previous phases of the study involved over 2,700 women between ages 18 and 45, all of whom had partners with genital herpes. Approximately 73% of the women who received the vaccine in these phases were protected against the disease.

- Practice strict handwashing.
- Avoid sexual intercourse during the active stage of this disease (while lesions are present) and use condoms during all sexual exposures.
- Urge her sexual partners to seek medical examination.

Other considerations include:

- reassuring the patient that intimate relationships are appropriate and that she may still have children
- advising the female patient to have a Papanicolaou test every 6 months.

Genital warts

A common and highly contagious sexually transmitted disease (STD), genital warts are caused by the human papillomavirus (HPV). The wart (papilloma) consists of fibrous tissue overgrowth from the dermis and thickened epithelial coverings. These tiny benign growths usually appear in the genital and anal areas. Also known as *venereal warts, HPV,* or *condylomata acuminata*, these growths are one of the most common STDs in the United States. Although generally benign, genital warts may lead to an increased risk of anogenital cancer. (Studies show an association between HPV types 11, 16, and 18 and cervical dysplasia and cancer.)

The Centers for Disease Control and Prevention reports that the disease affects more women than men. In women, the highest incidence is found in those between the ages of 15 and 25. In addition, Blacks have a rate of infection 1½ times higher than Whites.

Causes

Genital warts result from infection with one of the more than 30 known strains of HPV. Transmitted by sexual contact, HPV incubates from 1 to 6 months (the average is 2 months) before warts erupt.

Signs and symptoms

The patient's health history may include unprotected sexual contact with a partner with a known infection, a new partner, or many partners. Genital warts are usually firm, rough, and flesh-colored bumps. In women, these warts may be found in the vulvar region, inside of the vagina, on the cervix, or on and around the anus. In men, they may be found on the penile shaft or tip, scrotum, or urethra or around the anus. In both sexes, papillomas spread to the perineum and the perianal area. On inspection, you may find warts that begin as tiny red or pink swellings. These warts may grow as large as 4″ (10 cm) and may become pedunculated. Multiple swellings have a cauliflower-like appearance. Most patients report no symptoms; a few complain of itching, pain, mild irritation, burning, foul smell, pain with intercourse, increased vaginal discharge, or bleeding.

During pregnancy, genital warts in the vaginal and cervical walls may grow so large that they impede vaginal delivery. Other complications include possible genital tract dysplasia or cancer. Although rare, the mother may infect the child either during gestation or during delivery. Some neonates may develop laryngeal papillomatosis (throat warts), which may be fatal if the warts block the neonate's airways.

Diagnosis

Genital warts on the skin may be seen and generally recognized. Tests such as dark-field microscopy of wart-cell scrapings, which shows marked epidermal cell vascularization, may confirm the diagnosis. This differentiates genital warts from condylomata lata associated with second-stage syphilis. Another test involves applying 5% acetic acid (white vinegar) to the warts, which will turn white if they're papillomas.

Treatment

Frequently used therapies include cryosurgery, application of caustic agents, electrocautery, surgical excision, and laser ablation. Topical antimetabolites, such as 5-fluorouracil and podophyllin resin, have also been used. Topical interferon has been shown effective. Vaccine preparations show promise in preventing papillomavirus.

Warts that grow larger than 1″ (2.5 cm) are usually removed by carbon dioxide laser, cryosurgery, electrocautery, or fluorouracil cream debridement. Conventional surgery may be recommended to remove perianal warts.

Genital warts may be treated and removed successfully; however, some patients may have a recurrence. If warts reappear, the patient will have to undergo retreatment. If she continues to have recurrences despite retreatment, immune therapy (excising the warts and using them to prepare a vaccine to stimulate antibodies in the body) or interferon therapy (injections of protein to boost the body's immune response and prevent the virus from multiplying) may be prescribed. A vaccine is currently under investigation for papillomavirus in healthy individuals. (See *HPV vaccine,* page 298.)

Special considerations

- Use standard precautions when examining the patient, collecting a specimen, or performing associated procedures.
- Provide a nonthreatening, nonjudgmental atmosphere that encourages

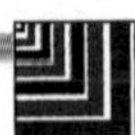

CUTTING EDGE

HPV VACCINE

A vaccine for human papillomavirus (HPV) has been proven safe in a phase I study with healthy volunteers. The vaccine is composed of stripped-down HPV that was available through molecular genetic and tissue culture manipulations. The vaccine was given at 0, 4, and 16 weeks of the study and the patients were observed for 48 weeks following the first dose. Patients received a dose of 3, 9, 30, or 100 mg of the virus at each immunization.

HPV has more than 70 different genotypes, such as HPV-11 and HPV-6, which produce visible anogenital warts, and HPV-16 and HPV-18, which are linked to cervical cancer. Thus, an HPV multivalent vaccine is being developed, which has prevented infection in animal trials.

the patient to verbalize her feelings about perceived changes in sexual identity and behavior.

PREVENTION POINTER

Recommend sexual abstinence until healing is complete. Use a condom during all sexual activity; however, warn the patient that genital warts may spread via contact with the perineum, anus, and the entire area between the legs, thus condoms only provide some protection.

- Advise the patient to inform her sexual partners about the risk of genital warts and their need for evaluation.
- Urge the patient to be tested for human immunodeficiency virus infection and other STDs.
- Emphasize that genital warts can recur and that the virus can mutate, causing infection with warts of a different strain.
- Remind the patient to report for weekly treatments until all warts are removed. Instruct her to schedule a checkup 3 months after all warts are gone.

PREVENTION POINTER

Encourage female patients to have a Papanicolaou test every 6 months because genital warts on the cervix may lead to an increased risk of cervical cancer.

Gonorrhea

A common but curable sexually transmitted disease, gonorrhea is an infection of the genitourinary tract (especially the urethra and cervix) and, occasionally, the rectum, pharynx, and eyes. Untreated gonorrhea can spread through the blood to the joints, tendons, meninges, and endocardium; in females, it can also lead to chronic pelvic inflammatory disease (PID) and can cause ectopic pregnancy and infertility in as many as 10% of infected women. After adequate treatment, the prognosis for both males and females is excellent, although reinfection is common.

Gonorrhea is especially prevalent among young people and in people with multiple sexual partners, particularly those between ages 19 and 25. The highest rates of infection are found in women ages 15 to 19 and men ages 20 to 24.

Causes

Transmission of *Neisseria gonorrhoeae,* the organism that causes gonorrhea, almost always follows sexual contact with an infected person. Pregnant women infected with gonorrhea can pass the disease to their neonate during delivery through the birth canal. Neonates born of infected mothers can contract gonococcal ophthalmia neonatorum. Also, children and adults with gonorrhea can contract gonococcal conjunctivitis by touching their eyes with contaminated hands.

Signs and symptoms

Although most males infected with gonorrhea remain asymptomatic, some may develop mild symptoms after a 2- to 10-day incubation period. Most infected females remain asymptomatic. Those with symptoms may complain of bleeding during intercourse, yellow or bloody vaginal discharge (probably the most common symptom in females), or pain or burning during urination. Their symptoms may progress to cramping, bleeding between menstrual periods, vomiting, and pain, indicating the development of PID. (See *What happens in gonorrhea,* page 300.) Other possible symptoms include pharyngitis, tonsillitis, and rectal burning, itching, and bloody mucopurulent discharge.

Other clinical features vary according to the site involved:

- *urethra* — dysuria, urinary frequency and incontinence, purulent discharge, itching, and red, edematous meatus
- *vulva* — occasional itching, burning, and pain due to exudate from an adjacent infected area (with symptoms that tend to be more severe before puberty or after menopause)
- *vagina* (most common site in children over age 1) — engorgement, redness, swelling, and profuse, purulent discharge
- *liver* — right upper quadrant pain in patients with perihepatitis
- *pelvis* — severe pelvic and lower abdominal pain, muscle rigidity, tenderness, and abdominal distention as well as nausea, vomiting, fever, and tachycardia in patients with salpingitis or PID as the infection spreads

Possible complications of gonorrhea include gonococcal septicemia and, if the women is pregnant, gonococcal ophthalmia neonatorum of the neonate after birth.

Gonococcal septicemia is more common in females than in males. Its characteristic signs include tender papillary skin lesions on the hands and feet; these lesions may be pustular, hemorrhagic, or necrotic. Gonococcal septicemia may also produce migratory polyarthralgia and polyarthritis and tenosynovitis of the wrists, fingers, knees, or ankles. Untreated septic arthritis leads to progressive joint destruction.

Signs of gonococcal ophthalmia neonatorum include lid edema, bilat-

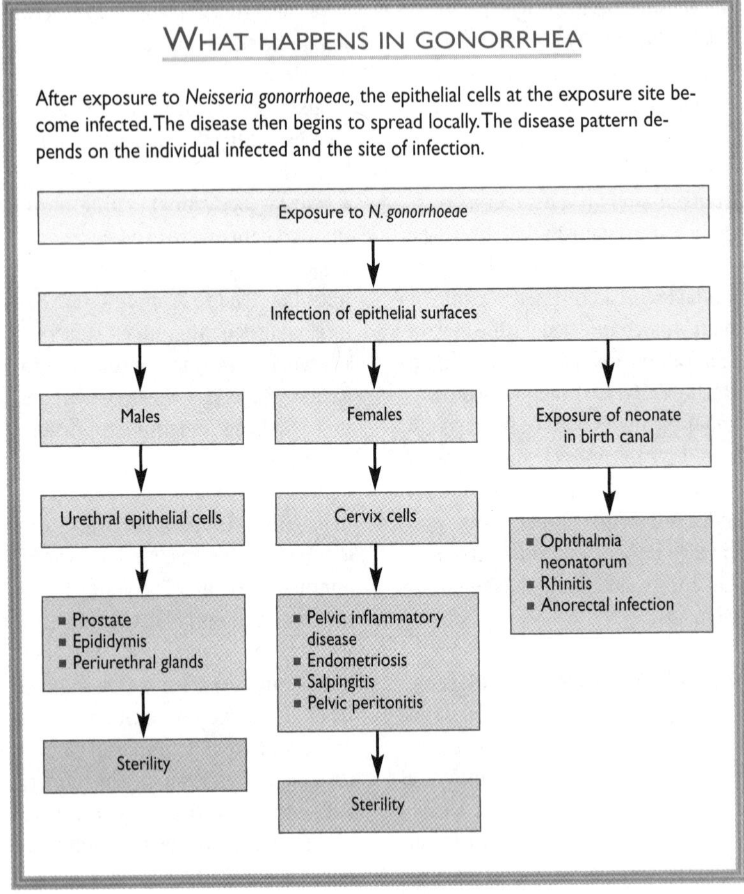

eral conjunctival infection, and abundant purulent discharge 2 to 3 days after birth. Adult conjunctivitis, most common in men, causes unilateral conjunctival redness and swelling. Untreated gonococcal conjunctivitis can progress to corneal ulceration and blindness.

Other possible complications of gonorrhea include infections, arthritis, PID, endocarditis, and infertility in women.

Diagnosis

A culture from the site of infection (urethra, cervix, rectum, or pharynx), grown on a Thayer-Martin or Transgrow medium, is the gold standard for diagnosing women by isolating *N. gonorrhoeae.* (See Neisseria gonorrhoeae.) A Gram stain showing gram-negative diplococci supports the diagnosis and may be sufficient to confirm gonorrhea in males.

Confirmation of gonococcal arthritis requires identification of gram-negative diplococci on smears made from joint fluid and skin lesions. Complement fixation and immunofluorescent assays of serum reveal antibody titers four times the normal rate. Culture of conjunctival scrapings confirms gonococcal conjunctivitis.

Treatment

For adults and adolescents, the recommended treatment for uncomplicated gonorrhea caused by susceptible non-penicillinase-producing *N. gonorrhoeae* is a single dose of ceftriaxone (Rocephin), 125 mg I.M. Other treatments include a single dose of ciprofloxacin (Cipro), ofloxacin (Floxin), or levofloxacin (Levaquin). Gonorrhea and chlamydial infections commonly infect people at the same time. Thus, for presumptive treatment of concurrent *Chlamydia trachomatis* infection, the clinician may prescribe doxycycline (Vibramycin) or azithromycin (Zithromax) with the ceftriaxone. A single dose of ceftriaxone and erythromycin (Erythrocin) for 7 days is recommended for pregnant women and patients allergic to penicillin. Ciprofloxacin and ofloxacin are contraindicated for children and pregnant or breast-feeding women.

If left untreated, gonorrhea can spread to the reproductive tract and even into the blood stream, infecting the heart, brain, and joints.

Treatment of gonococcal conjunctivitis requires a single dose of ceftriaxone, 1 g I.M., and lavage of the infected eye with saline solution once. Routine instillation of 1% silver nitrate drops or erythromycin ointment (Ilotycin) into neonates' eyes soon after delivery has greatly reduced the incidence of gonococcal ophthalmia neonatorum.

Neisseria gonorrhoeae

In gonorrhea, microscopic examination reveals gram-negative diplococcus *N. gonorrhoeae,* the causative organism.

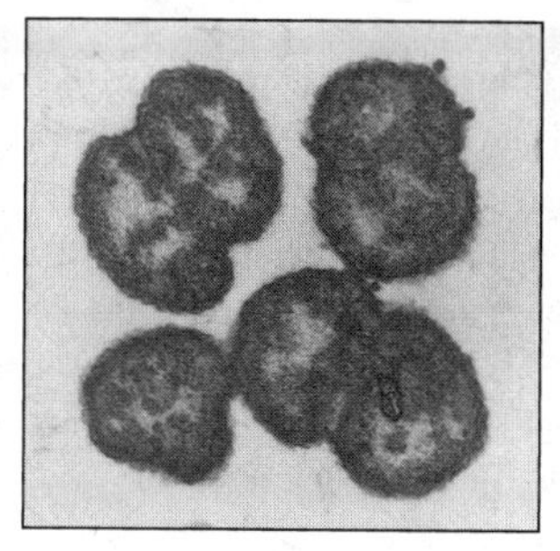

Special considerations

- Before treatment, establish whether the patient has any drug sensitivities, and watch closely for adverse drug reactions during therapy.
- Warn the patient that, until cultures prove negative, she's still infectious and can transmit gonococcal infection.
- Practice standard precautions.
- If the patient has gonococcal arthritis, apply moist heat to ease pain in affected joints.
- Urge the patient to inform sexual contacts of her infection so that they can seek treatment, even if cultures are negative. Advise her to avoid sexu-

al intercourse until treatment is complete.

- Report all cases of gonorrhea to local public health authorities for follow-up on sexual contacts. Examine and test all people exposed to gonorrhea as well as children of infected mothers.
- Routinely instill two drops of 1% silver nitrate solution or erythromycin ointment in the eyes of all neonates immediately after birth. Check neonates of infected mothers for signs of infection. Take specimens for culture from the newborn infant's eyes, pharynx, and rectum.

PREVENTION POINTER

To prevent gonorrhea, tell patients to avoid oral or sexual intercourse with anyone *suspected* of being infected, use condoms during intercourse, wash genitals with soap and water before and after intercourse, and avoid sharing washcloths or douche equipment.

- Report all cases of gonorrhea in children to child abuse authorities.

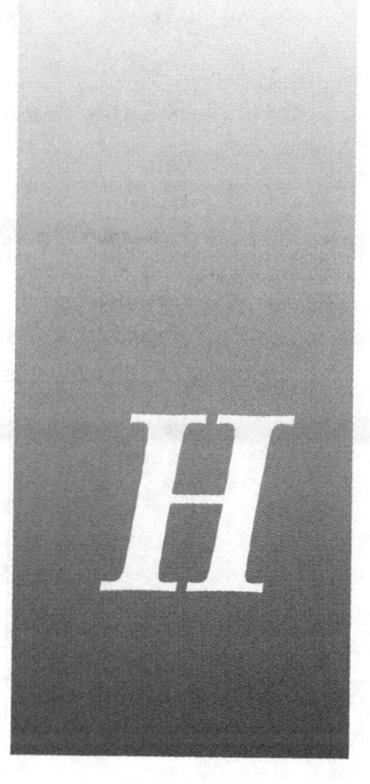

Herpes zoster

Herpes zoster, also known as *shingles,* is an acute unilateral and segmental inflammation of the dorsal root ganglia. It produces localized vesicular skin lesions confined to a dermatome. The patient with shingles may have severe neuralgic pain in the areas bordering the inflamed nerve root ganglia. (See *Tracing the path of herpes zoster,* pages 304 and 305.) The infection occurs only in someone who has had a previous infection of chickenpox, usually as a child, and is found primarily in adults over age 50; it seldom recurs. Herpes zoster may be more prevalent in people who had chickenpox at a very young age than in those who contracted chickenpox in adulthood. Herpes zoster is more common and severe in elderly, insulin-dependent patients and immunocompromised patients but is seldom fatal. It's also more severe in pregnant women than others of the same age, probably because of the mild immunosuppression and other factors associated with pregnancy. The prognosis is good and most patients recover completely unless the infection spreads to the brain.

(Text continues on page 306.)

Tracing the path of herpes zoster

The herpes zoster virus infects the nerves that innervate the skin, eyes, and ears. Each nerve (tagged for its corresponding vertebral source) emanates from the spine, banding and branching around the body to innervate a skin area called a *dermatome*. The herpes zoster rash erupts along the course of the affected nerve

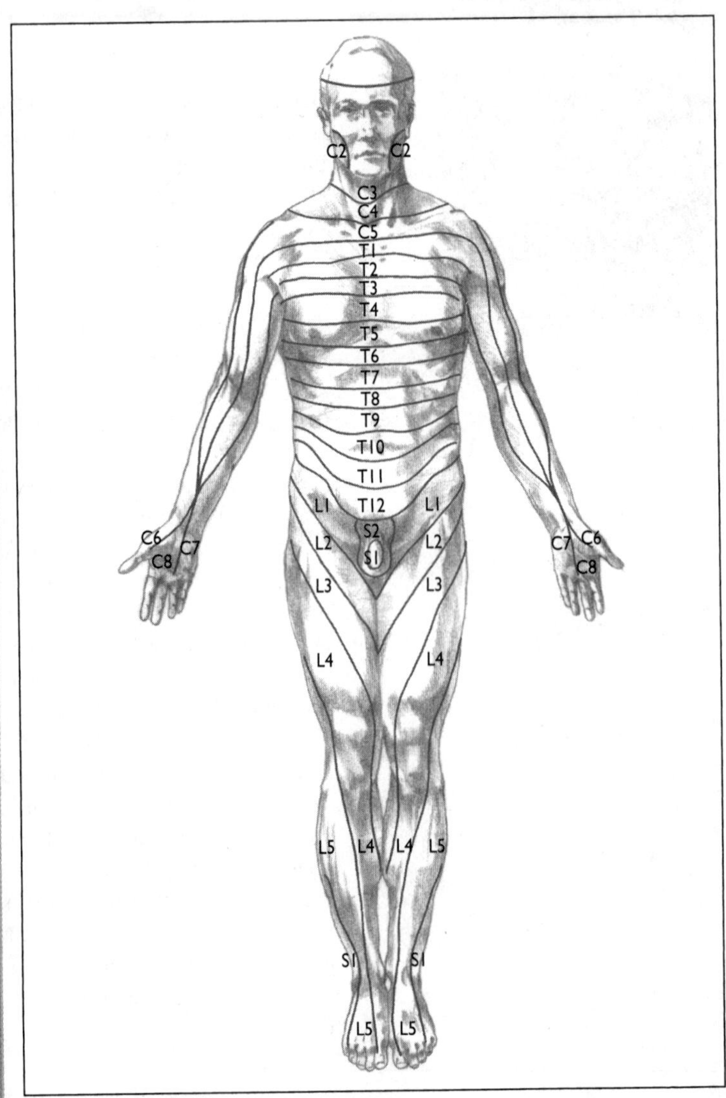

fibers, covering the skin in one or several of the dermatomes (as shown).

The thoracic (T) and lumbar (L) dermatomes are the most commonly affected but others, such as those covering the cervical (C) and sacral (S) areas, may also be affected. Dermatome levels can vary and overlap.

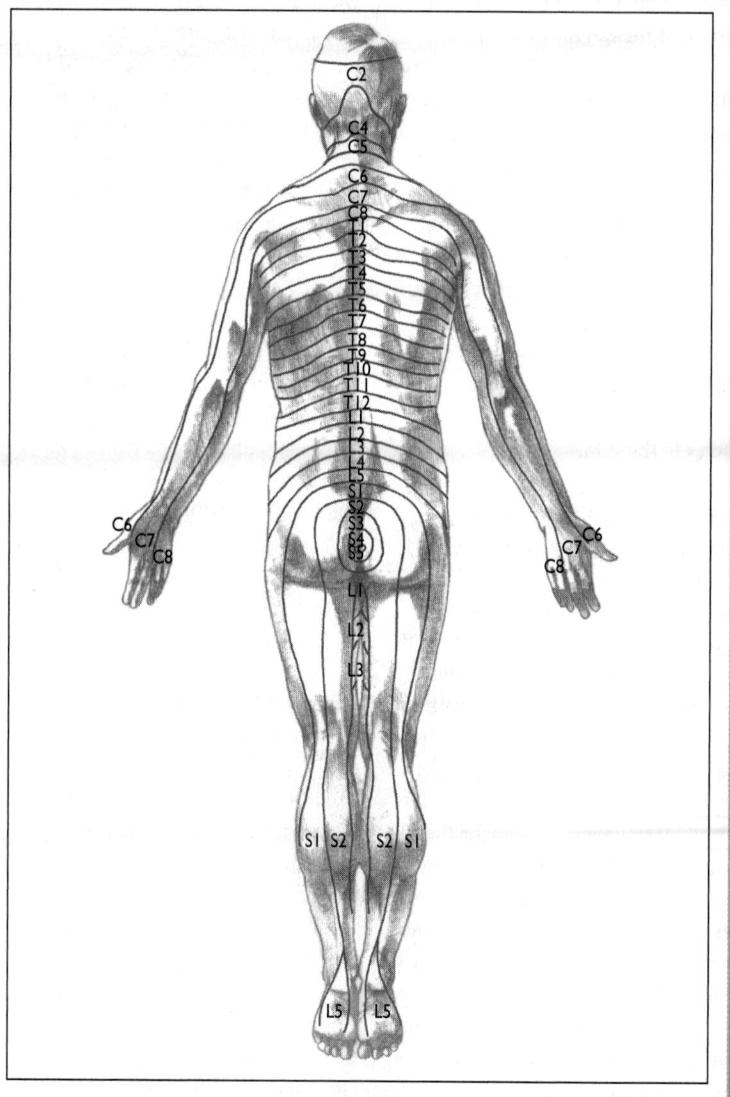

Causes

Herpes zoster is an infection caused by reactivation of the varicella-zoster virus (VZV), the same herpesvirus that causes chickenpox, which lies dormant in the cerebral ganglia (extramedullary ganglia of the cranial nerves) or the ganglia of posterior nerve roots. Although the cause for reactivation is unknown, it's thought to be associated with increasing age, stress, illness or infection, and debilitation. Although the process is unclear, the virus may multiply as it reactivates, and antibodies remaining from the initial infection may neutralize it. Without opposition from effective antibodies, the virus continues to multiply in the ganglia, destroys neurons, and spreads down the sensory nerves to the skin.

Signs and symptoms

The typical patient reports no history of exposure to others with VZV. She may complain initially of fever, malaise, unilateral stabbing pain that mimics appendicitis, tingling, itching, pleurisy, musculoskeletal pain, or other conditions. In 2 to 4 days, she may report severe, deep pain; reddening of the skin that's followed by blisters; and paresthesia or hyperesthesia (usually affecting the trunk and occasionally the arms and legs). Pain — described as intermittent, continuous, or debilitating — usually lasts from 1 to 4 weeks.

During examination of the patient within 2 weeks after her initial symptoms, you may observe small, red, nodular skin lesions spread unilaterally around the thorax or vertically over the arms or legs. Alternatively, instead of nodules, you may see vesicles filled with clear fluid or pus. About 7 to 10 days after they appear, these vesicles rupture and then dry, forming scabs. The lesions are most vulnerable to infection after rupture; some even become gangrenous. During palpation, you may detect enlarged regional lymph nodes. Herpes zoster may involve the cranial nerves (especially the trigeminal and geniculate ganglia or the oculomotor nerve). With geniculate involvement, you may observe vesicle formation in the external auditory canal and ipsilateral facial palsy. The patient may complain of hearing loss, dizziness, and loss of taste. With trigeminal involvement, the patient may complain of eye pain. She may also have corneal and scleral damage and impaired vision. Rarely, oculomotor involvement causes conjunctivitis, extraocular weakness, ptosis, and paralytic mydriasis.

Herpes zoster ophthalmicus may result in vision loss. Complications of generalized infection may involve acute urine retention and unilateral paralysis of the diaphragm. Another complication may be postherpetic neuralgia (most common in elderly patients), described as intractable neurologic pain that persists despite wound healing and that lasts more than 1 to 3 months after disease onset. In rare cases, herpes zoster may be complicated by generalized central nervous system (CNS) infection, muscle atrophy, motor paralysis (usually transient), acute transverse myelitis, and ascending myelitis. (See *Postherpetic neuralgia.*)

Diagnosis

Diagnosis is usually based on appearance of the skin lesions and a patient's past medical history of chickenpox. Tests, although usually unnecessary, may include viral culture of vesicular fluid and infected tissue analyses, which typically show eosinophilic intranuclear inclusions and varicella virus. Differentiation of herpes zoster from localized herpes simplex requires staining antibodies from vesicular fluid and identification under fluorescent light. Usually, though, the locations of herpes simplex and herpes zoster lesions are distinctly different. With CNS involvement, results of a lumbar puncture indicate increased pressure, and cerebrospinal fluid analysis demonstrates increased protein levels and, possibly, pleocytosis.

Treatment

Early treatment for herpes zoster, ideally within 48 to 72 hours of onset, provides the best chance of minimizing neurologic sequelae. Primary therapeutic goals include relief of itching with cool compresses and antipruritics (such as calamine lotion), relief of neuralgic pain with analgesics (such as aspirin [Bayer], acetaminophen [Tylenol] and, possibly, codeine), and preventing postherpetic neuralgia. A similar goal involves preventing secondary infection by applying a demulcent and skin protectant (such as collodion, compound benzoin tincture, and sulfonamide cream) to unbroken lesions. Other treatment measures include:

- Starting antiviral therapy within 2 to 3 days of onset usually provides early resolution of the skin blisters

Postherpetic Neuralgia

Postherpetic neuralgia occurs in approximately 20% of all herpes zoster cases. It's uncommon in young people but occurs in older adults, especially those over age 60. Postherpetic neuralgia is the unrelenting and sometimes debilitating pain that may persist for more than 1 month after the initial herpes zoster rash has faded and healed. The pain may develop days, weeks, or months after the rash is gone and can be described as a constant aching and burning, a cutting or stabbing pain, or allodynia, which is a feeling of heightened sensitivity to very minimal stimuli (such as a light breeze and clothing). The pain may be accompanied by a loss of sensation or numbness to the affected area. Symptoms usually last for months but, in some cases, may last for years or be lifelong.

There's no conventional treatment and sometimes even the strongest pain medications aren't helpful. Antiseizure medications such as gabapentin, antidepressants such as amitriptyline, and lidocaine patches have been found effective in some but not all patients. The best treatment for postherpetic neuralgia is prevention — early treatment with antiviral medications to speed recovery from herpes zoster and prevent the development of postherpetic neuralgia.

and shortens the duration of neurologic symptoms. Oral acyclovir therapy accelerates healing of lesions and resolution of zoster-associated pain. Famciclovir and valacyclovir have been effective and may be more effective than acyclovir. In the immunocompromised patient, herpes zoster should be treated with I.V. acyclovir.

- If bacteria infect ruptured vesicles, treatment includes an appropriate systemic antibiotic. Herpes zoster affecting trigeminal and corneal structures calls for instillation of idoxuridine ointment or another antiviral agent.
- To help a patient cope with the intractable pain of postherpetic neuralgia, a systemic corticosteroid, such as cortisone or corticotropin, may be ordered to reduce inflammation. The physician may also order tranquilizers, sedatives, or tricyclic antidepressants with phenothiazines.
- As a last resort for pain relief, transcutaneous peripheral nerve stimulation, patient-controlled analgesia, or a small dose of radiotherapy may be considered.

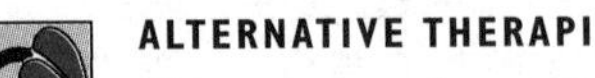

ALTERNATIVE THERAPIES

Although the safety and effectiveness of acupuncture and herbal remedies have not been adequately studied and herbal remedies aren't regulated by the FDA, some patients with herpes zoster have stated that acupuncture and herbal tonics were effective in relieving their pain. According to acupuncturists, therapy must start soon after the eruptions break out to prevent nerve damage, along with megadoses of vitamin B complexes and vitamin C to support the nervous system.

Special considerations

- Administer topical therapies. If the physician orders calamine lotion, apply it liberally to the patient's lesions. Avoid blotting contaminated swabs on unaffected skin areas. Be prepared to administer drying therapies, such as oxygen, if the patient has severe disseminated lesions. Use silver sulfadiazine to soften and debride infected lesions.
- Give analgesics exactly as scheduled to minimize severe neuralgic pain. For a patient with postherpetic neuralgia, consult with a pain specialist, and follow his recommendations to maximize pain relief without risking tolerance to the analgesic.
- Maintain meticulous hygiene to prevent spreading the infection to other parts of the patient's body.
- Monitor the patient for complications associated with herpes zoster.
- Inspect the patient's skin lesions daily for signs of healing or infection.
- To decrease discomfort from oral lesions, instruct the patient to use a soft toothbrush, eat soft foods, and use a saline- or bicarbonate-based mouthwash and oral anesthetics.
- Stress the need for adequate rest during the acute phase.

PREVENTION POINTER

Reassure the patient that herpes zoster isn't contagious to those who have already had chickenpox. However, warn her that it's contagious by direct contact with

CUTTING EDGE

Vaccinate or not?

A varicella vaccination was approved by the Food and Drug Administration in 1995 for use in children over age 1 and is now required for school entry. However, much controversy still exists surrounding this vaccine.

Promising results?

The vaccination is a live attenuated vaccine that provides long-lasting resistance to varicella. Preliminary studies show that when elderly people (who are the most affected with shingles) already harboring the dormant varicella-zoster virus receive what amounts to a booster vaccination, they significantly benefit. The booster increases cell-mediated and humoral immunity to protect the patient against viral reappearance, thus, decreasing the incidence and complications of herpes zoster. More studies, however, are needed before a booster vaccination is approved and used in elderly patients.

Increasing risk?

Recently, however, other researchers argue that the varicella vaccination could actually increase the risk of shingles in adults. Britain's Public Health Laboratory Service postulates that, although the vaccination may save thousands of lives, thousands more elderly people may die from the complications of herpes zoster. They reason that adults who live with children have more exposure to the varicella virus and, thereby, are protected against shingles because being close to the children would act like a booster vaccine. However, if all children were vaccinated, then adults who have had chickenpox would no longer have that protection or booster. Regardless, more information and data are necessary before determining the impact of the vaccine and the immunization schedule of all children in the United States.

blister fluid and may cause a person who hasn't had chickenpox previously to develop the infection. Warn her to stay away from nonimmune children, pregnant women, and elderly and immunocompromised persons until the blisters clear. (See *Vaccinate or not?*)

- Stress the need for meticulous hygiene to prevent spreading infection to other body parts.
- Repeatedly reassure the patient that herpetic pain will eventually subside. Suggest diversionary or relaxation activities to take her mind off the pain and pruritus.

Hirsutism

A distressing disorder usually found in women and children, hirsutism is the excessive growth of body hair, typically in an adult male distribution pattern. This condition commonly occurs spontaneously but may also develop as a secondary disorder of various underlying diseases. It must always be distinguished from hypertrichosis. The prognosis varies with the cause and the effectiveness of treatment.

Hypertrichosis

Hypertrichosis is a localized or generalized condition in males and females that is marked by excessive hair growth. Localized hypertrichosis usually results from local trauma, chemical irritation, or hormonal stimulation; pigmented nevi (Becker's nevus, for example) may also contain hairs. Generalized hypertrichosis results from neurologic or psychiatric disorders, such as encephalitis, multiple sclerosis, concussion, anorexia nervosa, or schizophrenia. Contributing factors include juvenile hypothyroidism, porphyria cutanea tarda, and the use of drugs such as phenytoin.

Hypertrichosis lanuginosa is a generalized proliferation of fine, lanugo-type hair (sometimes called *down,* or *woolly hair*). Such hair may be present at birth but generally disappears shortly thereafter. This condition may become chronic, with persistent lanugo-type hair growing over the entire body, or may develop suddenly later in life. It's rare and usually results from malignancy.

Causes

Idiopathic or familial hirsutism probably stems from a hereditary trait because the patient usually has a family history of the disorder. Causes of secondary hirsutism include endocrine abnormalities related to pituitary dysfunction (acromegaly, precocious puberty), adrenal dysfunction (Cushing's disease, congenital adrenal hyperplasia, or Cushing's syndrome), or ovarian lesions (such as polycystic ovary syndrome); and iatrogenic factors (such as the use of minoxidil, androgenic steroids, testosterone, diazoxide, glucocorticoids, and oral contraceptives). Other kinds of hirsutism have been reported. (See *Hypertrichosis.*)

Signs and symptoms

Hirsutism typically produces enlarged hair follicles as well as enlargement and hyperpigmentation of the hairs themselves. Excessive facial hair growth is the complaint for which most patients seek medical help. Generally, hirsutism involves the appearance of thick, pigmented hair in the beard area, upper back, shoulders, sternum, axillae, and pubic area. Frontotemporal scalp hair recession is often a coexisting condition. Patterns of hirsutism vary greatly, depending on the patient's race and age. Elderly women commonly show increased hair growth on the chin and upper lip. In secondary hirsutism, signs of masculinization may appear — deepening of the voice, increased muscle mass, increased size of genitalia, menstrual irregularity, and decreased breast size.

Diagnosis

A family history of hirsutism, absence of menstrual abnormalities, signs of masculinization, and a normal pelvic examination strongly suggest idiopathic hirsutism. Tests for secondary hirsutism depend on associated symptoms that suggest an underlying disorder. About 90% of women with hirsutism have an elevated free testosterone level.

Treatment

At the patient's request, treatment of idiopathic hirsutism consists of eliminating excess hair by scissors, shaving, or depilatory creams, or removal of the entire hair shaft with tweezers or wax. Bleaching the hair with hydrogen peroxide may also provide satisfactory results. Electrolysis can destroy hair bulbs permanently, but it works best when only a few hairs need to be removed. (A patient history of keloid formation contraindicates this procedure.) Hirsutism caused by elevated androgen levels may require low-dose dexamethasone or prednisone, oral contraceptives, or androgen receptor-competitive inhibitors, such as spironolactone, cyproterone acetate, or cimetidine; however, these drugs vary in effectiveness. Treatment of secondary hirsutism depends on the underlying disorder.

Special considerations

Care for patients with idiopathic hirsutism focuses on emotional support and patient teaching; care for patients with secondary hirsutism depends on the treatment of the underlying disease:

- Provide emotional support and be sensitive to the patient's feelings about her appearance.
- Watch for signs of contact dermatitis in patients being treated with depilatory creams, especially elderly patients. Also watch for infection of hair follicles after hair removal with tweezers or wax.
- Suggest consulting a cosmetologist about makeup or bleaching agents.

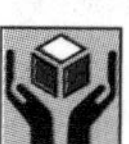

SPECIAL NEEDS

Remember that antiandrogen treatments should be avoided in pregnant women. In addition, counsel women of childbearing age to use effective contraceptive methods during therapy because treatment during pregnancy may cause malformation and pseudohermaphroditism in male infants.

HIV and AIDS

The Centers for Disease Control and Prevention (CDC) first recognized human immunodeficiency virus (HIV) and acquired immunodeficiency syndrome (AIDS) in 1981. One of the most widely publicized diseases, AIDS is characterized by progressive immunodeficiency. Although it's characterized by progressive destruction of cell-mediated (T-cell) immunity, it also affects humoral immunity, and even autoimmunity because of the central role of $CD4^+$ T cells in immune reactions. The resultant immunodeficiency makes the patient susceptible to opportunistic infections, unusual cancers, and other abnormalities that define AIDS. (See *Common AIDS infections and neoplasms*, page 312.)

A retrovirus — HIV, type I — is the primary etiologic agent. Transmission of HIV occurs by contact with infected blood or body fluids and is associated with identifiable high-risk behaviors. As a result, HIV incidence is disproportionately high in I.V. drug users, homosexual and bisexual men, neonates of HIV-infected women, recipients of contaminated blood or

Common AIDS infections and neoplasms

Infections and neoplasms commonly seen in patients with acquired immunodeficiency syndrome (AIDS) are listed here.

Infections

Common infections in AIDS may be protozoal, fungal, mycobacterial, or viral.

Protozoal

Cryptosporidium
Pneumocystis carinii
Toxoplasma gondii

Fungal

Candida species
Cryptococcus neoformans
Histoplasmosis

Mycobacterial

Mycobacterium avium-intracellulare
M. tuberculosis

Viral

Cytomegalovirus
Herpesvirus

Neoplasms

Hodgkin's disease
Kaposi's sarcoma
Malignant lymphoma

blood products (dramatically decreased since the mid-1980s), and heterosexual partners of people in the former groups. Because of similar routes of transmission, AIDS shares epidemiologic patterns with hepatitis B and sexually transmitted diseases. Thus, the number of women with HIV and AIDS is rising steadily, and HIV infection is now the third leading cause of death among women ages 25 to 44. HIV and AIDS also disproportionately affect minority women in the United States, making them the leading cause of death among Black women in this age group and Hispanic women in general. These two minority groups account for over 80% of women affected with HIV and AIDS in the United States. Also, because women in general have poorer access to or fail to use health care and social services, HIV-infected women are one-third more likely to die sooner than HIV-infected men.

The natural history of AIDS infection begins with infection by the HIV retrovirus, which is detectable only by laboratory tests, and ends with the severely immunocompromised, terminal stage of this disease. Depending on individual variations and the presence of cofactors that influence progression, the time elapsed from acute HIV infection to the appearance of symptoms (mild to severe), to diagnosis of AIDS and, eventually, to death varies greatly. More recently, dramatic advances in antiretroviral therapy and treatment and prophylaxis of common opportunistic infections have delayed the natural progression of HIV infection and prolonged survival.

Causes

AIDS results from infection with HIV, which strikes cells bearing the CD4 antigen; the latter (normally a receptor for major histocompatibility complex molecules) serves as a receptor for the retrovirus and lets it enter the cell. HIV prefers to infect the $CD4^+$ lymphocyte but may also infect other

$CD4^+$ antigen-bearing cells in the GI tract and uterine cervix as well as neuroglial cells. After invading a cell, the HIV replicates, leading to cell death, or becomes latent. HIV infection leads to profound pathology either directly, through destruction of $CD4^+$ cells, other immune cells, and neuroglial cells, or indirectly, through the secondary effects of $CD4^+$ T-cell dysfunction and resultant immunosuppression.

The infection process takes three forms:

- immunodeficiency (opportunistic infections and unusual cancers)
- autoimmunity (lymphoid interstitial pneumonitis, arthritis, hypergammaglobulinemia, and production of autoimmune antibodies)
- neurologic dysfunction (AIDS dementia complex, HIV encephalopathy, and peripheral neuropathies).

HIV is transmitted by direct inoculation during intimate sexual contact, especially associated with the mucosal trauma of receptive rectal intercourse, transfusion of contaminated blood or blood products (a risk diminished by routine testing of all blood products), sharing of contaminated needles, or transplacental or postpartum transmission from infected mother to fetus (by cervical or blood contact at delivery and in breast milk). For women, transmission through heterosexual intimate contact is the leading cause of transmission. Accumulating evidence suggests that casual household or social contact doesn't transmit HIV. The average time between exposure to the virus and diagnosis of AIDS is 8 to 10 years, but shorter and longer incubation times have also been recorded.

Signs and symptoms

HIV infection manifests in many ways. After a high-risk exposure and inoculation, the infected person usually experiences a mononucleosis-like syndrome, which may be attributed to the flu or another virus. The patient then may remain asymptomatic for years. In this latent stage, the only sign of HIV infection is laboratory evidence of seroconversion. When symptoms appear, they may take many forms, such as persistent generalized adenopathy, nonspecific signs and symptoms (weight loss, fatigue, night sweats, and fevers), neurologic symptoms resulting from HIV encephalopathy, an opportunistic infection, or cancer.

In addition to the symptoms common to men and women, women also experience HIV-gynecologic problems, such as recurrent vaginal yeast infections, other vaginal infections, severe herpes simplex virus ulcers, idiopathic genital ulcers, human papillomavirus infections, pelvic inflammatory disease, and menstrual irregularities.

The clinical course of HIV and AIDS varies slightly in children. Apparently, incubation time is shorter, with a mean of 17 months. Signs and symptoms resemble those in adults, except for findings related to sexually transmitted disease. Children show virtually all of the opportunistic infections observed in adults, with a higher incidence of bacterial infections, including otitis media, pneumonias other than that caused by *Pneumocystis carinii*, sepsis, chronic salivary gland enlargement, and lymphoid interstitial pneumonia.

Diagnosis

The CDC defines AIDS as an illness characterized by one or more "indicator" diseases that coexist with laboratory evidence of HIV infection and other possible causes of immunosuppression. The CDC's current AIDS surveillance case definition requires laboratory confirmation of HIV infection in people who have a CD4+ T-lymphocyte count of greater than 200 cells/μl or who have an associated clinical condition or disease.

The most commonly performed tests, antibody tests, indicate HIV infection indirectly by revealing HIV antibodies. The recommended protocol requires initial screening of individuals and blood products with an enzyme-linked immunosorbent assay (ELISA). A positive ELISA should be repeated and then confirmed by an alternate method, usually the Western blot or an immunofluorescence assay. The radioimmunoprecipitation assay is considered more sensitive and specific than the Western blot. Because it requires radioactive materials, it's a poor choice for routine screening. In addition, antibody testing isn't reliable. Because people produce detectable levels of antibodies at different rates — a "window" varying from a few weeks to as long as 35 months in one documented case — an HIV-infected person can test negative for HIV antibodies. Antibody tests are also unreliable in neonates because transferred maternal antibodies persist for 6 to 10 months. To overcome these problems, direct tests are used, including antigen tests (p24 antigen), HIV cultures, nucleic acid probes of peripheral blood lymphocytes, and the polymerase chain reaction. (See *HIV laboratory tests.*)

Additional tests to support an HIV diagnosis and help evaluate the severity of immunosuppression include $CD4^+$ and $CD8^+$ T-lymphocyte subset counts, erythrocyte sedimentation rate, complete blood cell count, serum $beta_2$-microglobulin, p24 antigen, neopterin levels, and anergy testing. Because many opportunistic infections in AIDS patients are reactivations of previous infections, patients are also tested for syphilis, hepatitis B, tuberculosis, toxoplasmosis and, in some areas, histoplasmosis.

Treatment

To date, there's no known cure for AIDS; however, in 1998, the CDC recommended that all people who have symptomatic or HIV infection receive aggressive antiviral therapy. In July of 2003, the CDC revised its guidelines for initiating treatment of antiretroviral therapy. (See *New guidelines for antiretroviral therapy,* pages 316 and 317.)

Treatment for HIV infection can be divided into four categories: prevention and therapy for opportunistic infections and malignancies, antiretroviral treatment, and hematopoietic stimulating factors.

HIV LABORATORY TESTS

This chart lists laboratory tests used for diagnosing and tracking human immunodeficiency virus (HIV) and assessing the patient's immune status.

Test	Findings in HIV infection
HIV antibody tests	
▪ Enzyme-linked immunosorbent assay	▪ Positive test results that must be confirmed by Western blot
▪ Western blot	▪ Positive
▪ Indirect immunofluorescence assay	▪ Positive test results that must be confirmed by Western blot
▪ Radioimmunoprecipitation assay	▪ Positive, more sensitive and specific than Western blot
HIV tracking	
▪ p24 antigen	▪ Positive for free viral protein
▪ Polymerase chain reaction	▪ Detection of HIV RNA or DNA
▪ Branch DNA	▪ Detection of HIV RNA
▪ Nucleic acid sequence-based amplification	▪ Detection of HIV RNA
▪ Peripheral blood mononuclear cell culture for HIV-1	▪ Positive when two consecutive assays detect reverse transcriptase or p24 antigen in increasing magnitude
▪ Quantitative cell culture	▪ Indication of viral load within cells
▪ Quantitative plasma culture	▪ Indication of viral load by free infectious virus in the plasma
▪ β_2 microglobulin	▪ Increased protein with disease progression
▪ Serum neopterin	▪ Increased levels seen with disease progression
Immune status	
▪ $CD4^+$ cell count	▪ Decreased
▪ $CD4^+$ cell percentage	▪ Decreased
▪ Ratio of $CD4^+$ cells to $CD8^+$ cells	▪ Decreased ratio of $CD4^+$ cells to $CD8^+$ cells
▪ White blood cell count	▪ Normal to decreased
▪ Immunoglobulin levels	▪ Increased
▪ $CD4^+$ cell function tests	▪ $CD4^+$ cells have decreased ability to respond to antigen
▪ Skin test sensitivity reaction	▪ Decreased to absent

Nucleoside analogues (sometimes called *reverse transcriptase inhibitors*) have been the mainstay of AIDS therapy in recent years. These drugs, which include zidovudine (AZT), lamivudine, didanosine, stavudine, abacavir, and zalcitabine, interfere with viral reverse transcriptase, which impairs

NEW GUIDELINES FOR ANTIRETROVIRAL THERAPY

The optimal time to initiate antiretroviral therapy is unknown among asymptomatic persons with HIV disease and CD4+ T-cell count of > 200 cells/µl. This table provides general guidance rather than absolute recommendations for an individual patient. All decisions regarding therapy should consider prognosis determined by the CD4+ T-cell count and level of plasma HIV RNA and the po-

Clinical category	CD4+ T-cell count	Plasma HIV RNA
Symptomatic (AIDS or severe symptoms)	Any value	Any value
Asymptomatic, AIDS	CD4+ T cells < 200/µl	Any value
Asymptomatic	CD4+ T cells > 200/µl but ≤ 350/µl	Any value
Asymptomatic	CD4+ T cells > 350/µl	> 55,000 (by RT-PCR or bDNA)**
Asymptomatic	CD4+ T cells > 350/µl	< 55,000 (by RT-PCR or bDNA)**

*Clinical benefit has been demonstrated in controlled trials only for patients with CD4+ T-cell count < 200/µl; however, the majority of physicians would offer therapy at a CD4+ T-cell threshold < 350/µl. A recent evaluation of data from the Multicenter AIDS Cohort Study (MACS) of 232 persons with CD4+ T-cell counts > 200 and < 350 cells/µl demonstrated that of 40 (17%) persons with plasma HIV RNA < 10,000 copies/ml, none progressed to AIDS by 3 years. (Source: Phair J.P., et al. "Virologic and immunologic values allowing safe deferral of antiretrovrial therapy," *AIDS* 16 (918): 2455-59. 2002) Of 28 persons (29%) with plasma viremia of 10,000 to 20,000 copies/ml, 4% and 11% progressed to AIDS at 2 and 3 years respectively. Plasma HIV RNA was calculated as RT-PCR values from measured bDNA values. (For additional information see *Considerations for Initiating Therapy for the Patient with Asymptomatic HIB-12 Infection.*)

tential benefits and risks of therapy, as indicated in this table, as well as the willingness of the patient to accept therapy.

Recommendation
Offer treatment.
Offer treatment.
Treatment should be offered, although it's controversial.*
Some experienced physicians recommend initiating therapy, recognizing that the 3-year risk for untreated patients to develop AIDS is > 30%. In the absence of increased levels of plasma HIV RNA, other physicians recommend deferring therapy and monitoring the CD4+ T-cell count and level of plasma HIV RNA more frequently. Clinical outcome data after initiating therapy are lacking.
Most experienced physicians recommend deferring therapy and monitoring the CD4+ T-cell count, recognizing that the 3-year risk for untreated patients to experience AIDS is < 15%.

**Although a 2- to 2.5-fold difference existed between RT-PCR and the first bDNA assay (version 2.0), with the 3.0 version bDNA assay, values obtained by bDNA and RT-PCR are similar except at the lower end of the linear range (< 1,500 copies/ml).

HIV's ability to turn its ribonucleic acid into deoxyribonucleic acid for insertion into the host cell.

Antiretroviral therapy typically begins when the patient's CD4+ T-cell count drops to less than 350/µl or when the patient develops an opportunistic infection. Most clinicians recommend starting the patient on a combination of these drugs in an attempt to gain the maximum benefit and inhibit the production of resistant mutant strains of HIV. The drug combinations and dosages are then altered, depending on the patient's response.

Increasingly, physicians are basing changes in therapy on the patient's viral load rather than on her CD4+ T cell count. Because the CD4+ count is influenced by the total white blood cell count, changes in the CD4+ count may have nothing to do with changes in the patient's HIV status. Many physicians recommend that a patient on antiretroviral therapy should have her viral load checked every 3 months.

Protease inhibitors, another class of antiretroviral agents, have greatly increased the life expectancy of AIDS patients. These drugs (which include ritonavir, indinavir, nelfinavir, and saquinavir) block the enzyme protease, which HIV needs to produce virions, the viral particles that spread the virus to other cells. The use of protease inhibitors dramatically reduces viral load — sometimes to undetectable levels — while producing a corresponding increase in the CD4+ T-cell count and, because they act at a different site than nucleoside analogues, protease inhibitors don't produce additional adverse effects when added to a patient's regimen.

After antiviral therapy is initiated, treatment should be aggressive. Initially, highly active antiviral therapy, consisting of a triple drug therapy regimen — a protease inhibitor and two non-nucleoside reverse transcriptase inhibitors — is recommended. In addition to these primary treatments, anti-infectives are used to combat opportunistic infections (or, with some patients, prophylactically to help resist opportunistic infections), and antineoplastic drugs are used to fight associated neoplasms. Supportive treatments help maintain nutritional status and relieve pain and other distressing physical and psychological symptoms.

Special considerations

- Advise health care workers and the public to use precautions in all situations that risk exposure to blood, body fluids, and secretions. Diligently practicing standard precautions can prevent the inadvertent transmission of AIDS and other infectious diseases transmitted by similar routes.
- Recognize that a diagnosis of AIDS is profoundly distressing because of the disease's social impact and discouraging prognosis. The patient may lose her job and financial security as well as the support of family and friends. Do your best to help the patient cope with an altered body image, the emotional burden of serious illness, and the threat of death, and encourage and assist the patient in learning about AIDS societies and support programs.
- Encourage HIV-positive women to have a complete gynecologic evaluation, including a Papanicolaou smear initially, during prenatal care, and then annually (every 6 months for those who are symptomatic).

Hyperparathyroidism

Hyperparathyroidism results from excessive secretion of parathyroid hormone (PTH) from one or more of the four parathyroid glands. PTH promotes bone resorption, and hypersecretion leads to hypercalcemia and hypophosphatemia. Overproduction of PTH by a tumor or hyperplastic tissue increases intestinal calcium absorption, reduces renal calcium clearance, and increases bone calcium release. Response to this excess varies for each patient for an unknown reason. It's three times more common in women than in men and the frequency increases with age.

Causes

Hyperparathyroidism may be primary or secondary. Although the exact cause is unknown, it's thought that primary hyperparathyroidism may be caused by:

- increased secretion of PTH (which can lead to increased serum calcium levels) by one or more enlarged parathyroid glands (most commonly caused by a single adenoma, but may

be a component of multiple endocrine neoplasia, which usually involves all four glands)
- parathyroid carcinoma
- previous exposure to radiation in the face or neck
- certain medications, such as thiazide diuretics and lithium
- heredity.

Secondary hyperparathyroidism occurs when the parathyroid gland chronically releases excessive PTH. A hypocalcemic state (decrease in circulating calcium) causes this release. Causes include:
- rickets
- chronic renal failure
- vitamin D deficiency
- malabsorption syndrome
- osteomalacia due to phenytoin (Dilantin).

Signs and symptoms

Signs and symptoms of primary hyperparathyroidism result from hypercalcemia and are typically present in several body systems. They may include:
- *renal and urinary systems* — polyuria, nephrocalcinosis, nocturia, polydipsia, dehydration, uremia symptoms, renal colic pain, nephrolithiasis, and renal insufficiency
- *musculoskeletal system* — vague aches and pains; arthralgias; localized swellings; chronic lower back pain and easy fracturing due to bone degeneration; bone tenderness; chondrocalcinosis (decreased bone mass); osteopenia and osteoporosis, especially affecting the vertebrae; erosions of the juxta-articular (adjoining joint) surface; subchondral fractures; traumatic synovitis; pseudogout (skeletal and articular systems); and muscle weakness and atrophy, particularly in the legs
- *gastrointestinal system* — pancreatitis causing constant, severe epigastric pain that radiates to the back; peptic ulcers causing abdominal pain, anorexia, nausea, and vomiting
- *central nervous system* — psychomotor and personality disturbances, emotional lability, depression, slow mentation, poor memory, drowsiness, ataxia, overt psychosis, stupor and, possibly, coma
- *integumentary system* — skin necrosis and pruritus caused by ectopic calcifications in the skin
- *other systems* — calcium microthrombi to lungs and pancreas, cataracts, anemia, and subcutaneous calcification.

Secondary hyperparathyroidism may produce the same features of calcium imbalance with skeletal deformities of the long bones (such as rickets) as well as symptoms of the underlying disease.

Complications of hyperparathyroidism include:
- pathologic fractures
- renal damage
- urinary tract infections
- hypertension
- arrhythmias
- insulin hypersecretion, decreased insulin sensitivity
- pseudogout.

Diagnosis

Primary hyperparathyroidism is commonly diagnosed based on elevated calcium levels (more than 10.5 mg/dl) in asymptomatic patients. Findings differ in primary and secondary disease. In primary disease, diagnosis also may be based on:

- hypercalcemia and high concentrations of serum PTH on radioimmunoassay, which confirms the diagnosis (Immunoradiometric assay [IRMA] is specific and sensitive in distinguishing primary hyperparathyroidism from other causes of hypercalcemia.)
- X-rays showing diffuse demineralization of bones, bone cysts, outer cortical bone absorption, and subperiosteal erosion of the phalanges and distal clavicles
- microscopic bone examination by X-ray spectrophotometry typically showing increased bone turnover
- elevated urine and serum calcium, chloride, and alkaline phosphatase levels; decreased serum phosphorus levels
- elevated uric acid and creatinine levels, which may also increase basal gastric acid secretion and serum immunoreactive gastrin
- increased serum amylase levels (may indicate acute pancreatitis).

Diagnosis of secondary disease is based on:

- normal or slightly decreased serum calcium level, variable serum phosphorus level, especially when the cause is rickets, osteomalacia, or kidney disease
- patient history possibly showing familial kidney disease, seizure disorders, or drug ingestion.

Treatment

Effective treatment varies, depending on the cause of the disease. In primary hyperparathyroidism, surgery is the only definitive therapy. In mild hyperparathyroidism, the only effective long-term medical therapy is maintaining hydration.

Treatment of primary disease includes:

- surgery to remove the adenoma or, depending on the extent of hyperplasia, all but one-half of one gland, to provide normal PTH levels (may relieve bone pain within 3 days, but renal damage may be irreversible)
- decreasing calcium levels using such methods as forcing fluids, limiting dietary intake of calcium, and promoting sodium and calcium excretion through forced diuresis (causing as much as 6 qt [6 L] of urine output in life-threatening circumstances), and use of furosemide (Lasix) or ethacrynic acid (Edecrin) (preoperatively or if surgery isn't feasible or necessary)
- oral sodium or potassium phosphate, subcutaneous calcitonin (Calcimar), I.V. plicamycin
- I.V. magnesium and phosphate or sodium phosphate solution by mouth or retention enema (for potential postoperative magnesium and phosphate deficiencies), possibly supplemental calcium, vitamin D, or calcitriol (Calcijex) (serum calcium level decreases to low-normal range during the first 4 to 5 days after surgery).

Treatment of secondary disease includes:

- vitamin D to correct the underlying cause of parathyroid hyperplasia; aluminum hydroxide preparation to correct hyperphosphatemia in the patient with kidney disease
- dialysis in the patient with renal failure to decrease phosphorus levels (may be lifelong)
- decreasing calcium levels, although enlarged glands may not revert to normal size and function even after calcium levels have been controlled in the patient with chronic secondary hyperparathyroidism
- for severe hypercalcemia (serum calcium greater than 14 mg/dl) or for the patient with severe symptoms, administration of calcitonin, a rapid-acting agent, along with hydration; possible initiation of pamidronate, a slower-acting agent, to provide a longer-lasting effect.

Special considerations

Care emphasizes prevention of complications from the underlying disease and its treatment:

- Obtain pretreatment baseline serum potassium, calcium, phosphate, and magnesium levels because these values may change abruptly during treatment.
- During hydration to reduce serum calcium level, record intake and output accurately. Strain urine to check for calculi. Provide at least 3 qt (3 L) of fluid per day, including cranberry or prune juice to increase urine acidity and help prevent calculus formation. As ordered, obtain blood samples and urine specimens to measure sodium, potassium, and magnesium levels, especially for the patient taking furosemide.

PREVENTION POINTER

Because the patient is predisposed to pathologic fractures, take safety precautions to minimize the risk of injury. Assist her with walking, keep the bed at its lowest position, and raise the side rails. Lift the immobilized patient carefully to minimize bone stress. Schedule care to allow as much rest as possible for the patient with muscle weakness.

- Watch for signs of peptic ulcer and administer antacids as appropriate.

After parathyroidectomy:

- Check frequently for respiratory distress, and keep a tracheotomy tray at the bedside. Watch for postoperative complications, such as laryngeal nerve damage or, rarely, hemorrhage. Monitor intake and output carefully.
- Check for swelling at the operative site. Place the patient in semi-Fowler's position, and support the head and neck with sandbags to decrease edema, which may cause pressure on the trachea.
- Watch for signs of mild tetany, such as complaints of tingling in the hands and around the mouth. These symptoms should subside quickly but may be prodromal signs of tetany, so keep calcium gluconate or calcium chloride I.V. available for emergency administration. Watch for increased neuromuscular irritability and other signs of severe tetany, and report them immediately.

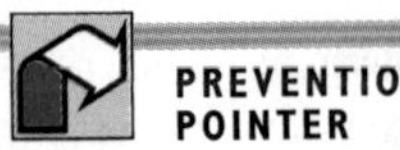

PREVENTION POINTER

Patient teaching for hyperparathyroidism

At discharge, instruct the patient to:
- drink enough fluids to avoid dehydration, which can increase blood calcium levels
- maintain regular exercise and avoid immobilization
- limit calcium intake to 1,200 mg per day
- avoid calcium-containing antacids
- avoid thiazide diuretics or any other medications that may further stimulate the parathyroid gland
- keep appointments for regular checkups for calcium monitoring.

- Ambulate the patient as soon as possible postoperatively, even though she may find this uncomfortable, because pressure on bones speeds up bone recalcification.
- Check laboratory results for low serum calcium and magnesium levels.
- Monitor for changes in mental status and watch for listlessness. In the patient with persistent hypercalcemia, check for muscle weakness and psychiatric symptoms. (Hypercalcemic states may cause anxiety, depression, psychosis, apathy, and fatigue.)
- At discharge, provide thorough patient-teaching to help avoid complications. (See *Patient teaching for hyperparathyroidism.*)

Hyperprolactinemia

Hyperprolactinemia, also known as *galactorrhea*, is inappropriate breast milk secretion. It generally occurs 3 to 6 months after the discontinuation of breast-feeding (usually after a first delivery). It may also follow an abortion or may develop in a female who hasn't been pregnant; it rarely occurs in males.

Causes

Hyperprolactinemia usually develops in a person with increased prolactin secretion from the anterior pituitary gland, with possible abnormal patterns of secretion of growth hormone, thyroid hormone, and corticotropin. However, increased prolactin serum concentration doesn't always cause hyperprolactinemia.

Additional factors that may precipitate this disorder include:
- *endogenous* — pituitary (high incidence with chromophobe adenoma), ovarian, or adrenal tumors and hypothyroidism; in males, pituitary, testicular, or pineal gland tumors
- *idiopathic* — possibly from stress or anxiety, which causes neurogenic depression of the prolactin-inhibiting factor
- *exogenous* — breast stimulation, genital stimulation, or drugs (such as hormonal contraceptives, meprobamate, and phenothiazines).

Signs and symptoms

In the female with hyperprolactinemia, milk continues to flow after the 21-day period that's normal after weaning. Hyperprolactinemia may also be spontaneous and unrelated to normal lactation, or it may be caused by manual expression. Such abnormal flow is usually bilateral and may be accompanied by amenorrhea.

Diagnosis

Characteristic clinical features and the patient history (including drug and sex histories) confirm hyperprolactinemia. Laboratory tests to help determine the cause include measurement of serum levels of prolactin, cortisol, thyroid-stimulating hormone, triiodothyronine, and thyroxine. A pregnancy test, computed tomography scan and, possibly, mammography may also be indicated.

Treatment

Treatment varies according to the underlying cause and ranges from simple avoidance of precipitating exogenous factors, such as drugs, to treatment of tumors with surgery, radiation, or chemotherapy.

Therapy for idiopathic hyperprolactinemia depends on whether the patient plans to have more children. If she does, treatment usually consists of bromocriptine; if she doesn't, oral estrogens (such as ethinyl estradiol) and progestins (such as progesterone) effectively treat this disorder. Idiopathic hyperprolactinemia may recur after discontinuation of drug therapy.

Special considerations

- Watch for central nervous system abnormalities, such as headache, failing vision, and dizziness.
- Maintain adequate fluid intake, especially if the patient has a fever. However, advise the patient to avoid tea, coffee, and certain tranquilizers that may aggravate engorgement.
- Instruct the patient to keep her breasts and nipples clean.
- Tell the patient who's taking bromocriptine to report nausea, vomiting, dyspepsia, loss of appetite, dizziness, fatigue, numbness, and hypotension. To prevent GI upset, advise her to eat small meals frequently and to take this drug with dry toast or crackers. After treatment with bromocriptine, milk secretion usually stops in 1 to 2 months, and menstruation recurs after 6 to 24 weeks.

Hypertension

Hypertension, an elevation in diastolic or systolic blood pressure, occurs as two major types: essential (primary) hypertension, occurring in 95% of cases with no identifiable cause, and secondary hypertension, occurring in 5% of cases as a result from renal disease or another identifiable cause. Malignant hypertension is a severe, fulminant form of hypertension common to both types. Hypertension is a major cause of stroke, heart disease, and renal failure.

Hypertension affects 15% to 20% of adults in the United States and the risk increases with age. Incidence is higher in those with less education and lower income.

SPECIAL NEEDS

Blacks are at an increased risk for primary hypertension when predisposition to low plasma renin levels diminishes the ability to excrete excess sodium. Hypertension develops at an earlier age in Blacks and tends to be more severe than in Whites.

Men have a higher incidence of hypertension from youth to middle adulthood; thereafter, women — in particular, postmenopausal women — have a higher incidence. According to Harvard Medical School, high blood pressure kills over 100,000 women annually and causes heart failure in 60% of affected women. Furthermore, high blood pressure poses a serious problem in pregnancy.

Essential hypertension usually begins insidiously as a benign disease that slowly progresses to a malignant state. If untreated, even mild cases can cause major complications and death. Carefully managed treatment, which may include lifestyle modifications and drug therapy, improves the prognosis. Untreated, it carries a high mortality rate. Severely elevated blood pressure (hypertensive crisis) may be fatal.

Causes

Risk factors for primary hypertension include:

- family history
- advancing age
- sleep apnea
- race (most common in blacks)
- obesity
- tobacco use
- high sodium intake
- high saturated fat intake
- excessive alcohol consumption
- sedentary lifestyle
- stress
- excess renin
- mineral deficiencies (calcium, potassium, and magnesium)
- diabetes mellitus.

Causes of secondary hypertension include:

- chronic renal disease (most common)
- coarctation of the aorta
- renal artery stenosis and parenchymal disease
- brain tumor, quadriplegia, and head injury
- pheochromocytoma, Cushing's syndrome, hyperaldosteronism, and thyroid, pituitary, or parathyroid dysfunction
- hormonal contraceptives, cocaine, epoetin alfa, sympathetic stimulants, monoamine oxidase inhibitors taken with tyramine, estrogen replacement therapy, and nonsteroidal anti-inflammatory drugs
- excessive alcohol consumption
- pregnancy-induced hypertension, also called *gestational hypertension* or *preeclampsia*. (For more details, see "Pregnancy-induced hypertension," page 398.)

Several theories help explain the development of hypertension, including:

Understanding blood pressure regulation

Hypertension may result from a disturbance in one of several intrinsic mechanisms listed here.

Renin-angiotensin system

The renin-angiotensin system acts to increase blood pressure through these mechanisms:

1. Sodium depletion, reduced blood pressure, and dehydration stimulate renin release.
2. Renin reacts with angiotensin, a liver enzyme, and converts it to angiotensin I, which increases preload and afterload.
3. Angiotensin I converts to angiotensin II in the lungs; angiotensin II is a potent vasoconstrictor that targets the arterioles.
4. Angiotensin II works to increase preload and afterload by stimulating the adrenal cortex to secrete aldosterone; this increases blood volume by conserving sodium and water.

Autoregulation

Several intrinsic mechanisms work to change an artery's diameter to maintain tissue and organ perfusion despite fluctuations in systemic blood pressure. These mechanisms include:

- stress relaxation, in which blood vessels gradually dilate when blood pressure increases to reduce peripheral resistance
- capillary fluid shift, in which plasma moves between vessels and extravascular spaces to maintain intravascular volume.

Sympathetic nervous system

When blood pressure drops, baroreceptors in the aortic arch and carotid sinuses decrease their inhibition of the medulla's vasomotor center. The consequent increases in sympathetic stimulation of the heart by norepinephrine increases cardiac output by strengthening the contractile force, raising the heart rate, and augmenting peripheral resistance by vasoconstriction. Stress can also stimulate the sympathetic nervous system to increase cardiac output and peripheral vascular resistance.

Antidiuretic hormone

The release of antidiuretic hormone can regulate hypotension by increasing reabsorption of water by the kidneys. With reabsorption, blood plasma volume increases, thus raising blood pressure.

- changes in the arteriolar bed, causing increased peripheral vascular resistance
- abnormally increased tone in the sympathetic nervous system that originates in the vasomotor system centers, causing increased peripheral vascular resistance
- increased blood volume resulting from renal or hormonal dysfunction
- an increase in arteriolar thickening caused by genetic factors, leading to increased peripheral vascular resistance
- abnormal renin release, resulting in the formation of angiotensin II, which constricts the arteriole and increases blood volume. (See *Understanding blood pressure regulation.*)

Signs and symptoms

Although hypertension is commonly asymptomatic, these signs and symptoms may occur:

- elevated blood pressure readings on at least two consecutive occasions after initial screening
- occipital headache (possibly worsening on rising in the morning as a result of increased intracranial pressure) with possible nausea and vomiting
- epistaxis possibly due to vascular involvement
- bruits (which may be heard over the abdominal aorta or carotid, renal, and femoral arteries) caused by stenosis or aneurysm
- dizziness, confusion, and fatigue caused by decreased tissue perfusion due to vasoconstriction of blood vessels
- blurry vision as a result of retinal damage
- nocturia caused by an increase in blood flow to the kidneys and an increase in glomerular filtration
- edema caused by increased capillary pressure.

SPECIAL NEEDS

Because many older adults have a wide auscultatory gap—the hiatus between the first Korotkoff sound and the next sound—failure to pump the blood pressure cuff up high enough can lead to missing the first beat and underestimating systolic blood pressure. To avoid missing the first Korotkoff sound when checking for elevated blood pressure, palpate the radial artery and inflate the cuff to approximately 20 mm beyond the point at which the pulse beat disappears.

If secondary hypertension exists, other signs and symptoms may be related to the cause. For example, Cushing's syndrome may cause truncal obesity and purple striae, whereas patients with pheochromocytoma may develop headache, nausea, vomiting, palpitations, pallor, and profuse perspiration.

Complications of hypertension include:

- hypertensive crisis, peripheral arterial disease, dissecting aortic aneurysm, coronary artery disease, angina, myocardial infarction (MI), heart failure, arrhythmias, and sudden death (see *What happens in hypertensive crisis*)
- transient ischemic attacks, stroke, retinopathy, and hypertensive encephalopathy
- renal failure.

Diagnosis

These tests help diagnose hypertensions:

- Serial blood pressure measurements of more than 140/90 mm Hg confirm hypertension.
- Urinalysis may show protein, casts, red blood cells, or white blood cells, suggesting renal disease; presence of catecholamines associated with pheochromocytoma; or glucose, suggesting diabetes.
- Laboratory tests may reveal elevated blood urea nitrogen and serum creatinine levels, suggesting renal disease, or hypokalemia indicating adrenal dysfunction (primary hyperaldosteronism).
- Complete blood count may reveal other causes of hypertension, such as polycythemia or anemia.

What happens in hypertensive crisis

Hypertensive crisis is a severe increase in arterial blood pressure caused by a disturbance in one or more of the regulating mechanisms. If untreated, hypertensive crisis may result in renal, cardiac, or cerebral complications and, possibly, death.

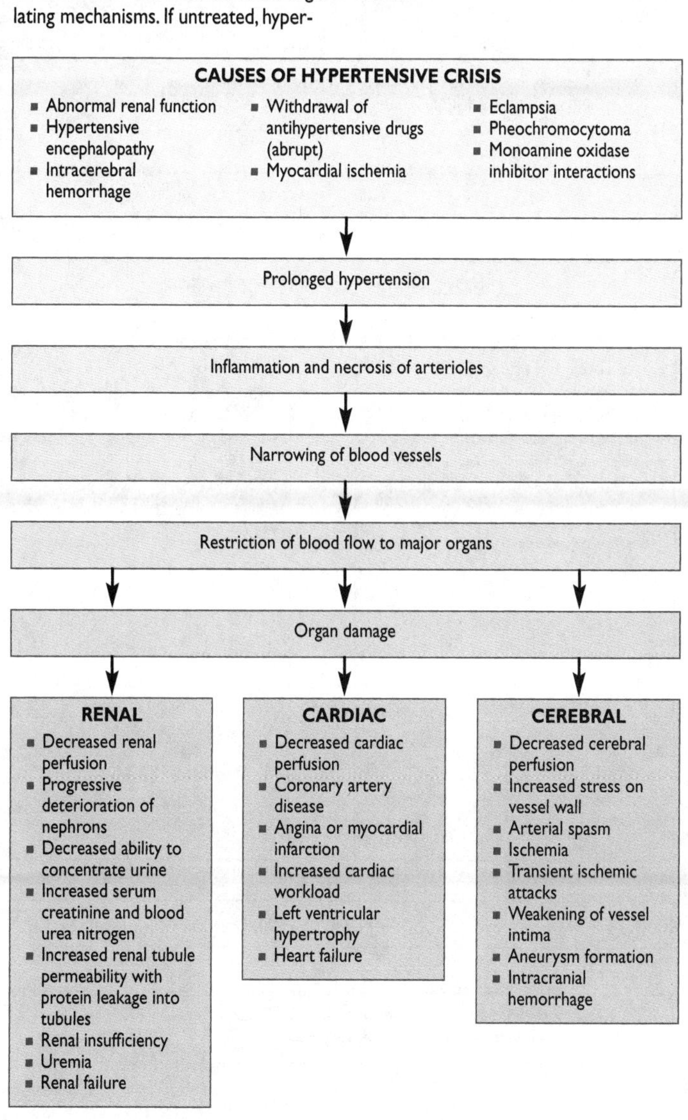

New blood pressure guidelines

This flowchart outlines guidelines for treatment stages in patients with hypertension.

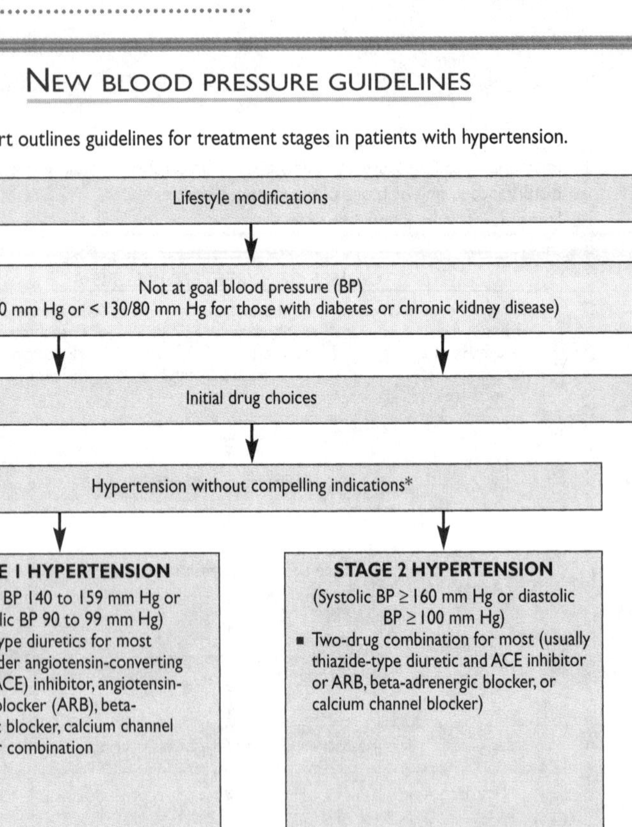

* Compelling indications include heart failure, post-myocardial infarction, high risk for coronary artery disease, diabetes, chronic kidney disease, and recurrent stroke prevention.

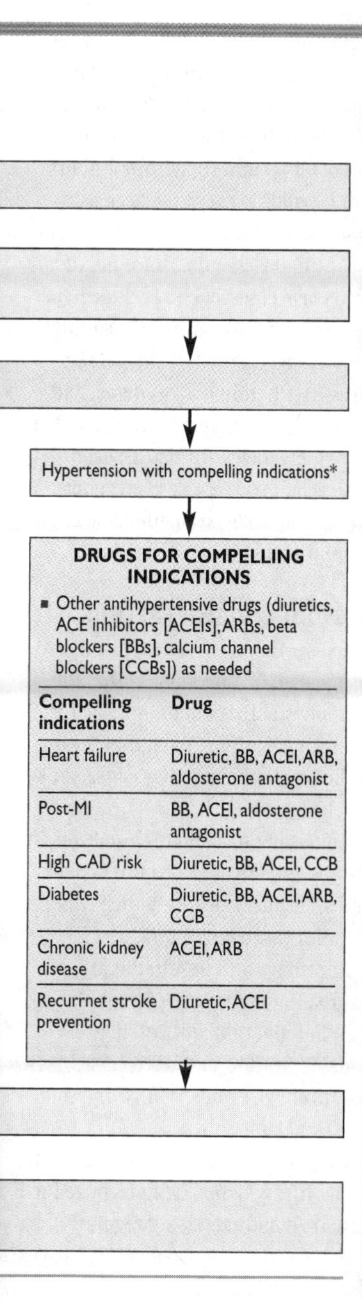

Compelling indications	Drug
Heart failure	Diuretic, BB, ACEI, ARB, aldosterone antagonist
Post-MI	BB, ACEI, aldosterone antagonist
High CAD risk	Diuretic, BB, ACEI, CCB
Diabetes	Diuretic, BB, ACEI, ARB, CCB
Chronic kidney disease	ACEI, ARB
Recurrnet stroke prevention	Diuretic, ACEI

- Excretory urography may reveal renal atrophy, indicating chronic renal disease. One kidney smaller than the other suggests unilateral renal disease.
- Electrocardiography may show left ventricular hypertrophy or ischemia.
- Chest X-rays may show cardiomegaly.
- Echocardiography may reveal left ventricular hypertrophy.

Treatment

In July of 2003, the U.S. Preventative Services Task Force strongly recommended blood pressure screening as the first step of treatment in all adults over age 18 because of evidence that early detection and treatment of high blood pressure can significantly reduce the risk of cardiovascular disease.

For treatment of high blood pressure, the National Heart, Lung, and Blood Institute, which is part of the National Institutes of Health, published new High Blood Pressure Guidelines in May of 2003. (See *New blood pressure guidelines.*) It recommends the following stepped-care approach:

- *Step 1* — Help the patient initiate necessary lifestyle modifications, including weight reduction, moderation of alcohol intake, regular physical exercise, reduction of sodium intake, and smoking cessation.
- *Step 2* — If the patient fails to achieve the desired blood pressure or make significant progress, continue lifestyle modifications and begin drug therapy. Drug therapy is individual-

ized and guided by associated diseases. Preferred drugs include thiazide diuretics, angiotensin-converting enzyme (ACE) inhibitors, or beta-adrenergic blockers. These drugs have been proven effective in reducing cardiovascular morbidity and mortality. If diuretics, ACE inhibitors, or beta-adrenergic blockers are ineffective or contraindicated, the physician may prescribe calcium antagonists, $alpha_1$-receptor blockers, or alpha-beta blockers. These drugs, although effective in reducing blood pressure, have yet to be proven effective in reducing morbidity and mortality.

- *Step 3* — If the patient fails to achieve the desired blood pressure or make significant progress, increase the drug dosage, substitute a drug in the same class, or add a drug from a different class.
- *Step 4* — If the patient fails to achieve the desired blood pressure or make significant progress, add a second or third agent or a diuretic (if one isn't already prescribed). Second or third agents may include vasodilators, $alpha_1$-antagonists, peripherally acting adrenergic neuron antagonists, ACE inhibitors, and calcium channel blockers.

Treatment of secondary hypertension focuses on correcting the underlying cause and controlling hypertensive effects.

Typically, hypertensive emergencies require parenteral administration of a vasodilator or an adrenergic inhibitor or oral administration of a selected drug, such as nifedipine, captopril, clonidine, or labetalol, to rapidly reduce blood pressure. The initial goal is to reduce mean arterial blood pressure by no more than 25% (within minutes to hours) and then reduce it to 160/110 mm Hg within 2 hours while avoiding excessive decreases that can precipitate renal, cerebral, or myocardial ischemia. Examples of hypertensive emergencies include hypertensive encephalopathy, intracranial hemorrhage, acute left-sided heart failure with pulmonary edema, and dissecting aortic aneurysm. Hypertensive emergencies are also associated with eclampsia or severe pregnancy-induced hypertension, unstable angina, and acute MI.

Special considerations

- To encourage adherence to antihypertensive therapy, suggest that the patient establish a daily routine for taking medication. Warn that uncontrolled hypertension may cause stroke and heart attack.
- Advise her to avoid high-sodium antacids and over-the-counter cold and sinus medications, which contain harmful vasoconstrictors.
- Encourage a change in dietary habits. Help the obese patient plan a weight-reduction diet; tell her to avoid high-sodium foods (pickles, potato chips, canned soups, and cold cuts) and table salt.
- Help the patient examine and modify her lifestyle (for example, by reducing stress and exercising regularly). (See *Lifestyle changes and DASH*, pages 332 and 333.)
- If a patient is hospitalized with hypertension, find out if she was taking

her prescribed medication. If she wasn't, ask why. If the patient can't afford the medication, refer her to an appropriate social service agency.

- When routine blood pressure screening reveals elevated pressure, make sure the cuff size is appropriate for the patient's upper arm circumference. Take the pressure in both arms in lying, sitting, and standing positions. Ask the patient if she smoked, drank a beverage containing caffeine, or was emotionally upset before the test. Advise the patient to return for blood pressure testing at frequent, regular intervals.
- To help identify hypertension and prevent untreated hypertension, participate in public education programs dealing with hypertension and ways to reduce risk factors. Encourage public participation in blood pressure screening programs. Routinely screen all patients, especially those at risk (including blacks and people with family histories of hypertension, stroke, or heart attack).

Hyperthyroidism

Hyperthyroidism (also known as *Graves' disease, von Basedow's disease,* or *thyrotoxicosis*) is a metabolic imbalance that results from thyroid hormone overproduction. The most common form of hyperthyroidism is Graves' disease, which increases thyroxine (T_4) production, enlarges the thyroid gland (goiter), and causes multiple system changes. With treatment, most patients can lead normal lives. However, if left untreated, hyperthyroidism may lead to a thyroid storm — an acute exacerbation of hyperthyroidism that constitutes a medical emergency that can lead to life-threatening cardiac, hepatic, or renal failure. (See *Other forms of hyperthyroidism,* page 334.)

Incidence of Graves' disease is highest between ages 30 and 40, especially in a patient with a family history of thyroid abnormalities. However, it may occur in young children and adolescents as well. It's more prevalent in women than in men by an 8 to 1 ratio.

Causes

Although the exact mechanism of hyperthyroidism isn't understood, it has a hereditary component and is usually associated with other autoimmune endocrinopathies.

Graves' disease is an autoimmune disorder characterized by the production of autoantibodies that attach to and then stimulate thyroid-stimulating hormone (TSH) receptors on the thyroid gland. A goiter is an enlarged thyroid gland, either the result of increased stimulation or a response to increased metabolic demand. Goiter occurs in iodine-deficient areas of the world, where the incidence increases during puberty (a time of increased metabolic demand). These goiters commonly regress to normal size after puberty in males, but not in females. The cause of sporadic goiter in non–iodine-deficient areas is unknown. Endemic and sporadic goiters are nontoxic and may be diffuse or nodular. Toxic goiters may be uni-

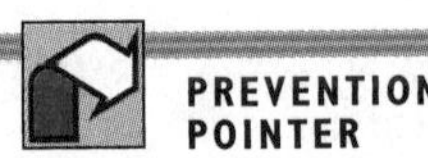

PREVENTION POINTER

LIFESTYLE CHANGES AND DASH

The National Heart, Lung, and Blood Institute published results from their PREMIER study in April of 2003. The study found that patients with high blood pressure can take behavioral steps along with dietary changes to prevent or control high blood pressure. These steps include:
- losing weight if overweight
- following a heart-healthy diet
- reducing salt and sodium intake
- increasing physical exercise

Food group	Daily servings	Serving sizes
Grains and grain products	7 to 8	▪ 1 slice of bread ▪ ½ cup dry cereal ▪ ½ cup cooked rice, pasta, or cereal
Vegetables	4 to 5	▪ 1 cup raw leafy vegetable ▪ ½ cup cooked vegetable ▪ 6 oz vegetable juice
Fruits	4 to 5	▪ 6 oz fruit juice ▪ 1 medium fruit ▪ ¼ cup dried fruit ▪ ½ cup fresh, frozen, or canned fruit
Low-fat or nonfat dairy foods	2 to 3	▪ 8 oz milk ▪ 1 cup yogurt ▪ 1½ oz cheese
Meats, poultry, and fish	2 or less	▪ 3 oz cooked meat, poultry, or fish
Nuts, seeds, and legumes	4 to 5 per week	▪ 1½ oz or ⅓ cup nuts ▪ ½ oz or 2 tbsp seeds ▪ ½ cup cooked legumes

nodular or multinodular and may secrete excess thyroid hormone.

Pituitary tumors with TSH-producing cells are rare, as is hypothalamic disease causing thyroid-releasing hormone (TRH) excess. Thyrotoxicosis may result from both genetic and immunologic factors, including:

- increased incidence in monozygotic twins, pointing to an inherited factor, probably an autosomal recessive gene
- occasional coexistence with other endocrine abnormalities, such as type 1 diabetes mellitus, thyroiditis, and hyperparathyroidism
- defect in suppressor T-lymphocyte function permitting production of au-

- limiting alcohol consumption
- quitting smoking.

Of the patients who followed the above steps along with the Dietary Approaches to Stop Hypertension (DASH) diet, 77% had the greatest decrease in blood pressure as compared to the 50% who received medication to lower their blood pressure. The DASH diet is a combination diet high in dietary fiber and fruits and vegetables, but low in saturated and total fat. Here are the DASH dietary guidelines:

Examples and notes	Significance to DASH diet
Whole-wheat bread, English muffin, pita bread, bagel, cereals, grits, oatmeal	Major sources of energy and fiber
Tomatoes, potatoes, carrots, squash, broccoli, turnip greens, collards, kale, spinach, artichokes, sweet potatoes, beans	Rich sources of potassium, magnesium, and fiber
Apricots, bananas, dates, oranges, orange juice, grapefruit, grapefruit juice, mangoes, melons, peaches, pineapples, prunes, raisins, strawberries, tangerines	Important sources of potassium, magnesium, and fiber
Skim or 1% milk, skim or low-fat buttermilk, nonfat or low-fat yogurt, part-skim mozzarella cheese, nonfat cheese	Major sources of calcium and protein
Select only lean; trim away visible fats; broil, roast, or boil instead of frying; remove skin from poultry	Rich sources of protein and magnesium
Almonds, filberts, mixed nuts, peanuts, walnuts, sunflower seeds, kidney beans, lentils	Rich sources of energy, magnesium, potassium, protein, and fiber

toantibodies (thyroid-stimulating immunoglobulin and TSH-binding inhibitory immunoglobulin)

- clinical thyrotoxicosis precipitated by excessive dietary intake of iodine or, possibly, stress (patients with latent disease)
- stress, such as surgery, infection, toxemia of pregnancy, or diabetic ketoacidosis, can precipitate thyroid storm (inadequately treated thyrotoxicosis)
- medications, such as lithium and amiodarone
- toxic nodules or tumors.

Other forms of hyperthyroidism

Other than primary hyperthyroidism, the disease can occur in many other forms, including:

- *Toxic adenoma,* a small, benign nodule in the thyroid gland that secretes thyroid hormone, is the second most common cause of hyperthyroidism. The cause of toxic adenoma is unknown; incidence is highest in elderly people. Clinical effects are essentially similar to those of Graves' disease, except that toxic adenoma doesn't induce ophthalmopathy, pretibial myxedema, or acropachy. Presence of adenoma is confirmed by radioactive iodine (^{131}I) uptake and thyroid scan, which show a single hyperfunctioning nodule suppressing the rest of the gland. Treatment involves ^{131}I therapy or surgery to remove adenoma after antithyroid drugs achieve a euthyroid state.
- *Thyrotoxicosis factitia* results from chronic ingestion of thyroid hormone for thyrotropin suppression in patients with thyroid carcinoma or from thyroid hormone abuse by people who are trying to lose weight.
- *Functioning metastatic thyroid carcinoma* is a rare disease that causes excess production of thyroid hormone.
- *Thyroid-stimulating hormone-secreting pituitary tumor* causes overproduction of thyroid hormone.
- *Subacute thyroiditis* is a virus-induced granulomatous inflammation of the thyroid, producing transient hyperthyroidism associated with fever, pain, pharyngitis, and tenderness in the thyroid gland.
- *Silent thyroiditis* is a self-limiting, transient form of hyperthyroidism, with histologic thyroiditis but no inflammatory symptoms.

Signs and symptoms

Signs and symptoms of hyperthyroidism include:

- enlarged thyroid (goiter)
- nervousness
- heat intolerance and sweating
- weight loss despite increased appetite
- frequent bowel movements
- tremor and palpitations
- exophthalmos (characteristic, but absent in many patients with thyrotoxicosis).

Because thyrotoxicosis profoundly affects virtually every body system, other common signs and symptoms include:

- *central nervous system* — difficulty concentrating due to accelerated cerebral function; excitability or nervousness caused by increased basal metabolic rate from T_4; fine tremor, shaky handwriting, and clumsiness from increased activity in the spinal cord area that controls muscle tone; emotional instability and mood swings ranging from occasional outbursts to overt psychosis (central nervous system)
- *integumentary system* — moist, smooth, warm, flushed skin (patient sleeps with minimal covers and little clothing); fine, soft hair; premature patchy graying and increased hair loss in both sexes; friable nails and onycholysis (distal nail separated from

the bed); pretibial myxedema (nonpitting edema of the anterior surface of the legs, dermopathy), producing thickened skin; accentuated hair follicles; sometimes itchy or painful raised red patches of skin with occasional nodule formation; microscopic examination showing increased mucin deposits (skin, hair, and nails)

- *cardiovascular system* — systolic hypertension; tachycardia; full, bounding pulse; wide pulse pressure; cardiomegaly; increased cardiac output and blood volume; visible point of maximal impulse; paroxysmal supraventricular tachycardia and atrial fibrillation (especially in elderly people); and occasional systolic murmur at the left sternal border
- *respiratory system* — increased respiratory rate and dyspnea on exertion and at rest, possibly due to cardiac decompensation and increased cellular oxygen use
- *gastrointestinal system* — excessive oral intake with weight loss; nausea and vomiting due to increased GI motility and peristalsis; increased defecation; soft stools or, in severe disease, diarrhea; liver enlargement
- *musculoskeletal system* — weakness, fatigue, and muscle atrophy; coexistence with myasthenia gravis (rare); possibly generalized or localized paralysis associated with hypokalemia; and, rarely, acropachy (soft-tissue swelling accompanied by underlying bone changes where new bone formation occurs)
- *reproductive system* — oligomenorrhea or amenorrhea, decreased fertility, increased incidence of spontaneous abortion (females), gynecomastia due to increased estrogen levels (males), diminished libido (both sexes)
- *special sensory organs* — exophthalmos due to combined effects of accumulated mucopolysaccharides and fluids in the retro-orbital tissues of the eyes, forcing the eyeball outward and causing lid retraction, thereby producing a characteristic staring gaze; occasional inflammation of conjunctivae, corneas, or eye muscles; diplopia; and increased tearing.

When thyrotoxicosis escalates to thyroid storm, a life-threatening medical emergency, possible symptoms include:

- high fever, possibly up to 106° F (41.1° C)
- tachycardia, pulmonary edema, hypertension, shock
- tremors, emotional lability, extreme irritability, confusion, delirium, psychosis, apathy, stupor, coma
- diarrhea, abdominal pain, nausea and vomiting, jaundice, hyperglycemia.

SPECIAL NEEDS

In elderly patients with atrial fibrillation or depression, consider apathetic thyrotoxicosis, a morbid condition resulting from overactive thyroid.

Possible complications of hyperthyroidism include:

- muscle wasting, atrophy, and paralysis
- visual loss or diplopia
- heart failure, arrhythmias
- hypoparathyroidism after surgical removal of thyroid

- hypothyroidism after radioiodine treatment.

Diagnosis

The diagnosis of hyperthyroidism is usually straightforward and depends on a careful clinical history and physical examination, a high index of suspicion, and routine hormone determinations. These tests confirm the disorder:

- Radioimmunoassay shows increased serum T_4 and triiodothyronine (T_3) concentrations.
- Thyroid scan reveals increased uptake of radioactive iodine (^{131}I). This test is contraindicated if the patient is pregnant.
- TSH levels are decreased.
- TRH stimulation test indicates hyperthyroidism if the TSH level fails to rise within 30 minutes after the administration of TRH.
- Ultrasonography confirms subclinical ophthalmopathy.

Treatment

The primary forms of therapy include:

- antithyroid drugs
- single oral dose of ^{131}I
- surgery.

Appropriate treatment depends on:

- severity of thyrotoxicosis
- causes
- patient age and parity
- how long surgery will be delayed (if the patient is an appropriate candidate for surgery).

Antithyroid therapy includes antithyroid drugs for children, young adults, pregnant women, and patients who refuse surgery or ^{131}I treatment. Antithyroid drugs are preferred in patients with new-onset Graves' disease because of spontaneous remission in many of these patients; they're also used to correct the thyrotoxic state in preparation for ^{131}I treatment or surgery. Treatment options include:

- thyroid hormone antagonists, including propylthiouracil (PTU) and methimazole (Tapazole), to block thyroid hormone synthesis (Hypermetabolic symptoms subside within 4 to 8 weeks after therapy begins, but remission of Graves' disease requires continued therapy for 6 months to 2 years.)
- propranolol (Inderal) until antithyroid drugs reach their full effect, to manage tachycardia and other peripheral effects of excessive hypersympathetic activity resulting from blocking the conversion of T_4 to the active T_3 hormone
- minimum dosage needed to keep maternal thyroid function within the high-normal range until delivery, and to minimize the risk of fetal hypothyroidism, with PTU as the preferred agent (during pregnancy)
- possibly antithyroid medications and propranolol for neonates for 2 to 3 months because most infants of hyperthyroid mothers are born with mild and transient thyrotoxicosis (neonatal thyrotoxicosis) caused by placental transfer of thyroid-stimulating immunoglobulins
- continuous control of maternal thyroid function because thyrotoxicosis is sometimes exacerbated in the puerperal period; antithyroid drugs gradually tapered and thyroid function re-

assessed after 3 to 6 months postpartum

- periodic checks of infant's thyroid function with a breast-feeding mother on low-dose antithyroid treatment due to the possible presence of small amounts of the drug in breast milk, which can rapidly lead to thyrotoxicity in the neonate
- single oral dose of ^{131}I (radioiodine ablation), the treatment of choice for patients not planning to have children (pregnancy is the sole contraindication for this treatment). (Patients of reproductive age must give informed consent for this treatment because ^{131}I concentrates in the gonads.)

During treatment with ^{131}I, the thyroid gland picks up the radioactive element as it would regular iodine. The radioactivity destroys some of the cells that normally concentrate iodine and produce T_4, thus decreasing thyroid hormone production and normalizing thyroid size and function.

In most patients, hypermetabolic symptoms diminish 6 to 8 weeks after such treatment (although some patients may require a second dose). However, a major and very common adverse effect of ^{131}I is hypothyroidism. In fact, most patients become hypothyroid, either immediately after treatment or shortly thereafter. These patients should expect lifelong thyroid replacement treatment with T_4 (thyroxine [Synthroid]).

Surgical treatment of hyperthyroidism involves subtotal thyroidectomy to decrease the thyroid gland's capacity for hormone production (in patients who refuse or aren't candidates for ^{131}I treatment). Treatment before and after surgery includes:

- iodides (Lugol's solution or saturated solution of potassium iodide), antithyroid drugs, and propranolol to relieve hyperthyroidism preoperatively (if patient doesn't become euthyroid, surgery should be delayed, and antithyroid drugs and propranolol given to decrease the systemic effects [cardiac arrhythmias] of thyrotoxicosis)
- lifelong regular medical supervision because most patients become hypothyroid, sometimes as long as several years after surgery.

Treatment of ophthalmopathy includes:

- local application of topical medications such as prednisone acetate suspension or, possibly, high doses of corticosteroids
- calcium channel blockers, such as diltiazem and verapamil, to block the peripheral effects of thyroid hormones
- external-beam radiation therapy or surgical decompression (for severe exophthalmos causing pressure on the optic nerve and orbital contents).

Emergency treatment of thyroid storm includes:

- antithyroid drug to stop conversion of T_4 to T_3 and to block sympathetic effect; corticosteroids to inhibit the conversion of T_4 to T_3; and iodide to block the release of thyroid hormone
- supportive measures, including the administration of nutrients, vitamins, fluids, oxygen, hypothermia blankets, and sedatives.

Special considerations

Patients with hyperthyroidism require vigilant care to prevent acute exacerbations and complications.

- Record vital signs and weight.
- Monitor serum electrolyte levels, and check periodically for hyperglycemia and glycosuria.
- Carefully monitor cardiac function if the patient is elderly or has coronary artery disease. If her heart rate is more than 100 beats/minute, check blood pressure and pulse rate often.
- Check level of consciousness and urine output.
- If the patient is pregnant, tell her to watch closely for signs of spontaneous abortion during the first trimester and report such signs immediately.
- Encourage bed rest and keep the patient's room cool, quiet, and dark. The patient with dyspnea will be most comfortable sitting upright or in high Fowler's position.
- Remember, extreme nervousness may produce bizarre behavior. Reassure the patient and family that such behavior will probably subside with treatment. Provide sedatives, as necessary.
- To promote weight gain, provide a balanced diet with six meals per day. If the patient has edema, suggest a low-sodium diet.
- If iodide is part of the treatment, mix it with milk, juice, or water to prevent GI distress and administer it through a straw to prevent tooth discoloration.
- Watch for signs of thyroid storm (tachycardia, hyperkinesis, fever, vomiting, hypertension).
- Check intake and output carefully to ensure adequate hydration and fluid balance.
- Closely monitor blood pressure, cardiac rate and rhythm, and temperature. If the patient has a high fever, reduce it with appropriate hypothermic measures. Maintain an I.V. line and give drugs, as ordered.
- If the patient has exophthalmos or another ophthalmopathy, suggest sunglasses or eye patches to protect her eyes from light. Moisten the conjunctivae often with isotonic eye drops. Warn the patient with severe lid retraction to avoid sudden physical movements that might cause the lid to slip behind the eyeball.
- Avoid excessive palpation of the thyroid to avoid precipitating thyroid storm.

Postoperative care

Thyroidectomy necessitates meticulous postoperative care to prevent complications:

- Check often for respiratory distress, and keep a tracheotomy tray at the bedside.
- Watch for evidence of hemorrhage into the neck, such as a tight dressing with no blood on it. Change dressings and perform wound care, as ordered; check the *back* of the dressing for drainage. Keep the patient in semi-Fowler's position, and support her head and neck with sandbags to ease tension on the incision.
- Check for dysphagia or hoarseness from possible laryngeal nerve injury.
- Watch for signs of hypoparathyroidism (tetany, numbness), a compli-

cation that results from accidental removal of the parathyroid glands during surgery.

- Stress the importance of regular medical follow-up after discharge because hypothyroidism may develop 2 to 4 weeks postoperatively.

Drug therapy monitoring

Drug therapy and ^{131}I therapy require careful monitoring and comprehensive patient teaching:

- After ^{131}I therapy, tell the patient not to expectorate or cough freely because her saliva will be radioactive for 24 hours. Stress the need for repeated measurement of serum T_4 levels.
- If the patient is taking propylthiouracil and methimazole, monitor complete blood count periodically to detect leukopenia, thrombocytopenia, and agranulocytosis. Instruct her to take these medications with meals to minimize GI distress and avoid over-the-counter cough preparations because many contain iodine.
- Tell her to report fever, enlarged cervical lymph nodes, sore throat, mouth sores, and other signs of blood dyscrasias and any rash or skin eruptions — signs of hypersensitivity.
- Watch the patient taking propranolol for signs of hypotension (dizziness, decreased urine output). Tell her to rise slowly after sitting or lying down to prevent orthostatic syncope.
- Instruct the patient receiving antithyroid drugs or ^{131}I therapy to report any symptoms of hypothyroidism.

Hypothyroidism

Hypothyroidism results from hypothalamic, pituitary, or thyroid insufficiency or resistance to thyroid hormone. The disorder can progress to life-threatening myxedema coma. Hypothyroidism is more prevalent in women than men; in the United States, the incidence is increasing significantly in people ages 40 to 50. Hypothyroidism occurs primarily after age 40. After age 65, the prevalence increases to as much as 10% in females (3% in males).

Causes

Hypothyroidism may reflect a malfunction of the hypothalamus, pituitary, or thyroid gland, all of which are part of the same negative-feedback mechanism. However, disorders of the hypothalamus and pituitary rarely cause hypothyroidism. Primary hypothyroidism, a disorder of the gland itself, is most common.

Chronic autoimmune thyroiditis, also called *chronic lymphocytic thyroiditis*, occurs when autoantibodies destroy thyroid gland tissue. Chronic autoimmune thyroiditis associated with goiter is called *Hashimoto's thyroiditis*. The cause of this autoimmune process is unknown. Even so, heredity has a role, and specific human leukocyte antigen subtypes are associated with greater risk.

Causes of hypothyroidism in adults include:

- inadequate production of thyroid hormone, usually after thyroidectomy or radiation therapy (particularly with radioactive iodine); inflamma-

Clinical findings in hypothyroidism

The health history and physical examination will reveal many signs and symptoms of acquired hypothyroidism. Typical clinical findings are listed here.

History

- Fatigue
  - Loss of energy
  - Muscle and joint pain
  - Extremity weakness
  - Lethargy
  - Somnolence
  - Depression
  - Emotional lability
- Forgetfulness
  - Impaired memory
  - Inability to concentrate
  - Mental impairment
  - Blurred vision
- Menstrual disturbance
- Fullness in throat
- Cold intolerance
- Hair loss
- Hoarseness
- Weight gain
- Decreased appetite

Physical examination

- Hypothermia
- Weight gain
- Dull facial expression
- Coarse facial features
- Eye puffiness
- Slow in movement
- Slow speech
- Hoarseness
- Goiter
- Bradycardia
- Hair loss
- Delayed relaxation of reflexes
- Dry skin
- Brittle hair
- Myxedema
- Constipation

tion; chronic autoimmune thyroiditis (Hashimoto's disease); or such conditions as amyloidosis and sarcoidosis (rare)

- pituitary failure to produce thyroid-stimulating hormone (TSH), hypothalamic failure to produce thyroid-releasing hormone (TRH), inborn errors of thyroid hormone synthesis, iodine deficiency (usually dietary), or use of such antithyroid medications as propylthiouracil.

Signs and symptoms

Typical, vague, early clinical features of hypothyroidism include weakness, fatigue, forgetfulness, sensitivity to cold, unexplained weight gain, and constipation. (See *Clinical findings in hypothyroidism.*) Other signs and symptoms include:

- characteristic myxedematous signs and symptoms of decreasing mental stability; coarse, dry, flaky, inelastic skin; puffy face, hands, and feet; hoarseness; periorbital edema; upper eyelid droop; dry, sparse hair; and thick, brittle nails (as disorder progresses)
- cardiovascular involvement, including decreased cardiac output, slow pulse rate, signs of poor peripheral circulation and, occasionally, an enlarged heart.
- anorexia, abdominal distention, menorrhagia, decreased libido, infer-

THYROID TEST RESULTS IN HYPOTHYROIDISM

This chart lists possible results of thyroid testing and what dysfunction is indicated by those results.

Thyrotropin-releasing hormone	Thyroid-stimulating hormone	Thyroid hormones (T_3 and T_4)	Dysfunction involves
Low	Low	Low	Hypothalamus
High	Low	Low	Pituitary gland
High	High	Low	Thyroid gland
High	Low or normal	T_3 and T_4 low, but reverse T_3 elevated	Peripheral conversion of thyroid hormone

tility, ataxia, and nystagmus; reflexes with delayed relaxation time (especially in the Achilles tendon)

- progression to myxedema coma, usually gradual but possibly developing abruptly, with stress aggravating severe or prolonged hypothyroidism, including progressive stupor, hypoventilation, hypoglycemia, hyponatremia, hypotension, and hypothermia.

Possible complications of hypothyroidism include:

- heart failure
- myxedema coma
- infection
- megacolon
- organic psychosis
- infertility.

Diagnosis

Diagnosis of hypothyroidism is based on:

- radioimmunoassay showing low triiodothyronine (T_3) and thyroxine (T_4) levels
- increased TSH level greater than 2.0 for primary hypothyroidism; decreased with hypothalamic or pituitary disorder
- thyroid panel differentiating primary hypothyroidism (thyroid gland hypofunction), secondary hypothyroidism (pituitary hyposecretion of TSH), tertiary hypothyroidism (hypothalamic hyposecretion of TRH), and euthyroid sick syndrome (impaired peripheral conversion of thyroid hormone due to a suprathyroidal illness such as severe infection) (see *Thyroid test results in hypothyroidism*)
- basal body temperature less than 97.8° F (36.6° C) (in women, axillary temperatures taken for 3 days starting in the morning on the second day of menstruation)
- elevated serum cholesterol, alkaline phosphatase, and triglyceride levels

- normocytic, normochromic anemia
- low serum sodium levels, decreased pH, and increased partial pressure of carbon dioxide, indicating respiratory acidosis (myxedema coma).

Treatment

Treatment of hypothyroidism includes:

- gradual thyroid hormone replacement with synthetic T_4 and, occasionally, T_3
- surgical excision, chemotherapy, or radiation for tumors.

SPECIAL NEEDS

Elderly patients should be started on a very low dose of T_4 to avoid cardiac problems. TSH levels guide gradual increases in dosage. (See *Hypothyroidism in children*.)

Special considerations

To manage treatment of the patient with hypothyroidism:

- Provide a high-bulk, low-calorie diet and encourage activity to combat constipation and promote weight loss. Administer cathartics and stool softeners as needed.
- After thyroid replacement begins, watch for symptoms of hyperthyroidism, such as restlessness, sweating, and excessive weight loss.
- Tell the patient to report any signs of aggravated cardiovascular disease, such as chest pain and tachycardia.
- To prevent myxedema coma, tell the patient to continue the course of thyroid medication even if symptoms subside.
- Warn the patient to report infection immediately and to make sure any physician who prescribes drugs for her knows about the underlying hypothyroidism.

Myxedema coma care

Treatment of myxedema coma requires supportive care:

- Check frequently for signs of decreasing cardiac output (such as decreased urine output).
- Monitor temperature until stable. Provide extra blankets and clothing and a warm room to compensate for hypothermia. Rapid rewarming may cause vasodilation and vascular collapse.
- Record intake and output and daily weight. As treatment begins, urine output should increase and body weight decrease; if not, report this immediately.
- Avoid sedation when possible or reduce dosage because hypothyroidism delays metabolism of many drugs.
- Maintain a patent I.V. line. Monitor serum electrolyte levels carefully when administering I.V. fluids.
- Monitor vital signs carefully when administering levothyroxine because rapid correction of hypothyroidism can cause adverse cardiac effects. Report chest pain or tachycardia immediately.

SPECIAL NEEDS

Watch for hypertension and heart failure in the elderly patient.

Hypothyroidism in children

A deficiency of thyroid hormone secretion during fetal development and early infancy results in infantile cretinism (congenital hypothyroidism). Hypothyroidism in infants is seen as respiratory difficulties, cyanosis, persistent jaundice, lethargy, excessive somnolence, large tongue, abdominal distention, poor feeding, abnormal deep tendon reflexes, and hoarse crying. Prompt treatment of hypothyroidism in infants prevents physical and mental retardation.

Older children who suffer from hypothyroidism have similar symptoms to those of adults, plus poor skeletal growth and late epiphyseal maturation and dental development. Sexual maturation may be accelerated in younger children and delayed in older children.

Cretinism is three times more common in girls than boys. Early diagnosis and treatment allow the best prognosis; infants treated before age 3 months usually grow and develop normally. Athyroid children who remain untreated after age 3 months and children with acquired hypothyroidism who remain untreated beyond age 2 years have irreversible mental retardation, although their skeletal abnormalities are reversible with treatment.

Special considerations

- Prevention, early detection, comprehensive parent teaching, and psychological support are essential. Know the early signs. Be especially wary if parents emphasize how good and how quiet their new baby is.
- Inform parents that the child will require lifelong treatment with thyroid supplements. Stress the need to comply with the treatment regimen to prevent further mental impairment.
- Provide support to help parents deal with a child who may be mentally retarded. Help them adopt a positive but realistic attitude and focus on their child's strengths rather than her weaknesses. Encourage them to provide stimulating activities to help the child reach her maximal potential. Refer them to appropriate community resources for support.
- To prevent infantile cretinism, emphasize the importance of adequate nutrition during pregnancy, including iodine-rich foods and the use of iodized salt or, in case of sodium restriction, an iodine supplement.

- Check arterial blood gas values for hypercapnia, metabolic acidosis, and hypoxia to determine whether the patient who's severely myxedematous requires ventilatory assistance.
- Administer corticosteroids as ordered.
- Because myxedema coma may have been precipitated by an infection, check possible sources of the infection, such as blood and urine, and obtain sputum cultures.

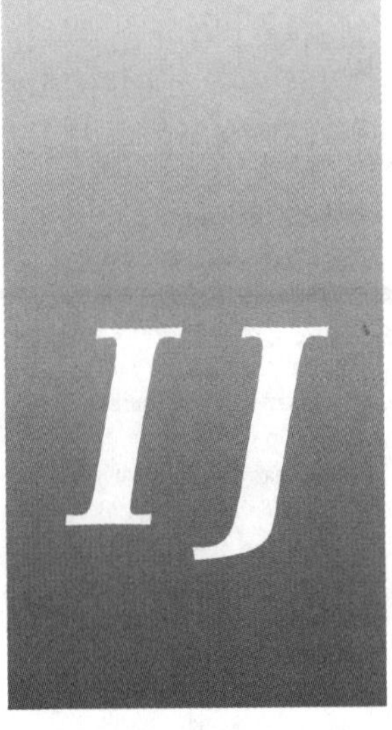

Infertility

Infertility affects approximately 10% to 15% of all couples in the United States. About 30% to 40% of all infertility is attributed to the female, and 30% to 40% to the male; about 20% is due to a combination of male and female factors. Following extensive investigation and treatment, approximately 50% of these infertile couples achieve pregnancy. Of the 50% who don't, 10% have no pathologic basis for infertility; the prognosis for this group becomes extremely poor if pregnancy isn't achieved within 3 years.

Causes

The causes of female infertility may be:

- *functional.* Complex hormonal interactions determine the normal function of the female reproductive tract and require an intact hypothalamic-pituitary-ovarian axis system that stimulates and regulates the production of hormones necessary for normal sexual development and function. Any defect or malfunction of this axis can cause infertility due to insufficient gonadotropin secretions (both luteinizing and follicle-stimulating hormones). The ovary controls, and is controlled by, the hypothalamus through a system of negative and positive feedback mediated by estrogen production. Insufficient gonadotropin levels may result from infections, tumors, or neurologic disease of the hypothalamus or pituitary gland. Hypothyroidism also impairs fertility.

- *anatomic.* Anatomic causes include:
  - ovarian factors, which are a major cause of infertility and are related to anovulation and oligo-ovulation (infrequent ovulation). Pregnancy or direct visualization provides irrefutable evidence of ovulation. Presumptive signs of ovulation include regular menses, cyclic changes reflected in basal body temperature readings, postovulatory progesterone levels, and endometrial changes due to the presence of progesterone. Absence of presumptive signs suggests anovulation. Ovarian failure, in which the ovaries produce no ova, may result from ovarian dysgenesis or premature menopause. Amenorrhea is commonly associated with ovarian failure. Oligo-ovulation may be due to a mild hormonal imbalance in gonadotropin production and regulation and may be caused by polycystic disease of the ovary or abnormalities in the adrenal or thyroid gland that adversely affect hypothalamic-pituitary function.
  - *uterine fibroids or uterine abnormalities,* which rarely cause infertility but may include a congenitally absent uterus, bicornuate or double uterus, leiomyomas, or Asherman's syndrome, in which the anterior and posterior uterine walls adhere because of scar tissue formation.
  - *tubal and peritoneal factors,* which are due to faulty tubal transport mechanisms and unfavorable environmental influences affecting the sperm, ova, or recently fertilized ovum. Tubal loss or impairment may occur secondary to ectopic pregnancy. Commonly, tubal and peritoneal factors result from anatomic abnormalities, such as bilateral occlusion of the tubes due to salpingitis (resulting from gonorrhea, tuberculosis, or puerperal sepsis), peritubal adhesions (resulting from endometriosis, pelvic inflammatory disease [PID], diverticulosis, or childhood rupture of the appendix), and uterotubal obstruction due to tubal spasm.
  - *cervical factors,* which may include malfunctioning cervix that produces deficient or excessively viscous mucus and is impervious to sperm, preventing entry into the uterus. In cervical infection, viscous mucus may contain spermicidal macrophages. The possible existence of cervical antibodies that immobilize sperm is also under investigation.

- *psychosocial problems.* Although relatively few cases of infertility can be attributed to psychosocial problems, occasionally, ovulation may stop under stress due to failure of luteinizing hormone release. The frequency of intercourse may also be related. More often, however, psychosocial problems result from, rather than cause, infertility.

Diagnosis

Inability to achieve pregnancy after having regular intercourse without contraception for at least 1 year suggests infertility. (In women over age 35, many physicians use 6 months rather than 1 year as a cutoff point.)

Diagnosis requires a complete physical examination and health history, including specific questions on the patient's reproductive and sexual function, past diseases, mental state, previous surgery, types of contraception used in the past, and family history. Irregular, painless menses may indicate anovulation. A history of PID may suggest fallopian tube blockage. Sometimes PID is silent and no history may be known.

These tests assess ovulation:

- *Basal body temperature graph* shows a sustained elevation in postovulation body temperature until just before onset of menses, indicating the approximate time of ovulation.
- *Endometrial biopsy*, done on or about day 5 after the basal body temperature rises, provides histologic evidence that ovulation has occurred.
- *Progesterone blood levels*, measured when they should be highest, can show a luteal phase deficiency or presumptive evidence of ovulation.

These procedures assess structural integrity of the fallopian tubes, the ovaries, and the uterus:

- *Urinary LH kits*, available without a prescription, can sensitively detect the LH surge about 24 hours preovulation.
- *Hysterosalpingography* provides radiologic evidence of tubal obstruction and abnormalities of the uterine cavity and cervix by injecting radiopaque contrast fluid through the cervix.
- *Endoscopy* confirms the results of hysterosalpingography and visualizes the endometrial cavity by hysteroscopy or explores the posterior surface of the uterus, fallopian tubes, and ovaries by culdoscopy. Laparoscopy, the final diagnostic tool, allows visualization of the abdominal and pelvic areas
- *Ultrasound* provides evidence of ovarian cysts and uterine fibroids.

Male-female interaction studies include:

- *Postcoital test* (Sims-Huhner test) examines the cervical mucus for motile sperm cells following intercourse that takes place at midcycle (as close to ovulation as possible).
- *Immunologic or antibody testing* detects spermicidal antibodies in the sera of the female. Further research is being conducted in this area.

Treatment

Treatment depends on identifying the underlying abnormality or dysfunction within the hypothalamic-pituitary-ovarian complex. In hyperactivity or hypoactivity of the adrenal or thyroid gland, hormone therapy is necessary; progesterone deficiency requires progesterone replacement. Anovulation necessitates treatment with clomiphene, human menopausal gonadotropins, or human chorionic gonadotropin; ovulation usually occurs several days after such administration. If mucus production decreases (an adverse effect of clomiphene),

OTHER INFERTILITY TREATMENT OPTIONS

Other options for treating infertility include in vitro fertilization (IVF), gamete intrafallopian tube transfer (GIFT), intracytoplasmic sperm injection (ICSI), intrauterine insemination (IUI), round spermatid nucleus injection (ROSNI), and zygote intrafallopian transfer (ZIFT). Each is explained here.

IVF

In IVF, removal of preovulatory oocytes from the ovaries and the fertilization with sperm occurs outside the womb in a laboratory. Follicular aspiration is done via the transvaginal route. The ova are scanned by microscope for the appearance of the corona cumulus complex. The sperm is washed and separated by centrifugation, leaving "mobile" sperm. The embryos are transferred into the womb 42 to 74 hours after fertilization.

GIFT

In GIFT, oocytes are retrieved from the woman and mixed with washed sperm in the laboratory. The gamete is placed in the fallopian tube near the fimbriae via laparoscopy.

ICSI

In ICSI, a single sperm is paralyzed and aspirated into a needle. The chosen oocyte's lining is chemically removed by the use of hyaluronidase. The sperm is injected into the ovum, resulting in fertilization. The fertilized egg is transferred into the woman's body via the transvaginal route.

IUI

In IUI, sperm is placed directly inside the uterus via a cannula.

ROSNI

ROSNI results in fertilization by removing immature cells from the testicles and injecting their nuclei into an oocyte. The fertilized egg is placed into the woman via the transvaginal route.

ZIFT

As in GIFT, ZIFT involves retrieving oocytes from the woman and mixing them with washed sperm in the laboratory. Unlike GIFT, however, the zygote is placed into the fallopian tube via laparoscopy 24 hours after fertilization occurs.

small doses of estrogen to improve the quality of cervical mucus may be given concomitantly; however, the success of this intervention remains unproven.

Surgical restoration may correct certain anatomic causes of infertility such as fallopian tube obstruction. Surgery may also be necessary to remove tumors located within or near the hypothalamus or pituitary gland. Endometriosis requires drug therapy (danazol or medroxyprogesterone, or noncyclic administration of oral contraceptives), surgical removal of areas of endometriosis, or a combination of both.

Other infertility treatment options, often controversial and involving emotional stress and financial cost, include surrogate mothering, frozen embryos, or in vitro fertilization (IVF). Due to the success rate of IVF (about 20%), it may be used instead of surgery in many cases. (See *Other infertility treatment options.*)

Special considerations

Management includes providing the infertile couple with emotional support and information about diagnostic and treatment techniques. An infertile couple may suffer loss of self-esteem. They may also feel angry, guilty, or inadequate, and the diagnostic procedures for this disorder may intensify their anxiety. You can help by explaining these procedures thoroughly. Above all, encourage the patient and her partner to talk about their feelings, and listen to what they have to say with a nonjudgmental attitude. If the patient requires surgery, tell her what to expect postoperatively, depending on which procedure is to be performed.

Irritable bowel syndrome

Irritable bowel syndrome (IBS) is marked by chronic symptoms of abdominal pain, alternating constipation and diarrhea, excess flatus, a sense of incomplete evacuation, and abdominal distention. Irritable bowel syndrome is a common, stress-related disorder. However, 20% of patients never seek medical attention. IBS is a chronic condition that has no anatomical abnormality or inflammatory component. It occurs in women twice as commonly as men.

Causes

IBS appears to reflect motor disturbances of the entire colon in response to stimuli. Some muscles of the small bowel are particularly sensitive to motor abnormalities and distention; others are particularly sensitive to certain foods and drugs. The patient may be hypersensitive to the hormones gastrin and cholecystokinin. The pain of IBS seems to be caused by abnormally strong contractions of the intestinal smooth muscle as it reacts to distention, irritants, or stress. (See *What happens in IBS.*) Causes include:

- ingestion of irritants (coffee, raw fruit, or vegetables)
- lactose intolerance
- abuse of laxatives
- hormonal changes (menstruation).

Signs and symptoms

Signs and symptoms of IBS include:

- cramping of the lower abdomen secondary to muscle contraction; usually occurring during the day and relieved by defecation or passage of flatus
- fever and chills
- pain that intensifies 1 to 2 hours after a meal from irritation of nerve fibers by causative stimulus
- constipation alternating with diarrhea, with one dominant; secondary to motor disturbances from causative stimulus
- mucus passed through the rectum from altered secretion in intestinal lumen due to motor abnormalities
- abdominal distention and bloating caused by flatus and constipation.

Diagnosis

- Stool samples for ova, parasites, bacteria, and blood rule out infection.
- Lactose intolerance test rules out lactose intolerance.

What happens in IBS

Typically, the GI tract of a patient with irritable bowel syndrome (IBS) appears normal. However, careful examination of the colon may reveal functional irritability—an abnormality in colonic smooth-muscle function marked by excessive peristalsis and spasms, even during remission.

Intestinal function

To understand what happens in IBS, consider how smooth muscle controls bowel function. Normally, segmental muscle contractions mix intestinal contents while peristalsis propels the contents through the GI tract. Motor activity is most propulsive in the proximal (stomach) and the distal (sigmoid) portions of the intestine. Activity in the rest of the intestines is slower, permitting nutrient and water absorption.

In IBS, the autonomic nervous system, which innervates the large intestine, fails to initiate the alternating contractions and relaxations that propel stools smoothly toward the rectum. The result is constipation or diarrhea or both.

Constipation

Some patients have spasmodic intestinal contractions that set up a partial obstruction by trapping gas and stools. This causes distention, bloating, gas pain, and constipation.

Diarrhea

Other patients have dramatically increased intestinal motility. Eating or cholinergic stimulation triggers the small intestine's contents to rush into the large intestine, dumping watery stools and irritating the mucosa. The result is diarrhea.

Mixed symptoms

If further spasms trap liquid stools, the intestinal mucosa absorbs water from the stools, leaving them dry, hard, and difficult to pass. The result: a pattern of alternating diarrhea and constipation.

- Barium enema may reveal colon spasm and tubular appearance of descending colon without evidence of cancers and diverticulosis.
- Sigmoidoscopy or colonoscopy may reveal spastic contractions without evidence of colon cancer or inflammatory bowel disease.
- Rectal biopsy rules out malignancy.

Treatment

Treatment of IBS may include:

- stress relief measures, including counseling or mild anti-anxiety agents
- investigation and avoidance of food irritants and gas-producing foods
- application of heat to the abdomen
- bulking agents to reduce episodes of diarrhea and minimize effect of nonpropulsive colonic contractions
- antispasmodics (propantheline [Pro-Banthine] or diphenoxylate with atropine [Lomotil]) for pain
- loperamide (Imodium A-D) (possibly) to reduce urgency and fecal soiling in patients with persistent diarrhea
- bowel training (if the cause of IBS is chronic laxative abuse) to regain muscle control.

Special considerations

Because the patient with IBS won't be hospitalized, focus your care on patient teaching.

- Tell the patient to avoid irritating or gas-producing foods and encourage her to develop regular bowel habits.
- Help the patient deal with stress associated with the disease's effects and warn against dependence on sedatives or antispasmodics.
- Encourage regular checkups because IBS is associated with a higher-than-normal incidence of diverticulitis and colon cancer. For patients over age 40, emphasize the need for an annual sigmoidoscopy and rectal examination.

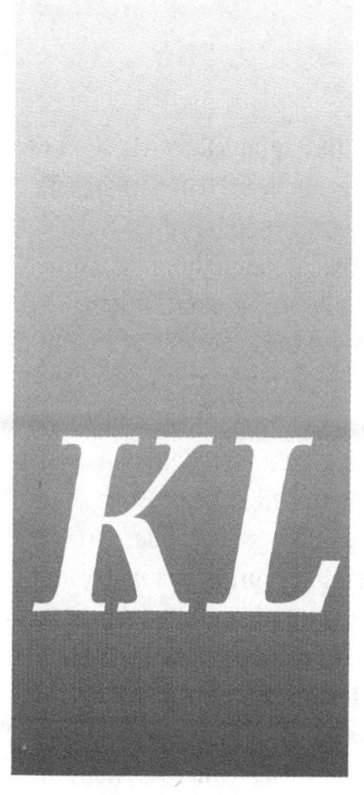

Kyphosis

The upper back or thoracic region is normally curved forward. If the curve exceeds 50 degrees, it's considered *kyphotic*. Kyphosis, also called *roundback* or *hunchback*, is an exaggerated anteroposterior curving of the spine that causes a bowing of the back, commonly at the thoracic but sometimes at the thoracolumbar or sacral level. Kyphosis occurs in children and adults. Symptomatic adolescent kyphosis is more prevalent in girls than in boys and typically occurs between ages 12 and 16. It can worsen during adolescence or can result from compression of vertebrae that occurs with aging, particularly in women with osteoporosis.

Causes

Congenital kyphosis is rare but usually severe, with resultant cosmetic deformity and reduced pulmonary function. Adolescent kyphosis (Scheuermann's disease, juvenile kyphosis, vertebral epiphysitis), the most common form of this disorder, may result from growth retardation or a vascular disturbance in the vertebral epiphysis (usually at the thoracic level) during periods of rapid growth or from congenital deficiency in the thickness of the vertebral plates. Other causes include infection, inflammation, aseptic necrosis, injuries (such as a car crash) and disk degeneration. The subsequent stress of weight bearing on the compromised vertebrae may result in the thoracic hump commonly seen in adolescents with kyphosis.

Adult kyphosis (adult roundback) may result from:

- aging and associated degeneration of intervertebral disks, atrophy, and osteoporotic collapse of the vertebrae
- endocrine disorders, such as hyperparathyroidism and Cushing's disease
- prolonged steroid therapy
- other conditions, such as arthritis, Paget's disease, polio, compression fracture of the thoracic vertebrae, metastatic tumor, plasma cell myeloma, or tuberculosis.

In addition, kyphosis may also occur in children and adults with poor posture. Disk lesions called *Schmorl's nodes* may develop in anteroposterior curving of the spine and are localized protrusions of nuclear material that extend through the cartilage plates and into the spongy bone of the vertebral bodies. If the anterior portions of the cartilage are destroyed, they're replaced by fibrocartilage, which then ossifies, causing ankylosis.

Signs and symptoms

Development of adolescent kyphosis is usually insidious, commonly occurring after a history of excessive sports activity, and may be asymptomatic except for the obvious curving of the back (sometimes more than 90 degrees). In some adolescents, kyphosis may produce mild pain at the apex of the curve (about 50% of patients), fatigue, tenderness or stiffness in the involved area or along the entire spine, and prominent vertebral spinous processes at the lower dorsal and upper lumbar levels, with compensatory increased lumbar lordosis, and hamstring tightness. Rarely, kyphosis may cause neurologic damage, such as spastic paraparesis secondary to spinal cord compression and herniated nucleus pulposus. In adolescent and adult forms of kyphosis that aren't due to poor posture alone, the spine won't straighten when the patient assumes a recumbent position.

Adult kyphosis produces a characteristic roundback appearance, possibly associated with pain, weakness of the back, and generalized fatigue. Unlike the adolescent form, adult kyphosis rarely produces local tenderness, except in osteoporosis with a recent compression fracture.

Diagnosis

Physical examination reveals curvature of the thoracic spine in varying degrees of severity. X-rays of the spine can confirm diagnosis and identify its underlying cause by showing vertebral wedging, Schmorl's nodes, irregular end plates, and possibly mild scoliosis of 10 to 20 degrees. Adolescent kyphosis must be distinguished from tuberculosis and other inflammatory or neoplastic diseases that cause vertebral collapse; the severe pain, bone destruction, or systemic symptoms associated with these diseases help rule out a diagnosis of kyphosis. Other sites of bone disease, primary sites of malignancy, and infection must be evaluated, possibly through vertebral biopsy. Magnetic resonance imaging or computed tomography scan can also assess lumbar anatomy.

Treatment

Congenital defects usually have to be repaired surgically. The procedures are complicated and lengthy. Typically, hardware is surgically placed to stabilize the back bone.

For kyphosis caused by poor posture alone, treatment may consist of therapeutic exercises, bed rest on a firm mattress (with or without traction), and a brace to straighten the kyphotic curve until spinal growth is complete. A brace, however, is a treatment modality reserved only for adolescents. Corrective exercises include pelvic tilt to decrease lumbar lordosis, hamstring stretch to overcome muscle contractures, and thoracic hyperextension to flatten the kyphotic curve. These exercises may be performed in or out of the brace. Lateral X-rays taken every 4 months evaluate correction. Gradual weaning from the brace can begin after maximum correction of the kyphotic curve, after vertebral wedging has decreased, and after the spine has reached full skeletal maturity. Loss of correction indicates that weaning from the brace has been too rapid, and time out of the brace is decreased accordingly.

Treatment for both adolescent and adult kyphosis also includes appropriate measures for the underlying cause and, possibly, spinal arthrodesis for relief of symptoms. Although rarely necessary, surgery may be recommended when kyphosis causes neurologic damage, a spinal curve greater than 60 degrees, or intractable and disabling back pain in a patient with full skeletal maturity. Preoperative measures may include halo-femoral traction. Corrective surgery includes a posterior spinal fusion with spinal instrumentation, iliac bone grafting, and plaster immobilization. Anterior spinal fusion followed by immobilization in plaster may be necessary when kyphosis produces a spinal curve greater than 70 degrees. Kyphosis caused by osteoporosis isn't treated except to prevent further bone softening.

Special considerations

Effective management of kyphosis necessitates first-rate supportive care for patients in traction or a brace, skillful patient teaching, and sensitive emotional support:

- Teach the patient with adolescent kyphosis caused by poor posture alone the prescribed therapeutic exercises and the fundamentals of good posture. Suggest bed rest when pain is severe. Encourage use of a firm mattress, preferably with a bed board. If the patient needs a brace, explain its purpose and teach her how and when to wear it.
- Teach good skin care. Tell the patient not to use lotions, ointments, or powders where the brace contacts the skin. Warn her that only the physician or orthotist should adjust the brace.

- If corrective surgery is needed, explain all preoperative tests thoroughly as well as the need for postoperative traction or casting, if applicable. After surgery, check neurovascular status every 2 to 4 hours for the first 48 hours, and report any changes immediately. Turn the patient often by logrolling and teach the patient how to logroll herself.
- Offer pain medication every 3 or 4 hours for the first 48 hours. Institute blood product replacement, if ordered. Accurately measure fluid intake and output, including urine specific gravity. Insert a nasogastric tube and an indwelling urinary catheter, if ordered; a rectal tube may also be necessary if paralytic ileus causes abdominal distention.
- Provide meticulous skin care. Check the skin at the cast edges several times per day; use heel and elbow protectors to prevent skin breakdown. Remove antiembolism stockings, if ordered, at least three times per day for at least 30 minutes.
- Provide emotional support. The adolescent patient is likely to exhibit mood changes and periods of depression. Maintain communication, and offer frequent encouragement and reassurance.
- Assist during removal of sutures and application of a new cast (usually about 10 days after surgery). Encourage gradual ambulation (usually with the use of a tilt table in the physical therapy department).
- At discharge, provide detailed, written cast care instructions. Tell the patient to immediately report pain, burning, skin breakdown, loss of feeling, tingling, numbness, or cast odor. Advise her to drink plenty of liquids to avoid constipation, and to report any illness (especially abdominal pain or vomiting) immediately. Arrange for home visits by a social worker and a home care nurse.

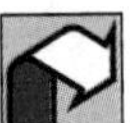

PREVENTION POINTER

Encourage women to start early with calcium supplementation and appropriate exercise, continuing throughout their lives. Studies have shown that high calcium intake can delay the onset of osteoporosis and, therefore, delay or prevent kyphosis.

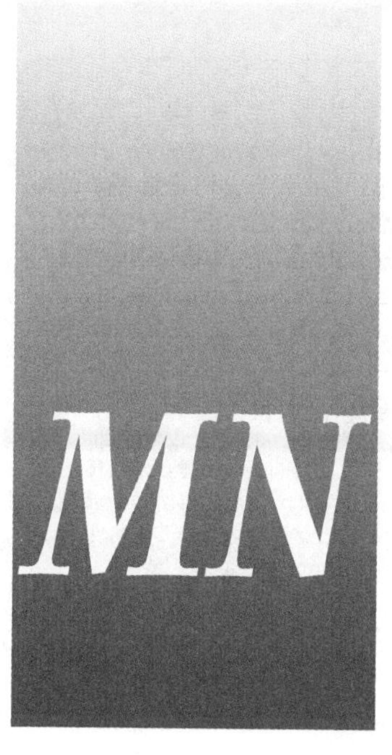

Melasma

A patchy, hypermelanotic skin disorder, melasma (also known as *chloasma* or *mask of pregnancy*) poses a serious cosmetic, although non–life-threatening problem. It darkens the facial skin, commonly affecting the cheeks, forehead, jaw line, and areas around the mouth. Although it tends to occur in all races, it's more common in darker skin types, especially Hispanics and Asians. Melasma affects females more often than males, occurring commonly in women during their reproductive years.

Causes

The cause of melasma is unknown. Genetics may play a large role as more than 30% of patients have a family history of melasma. Histologically, hyperpigmentation results from increased melanin production, although the number of melanocytes remains normal. Melasma may be related to the increased hormonal levels associated with pregnancy, menopause, ovarian cancer, and the use of hormonal contraceptives or hormonal replacement threapy. Progestational agents, phenytoin, and mephenytoin may also contribute to this disorder. Exposure to sunlight may stimulate melasma, but it may also develop without any apparent predisposing factor. Patients with acquired immunodeficiency syndrome have an increased incidence of similar hyperpigmentation. Another study found a fourfold increase in thyroid disease in patients with melasma. Thus, genetics and hormonal influences along with ultraviolet light are likely the major causes of melasma.

Signs and symptoms

Typically, melasma produces large, tan-brown, irregular patches, symmetrically distributed on the forehead, cheeks, and sides of the nose. Less commonly, these patches may occur on the neck, upper lip, and temples.

Diagnosis

Observation of characteristic dark patches on the face usually confirms melasma. The patient history may reveal predisposing factors.

Treatment

Treatment consists primarily of application of bleaching agents; the most commonly used agents contain 2% to 4% hydroquinone (Esoterica) to inhibit melanin synthesis. This medication is applied twice daily for up to 8 weeks. Combination sunscreen and hydroquinone products also have been effective. Tretinoin (Retin-A) can be used as monotherapy or with hydroquinone. Azelaic acid is as effective as hydroquinone in treating melasma. A new medication used for treating melasma, Tri-Luma, is a combination of hydroquinone, tretinoin, and fluocinolone acetonide (a potent topical steroid). Although Tri-Luma has been proven safe and effective, it's use is limited to no more than 8 weeks because it's a potent topical steroid that may cause skin atrophy.

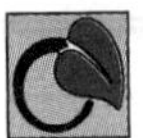

ALTERNATIVE THERAPIES

Some natural remedies are available, but their efficacy and safety haven't been fully evaluated and approved by the FDA. Kojic acid is a Japanese bleaching agent that's derived from fungal and organic plant materials. It helps reduce melanin formation and is widely used in Asian and ethnic bleaching products. Other natural remedies that have skin brightening qualities are bearberry and licorice extracts and vitamin C.

Some patients resort to removing superficial pigmented skin cells, through exfoliation, chemical peels, microdermabrasion, and light freezing of the skin with liquid nitrogen. However, these methods may cause excess irritation and actually may cause an increase in skin pigmentation.

Regardless of the form of treatment, patients with melasma must adhere to strict avoidance of exposure to sunlight, use of sunscreens, and discontinuation of hormonal contraceptives (if that's the underlying cause). Melasma associated with pregnancy usually clears within a few months after delivery.

Special considerations

- Advise the patient to avoid sun exposure by using sunscreens and wearing protective clothing. Bleaching agents may help but may require repeated treatments to maintain the desired effect. Cosmetics may help mask deep pigmentation.

- Reassure the patient that melasma is treatable. It may fade spontaneously postpartum, with protection from sunlight, and after discontinuing hormonal contraceptives. Caution the patient that treatment may take months and lightening of the pigment may be gradual.

Menopause

Menopause is the cessation of menstruation. It results from a complex syndrome of physiologic changes, called the *climacteric*, caused by declining ovarian function. The climacteric produces various body changes, the most dramatic being menopause.

Causes

Menopause occurs in three forms:

- *Physiologic menopause*, the normal decline in ovarian function due to aging, begins in most women between ages 40 and 50 and results in infrequent ovulation, decreased menstrual function and, eventually, cessation of menstruation (usually between ages 45 and 55).
- *Pathologic (premature) menopause*, the gradual or abrupt cessation of menstruation before age 40, occurs idiopathically in about 5% of women in the United States. However, certain diseases, especially severe infections and reproductive tract tumors, may cause pathologic menopause by seriously impairing ovarian function. Other factors that may precipitate pathologic menopause include malnutrition, debilitation, extreme emotional stress, excessive radiation exposure, and surgical procedures that impair ovarian blood supply.
- *Artificial menopause* may follow radiation therapy or surgical procedures such as oophorectomy.

Signs and symptoms

Many menopausal women are asymptomatic, but some have severe symptoms. The decline in ovarian function and consequent decreased estrogen level produce menstrual irregularities, such as a decrease in the amount and duration of menstrual flow, spotting, and episodes of amenorrhea and polymenorrhea (possibly with hypermenorrhea). Irregularities may last a few months or persist for several years before menstruation ceases permanently.

Artificial menopause produces symptoms within 2 to 5 years in 95% of women. Cessation of menstruation in pathologic and artificial menopause is commonly abrupt and may cause severe vasomotor and emotional disturbances. Menstrual bleeding after 1 year of amenorrhea may indicate organic disease.

These body system changes may occur (usually after the permanent cessation of menstruation):

- *Reproductive system* — Menopause may cause shrinkage of vulval structures and loss of subcutaneous fat, possibly leading to atrophic vulvitis; atrophy of vaginal mucosa and flattening of vaginal rugae, possibly causing bleeding after coitus or douching; vaginal itching and discharge from bacterial invasion; and loss of capillaries in the atrophying vaginal wall, causing the pink, rugal lining to become smooth and white. Menopause may also produce excessive vaginal dryness and dyspareunia due to decreased lubrication from the vaginal walls and decreased secretion from Bartholin's glands; smaller ovaries and oviducts; and progressive pelvic relaxation as the supporting structures lose their tone because of the absence of estrogen.

As a woman ages, atrophy causes the vagina to shorten and the mucous lining to become thin, dry, less elastic, and pale as a result of decreased vascularity. In addition, the pH of vaginal secretions increases, making the vaginal environment more alkaline. The type of flora also changes, increasing the older woman's chance of vaginal infections.

- *Urinary system* — Atrophic cystitis due to the effects of decreased estrogen levels on bladder mucosa and related structures may cause pyuria, dysuria, and urinary frequency, urgency, and incontinence. Urethral carbuncles from loss of urethral tone and mucosal thinning may cause dysuria, meatal tenderness, and hematuria.
- *Mammary system* — Breast size decreases due to decreasing size of mammary glands and ducts.
- *Integumentary system* — The patient may experience loss of skin elasticity and turgor due to estrogen deprivation, loss of pubic and axillary hair and, occasionally, slight alopecia.
- *Autonomic nervous system* — The patient may experience hot flashes and night sweats (in 60% of women), vertigo, syncope, tachycardia, dyspnea, tinnitus, emotional disturbances (irritability, nervousness, crying spells, fits of anger), and exacerbation of preexisting depression, anxiety, and compulsive, manic, or schizoid behavior.
- *Musculoskeletal system* — Menopause may also induce atherosclerosis, and a decrease in estrogen level contributes to osteoporosis.
- *Cardiovascular system* — Ovarian activity in younger women is believed to provide a protective effect for the cardiovascular system, and the loss of this function at menopause may partly explain the increased death rate from myocardial infarction in older women. Also, estrogen has been found to increase levels of high-density lipoprotein cholesterol.

Diagnosis

The patient history and typical clinical features suggest menopause. A Papanicolaou (Pap) test may show the in fluence of estrogen deficiency on vaginal mucosa. Radioimmunoassay shows these blood hormone levels:

- estrogen: 0 to 14 ng/dl
- plasma estradiol: 15 to 40 pg/ml
- estrone: 25 to 50 pg/ml.

Radioimmunoassay also shows these urine values:

- estrogen: 6 to 28 μg/24 hours
- pregnanediol (urinary secretion of progesterone): 0.3 to 0.9 mg/24 hours.

Follicle-stimulating hormone production may increase as much as 15 times its normal level; luteinizing hormone production, as much as 5 times.

Pelvic examination, endometrial biopsy, and dilatation and curettage may rule out organic disease in patients with abnormal menstrual bleeding.

Treatment

Estrogen is the treatment of choice in relieving vasomotor symptoms and symptoms caused by vaginal and urethral mucosal atrophy. It also improves mood, helps prevent osteoporosis, and reduces the morbidity and mortality associated with cardiovascular disease. Because recent studies have identified a possible link between estrogen replacement therapy (ERT) and breast cancer, the patient should first have a screening mammogram.

ERT may be administered cyclically or continuously. Patients usually receive the lowest dosage that effectively treats symptoms and prevents osteoporosis. Severe hot flashes may require a higher dosage for a limited period, followed by a gradual reduction in the standard dose.

In women who haven't had hysterectomies, the addition of a progestin (such as medroxyprogesterone [Provera]) during the last 12 days of estrogen administration lowers the incidence of hyperplasia and endometrial cancer. In women who have had hysterectomies, progestin's relationship to breast cancer is unknown.

The oral route is preferred for estrogen-progestin therapy; the transdermal route reduces GI adverse effects such as nausea, and topical estrogen relieves symptoms of vaginal atrophy. Regardless of the route, the patient must understand the risk of endometrial hyperplasia and have regular checkups to detect it early. (See *Estrogen-progestin guidelines*, page 360.)

Contraindications for ERT include unexplained vaginal bleeding, liver disease, recent vascular thrombosis, breast cancer, and endometrial cancer. If ERT is contraindicated, medroxyprogesterone, megestrol, and clonidine may reduce the incidence of hot flashes. Psychotherapy and drug therapy may relieve psychological disturbances. (For further details on estrogen and hormone replacement therapy, see chapter 4).

Special considerations

- Provide the patient with all the facts about ERT. Make sure she realizes the need for regular monitoring.
- Before ERT begins, have the patient undergo a baseline physical examination, Pap test, and mammogram.
- Advise the patient not to discontinue contraceptive measures until cessation of menstruation has been confirmed.
- Tell the patient to immediately report vaginal bleeding or spotting after menstruation has ceased.

Estrogen-progestin guidelines

If the patient is receiving sequential estrogen-progestin therapy, alert her to the possibility of monthly withdrawal bleeding after the cessation of progestin therapy, and tell her that such bleeding is benign. (If breakthrough bleeding occurs before day 6 of progestin therapy, an endometrial biopsy is needed to rule out hyperplasia.) Other adverse effects of progestin include breast tenderness, fluid retention, weight gain, dysmenorrhea, and depression.

Without progestin, however, long-term estrogen replacement therapy carries an increased risk of endometrial hyperplasia and, eventually, endometrial cancer. With this in mind, consider these guidelines:

- Symptoms associated with the progestin component may resolve when the daily dose of medroxyprogesterone is reduced from 10 mg to 5 mg. The lower dose, however, doesn't offer as much protection as the higher one.
- Withdrawal bleeding often can be eliminated by reducing the conjugated estrogen dose from 0.625 mg to 0.3 mg or by adding 2.5 mg of medroxyprogesterone daily. However, this lower dose of estrogen may be ineffective in relieving climacteric symptoms and in protecting against osteoporosis.
- If estrogen-only therapy is given, an endometrial biopsy should be performed before therapy begins and annually thereafter. If endometrial hyperplasia develops, the patient must either stop estrogen therapy or add progestin. In either case, a repeat biopsy is essential to ensure that the hyperplasia has resolved. Transvaginal ultrasonography can detect excessive endometrial proliferation.

Migraine headache

The most common patient complaint, headache usually occurs as a symptom of an underlying disorder. Ninety percent of all headaches are vascular, result from muscle contraction, or a combination; 10% are due to underlying intracranial, systemic, or psychological disorders. Migraine headaches, probably the most intensely studied, are throbbing, vascular headaches that usually begin to appear in childhood or adolescence and recur throughout adulthood. Affecting up to 10% of the United States population, they're more common in females and have a strong familial incidence.

Causes

Headaches are believed to be associated with constriction and dilation of intracranial and extracranial arteries. During a migraine attack, certain biochemical abnormalities are thought to occur. These abnormalities include local leakage of a vasodilator polypeptide called *neurokinin* through the dilated arteries and a decrease in the plasma level of serotonin.

Most chronic headaches result from tension (muscle contraction), which may be caused by:

- emotional stress or fatigue
- menstruation
- environmental stimuli (noise, crowds, or bright lights)

- vitamin A intake.

Other possible causes include:

- glaucoma
- inflammation of the eyes or mucosa of the nasal or paranasal sinuses
- diseases of the scalp, teeth, extracranial arteries, external or middle ear, or throat
- vasodilators (nitrates, alcohol, and histamines)
- systemic disease
- hypertension
- increased intracranial pressure (ICP)
- head trauma or tumor
- intracranial bleeding, abscess, or aneurysm
- hormone replacement therapy.

The evolution of a migraine headache has four distinct phases:

- *Normal* — Cerebral and temporal arteries are innervated extracranially; parenchymal arteries are noninnervated.
- *Vasoconstriction (aura)* — Stress-related neurogenic local vasoconstriction of innervated cerebral arteries reduces cerebral blood flow (localized ischemia). Systematically, the prostaglandin thromboxane causes increased platelet aggregation and release of serotonin, a potent vasoconstrictor and, possibly, other vasoactive substances.
- *Parenchymal artery dilation* — Noninnervated parenchymal vessels dilate in response to local acidosis and anoxia (ischemia). Neurogenic or biological factors may cause preformed arteriovenous shunts to open. Increased blood flow, increased internal pressure, and enhanced pulsations short-circuit the normal nutritive capillaries and cause pain.
- *Vasodilation (headache)* — Compensatory mechanisms cause marked vasodilation of the innervated arteries, resulting in headache. Systemic platelet aggregation decreases, and falling serotonin levels result in vasodilation. A painful, sterile perivascular inflammation develops and persists into the postheadache phase.

Signs and symptoms

Initially, migraine headaches usually produce unilateral, pulsating pain, which later becomes more generalized. They're commonly preceded by a scintillating scotoma, geometric visual patterns, unusual tastes or smell, hemianopsia, unilateral paresthesia, or speech disorders. The patient may experience irritability, sweating, anorexia, nausea, vomiting, and photophobia. (See *Clinical features of migraine headache*, page 362.)

Both muscle contraction and traction-inflammatory vascular headaches produce a dull, persistent ache, tender spots on the head and neck, and a feeling of tightness around the head, with a characteristic "hat-band" distribution. The pain is commonly severe and unrelenting. If caused by intracranial bleeding, headache may result in neurologic deficits, such as paresthesia and muscle weakness; narcotics may fail to relieve pain in these cases. If caused by a tumor, pain is most severe when the patient awakens.

Clinical features of migraine headache

This chart lists types of migraine headache along with the clinical features of each.

Type	Signs and symptoms
Common migraine (most prevalent)	
Usually occurs on weekends or holidays	▪ Prodromal symptoms, including fatigue, nausea, vomiting, and fluid imbalance, that precede headache by about 1 day ▪ Sensitivity to light and noise (most prominent feature) ▪ Headache pain (unilateral or bilateral, aching or throbbing)
Classic migraine	
Usually occurs in compulsive personalities or within families	▪ Prodromal symptoms, including vision disturbances, such as zigzag lines and bright lights (most common), sensory disturbances (tingling of face, lips, and hands), or motor disturbances (staggering gait) ▪ Recurrent, periodic headaches
Hemiplegic and ophthalmoplegic migraine (rare)	
Usually occurs in young adults	▪ Severe, unilateral pain ▪ Extraocular muscle palsies (involving third cranial nerve) and ptosis ▪ With repeated headaches, possible permanent injury to the third cranial nerve ▪ In hemiplegic migraine, neurologic deficits (hemiparesis, hemiplegia) that may persist after headache subsides
Basilar artery migraine	
Occurs in young women before their menstrual periods	▪ Prodromal symptoms, including partial vision loss followed by vertigo, ataxia, dysarthria, tinnitus and, sometimes, tingling of fingers and toes that lasts from several minutes to almost 1 hour ▪ Headache pain, severe occipital throbbing, vomiting

Complications may include:

- misdiagnosis of a more serious condition such as stroke
- status migraines
- drug dependency
- disruption of lifestyle.

Diagnosis

Diagnosis requires a history of recurrent headaches and physical examination of the head and neck. Such examination includes percussion, auscultation for bruits, inspection for signs of infection, and palpation for defects, crepitus, or tender spots (especially after trauma). Definitive diagnosis also requires a complete neurologic examination, assessment for other systemic diseases, and a psychosocial evaluation when such factors are suspected.

Diagnostic tests include cervical spine and sinus X-rays, EEG, computed tomography scan (performed before lumbar puncture to rule out increased ICP) or magnetic resonance imaging. A lumbar puncture isn't done if there's evidence of increased ICP or if a brain tumor is suspected because rapidly reducing pressure, by removing spinal fluid, can cause brain herniation.

Treatment

Depending on the type of headache, analgesics — ranging from aspirin (Bayer) to codeine or meperidine (Demerol) — may provide symptomatic relief. Other measures include identification and elimination of causative factors and, possibly, psychotherapy for headaches caused by emotional stress. Chronic tension headaches may also require muscle relaxants.

For migraine headaches, ergotamine (Migranal) alone or with caffeine may be an effective treatment. Remember that pregnant women can't take these medications because they stimulate uterine contractions. These drugs and others, such as metoclopramide (Reglan) or naproxen (Naprosyn), work best when taken early in the course of an attack. If nausea and vomiting make oral administration impossible, drugs may be given as rectal suppositories.

Drugs in the class of sumatriptan (Imitrex) are considered by many physicians to be the drug of choice for acute migraine attacks or cluster headaches. Drugs that can help prevent migraine headaches include propranolol (Inderal), atenolol (Tenormin), clonidine (Catapres), and amitriptyline.

Special considerations

Headaches seldom require hospitalization unless caused by a serious disorder. If that's the case, direct your care to the underlying problem. Otherwise, consider these patient care measures:

- Obtain a complete patient history, including duration and location of the headache, time of day it usually begins, nature of the pain, concurrence with other symptoms such as blurred vision, medications taken such as hormonal contraceptives, prolonged fasting, and precipitating factors, such as tension, menstruation, loud noises, menopause, or alcohol. Exacerbating factors can also be assessed through ongoing observation of the patient's personality, habits, activities of daily living, family relationships, coping mechanisms, and relaxation activities.
- Using the patient history as a guide, help the patient avoid exacerbating factors. Advise her to lie down in a dark, quiet room during an attack and to place ice packs on her forehead or a cold cloth over her eyes.
- Instruct the patient to take the prescribed medication at the onset of migraine symptoms; prevent dehydration by drinking plenty of fluids after nausea and vomiting subside, and use other headache relief measures.
- The patient with a migraine headache usually needs to be hospitalized only if nausea and vomiting are severe

enough to induce dehydration and possible shock.

Multiple sclerosis

Multiple sclerosis (MS) is a chronic, degenerative disease that causes demyelination of the white matter of the brain and spinal cord and damage to nerve fibers and their targets. Characterized by exacerbations and remissions, MS is a major cause of chronic disability in young adults. It usually becomes symptomatic between ages 20 and 40 (the average age of onset is 27). MS affects three women for every two men and five whites for every nonwhite. Incidence is generally higher among urban populations and upper socioeconomic groups. A family history of MS and living in a cold, damp climate increase the risk.

The prognosis varies. MS may progress rapidly, disabling the patient by early adulthood or causing death within months of onset. However, 70% of patients lead active, productive lives with prolonged remissions.

Several types of MS have been identified. Terms to describe MS types include:

- *Relapsing-remitting MS* demonstrates definite but unpredictable relapses (or acute attacks or exacerbations) during which new symptoms appear or existing symptoms become more severe and last for varying periods (days to months). Although patients recover fully from these acute attacks, they'll always have MS and its degenerative effects. (*Note:* The disease doesn't worsen between the attacks.)
- *Benign MS* involves one or two attacks after which recovery is complete and no any permanent disability remains. However, minimal disability occurs after 10 to 15 years of onset.
- *Primary-progressive MS* is a steady progression and worsening of symptoms from onset with minor recovery or plateaus. (This form is uncommon and may involve different brain and spinal cord damage than other forms.)
- *Secondary-progressive MS* begins as a pattern of clear-cut relapses and recovery with steadily progressive disability that worsens later in the course of the disease between acute attacks.

Causes

The exact cause of MS is unknown; however, current theories suggest that a slow-acting or latent viral infection triggers an autoimmune response. Other theories suggest that environmental and genetic factors may also be linked to MS.

Certain conditions appear to precede onset or exacerbation, including:

- emotional stress
- fatigue (physical or emotional)
- pregnancy
- acute respiratory infections.

In MS, sporadic patches of axon demyelination and nerve fiber loss occur throughout the central nervous system, inducing widely disseminated and varied neurologic dysfunction. New evidence of nerve fiber loss may provide an explanation for the neurologic deficits experienced by many patients with MS. The axons determine the presence or absence of function; loss of myelin doesn't correlate with loss of function.

Signs and symptoms

Signs and symptoms of MS depend on the extent and site of myelin destruction, the extent of remyelination, and the adequacy of subsequent restored synaptic transmissions. Flare-ups may be transient or last for hours or weeks, possibly waxing and waning with no predictable pattern. The patient may have difficulty describing the symptoms. Clinical effects may be so mild that the patient is unaware of them or so intense that they're debilitating. Typical first signs and symptoms related to conduction deficits and impaired impulse transmission along the nerve fiber and include:

- vision problems
- sensory impairment, such as burning and pins and needles, decreased ability to sense temperatures or vibrations, and decreased strength
- fatigue.

Other characteristic changes include:

- *ocular disturbances* — optic neuritis, diplopia, ophthalmoplegia, blurred vision, and nystagmus from impaired cranial nerve dysfunction and conduction deficits to the optic nerve
- *muscle dysfunction* — weakness, paralysis ranging from monoplegia to quadriplegia, spasticity, hyperreflexia, intention tremor, and gait ataxia from impaired motor reflex
- *urinary disturbances* — incontinence, frequency, urgency, and frequent infections from impaired transmission involving sphincter innervation
- *bowel disturbances* — involuntary evacuation or constipation from altered impulse transmission to internal sphincter
- *fatigue* — commonly the most debilitating symptom
- *speech problems* — poorly articulated or scanning speech and dysphagia from impaired transmission to the cranial nerves and sensory cortex.

Complications of MS may include:

- injuries from falls
- urinary tract infection
- constipation
- joint contractures
- pressure ulcers
- rectal distention
- pneumonia
- depression.

Diagnosis

Because early symptoms may be mild, years may elapse between onset and diagnosis. Diagnosis of this disorder requires evidence of two or more neurologic attacks. Periodic testing and close observation are necessary, perhaps for years, depending on the course of the disease. Spinal cord compression, foramen magnum tumor (which may mimic the exacerbations and remissions of MS), multiple small strokes, syphilis or another infection, thyroid disease, and chronic fatigue syndrome must be ruled out.

The following tests may be useful in diagnosing MS:

- Magnetic resonance imaging reveals multifocal white matter lesions.

- EEG reveals abnormalities in brain waves in one-third of patients.
- Lumbar puncture shows normal total cerebrospinal fluid (CSF) protein but elevated immunoglobulin (Ig) G (gamma globulin); IgG reflects hyperactivity of the immune system due to chronic demyelination. An elevated CSF IgG is significant only when serum IgG is normal. CSF white blood cell count may be elevated.
- CSF electrophoresis detects bands of IgG in most patients, even when the percentage of IgG in CSF is normal. Presence of kappa light chains provides additional support to the diagnosis.
- Evoked potential studies (visual, brain stem, auditory, and somatosensory) reveal slowed conduction of nerve impulses in most patients.

Treatment

The aim of treatment is threefold: Treat the acute exacerbation, treat the disease process, and treat the related signs and symptoms. These measures include:

- I.V. methylprednisolone (Depo-Medrol) followed by oral therapy reduces edema of the myelin sheath (speeds recovery from acute attacks). Other drugs, such as azathioprine (Imuran) or methotrexate (Rheumatrex) and misoprostol (Cytotec) may be used.
- Immune system therapy consisting of interferon beta-1a (Avonex), interferon beta-1b (Betaseron), and glatiramer (Copaxone), (a combination of four amino acids) reduces frequency and severity of relapses and may slow central nervous system damage.
- Stretching and range-of-motion exercises coupled with correct positioning may relieve the spasticity resulting from opposing muscle groups relaxing and contracting at the same time and may be helpful in relaxing muscles and maintaining function.
- Baclofen and tizanidine may be used to treat spasticity. For severe spasticity, botulinum toxin injections, intrathecal injections, nerve blocks, and surgery may be necessary.
- Frequent rest periods, aerobic exercise, and cooling techniques (air conditioning, breezes, water sprays) may minimize fatigue. Fatigue is characterized by an overwhelming feeling of exhaustion without obvious cause that can occur at any time of the day without warning. Changes in environmental conditions, such as heat and humidity, can aggravate fatigue.
- Amantadine (Symmetrel) treats stiffness; pemoline (Cylert) and methylphenidate (Ritalin) serve as antidepressants, which helps manage fatigue.
- Interferon beta-1a, the only proven therapy for the relapsing form of MS, decreases the number of flare-ups and slows the occurrence of the degenerative disabilities associated with MS.
- Bladder problems (failure to store urine, failure to empty the bladder or, more commonly, both) are managed by such strategies as drinking cranberry juice or insertion of an indwelling catheter and suprapubic tubes. Intermittent self-catheterization and postvoid catheterization programs are

helpful as well as anticholinergic medications for urge incontinence or urinary retention.

- Bowel problems (constipation and involuntary evacuation) are managed by such measures as increasing fiber intake, using bulking agents, and bowel-training strategies, including daily suppositories and rectal stimulation.
- Low-dose tricyclic antidepressants, phenytoin (Dilantin), or carbamazepine (Tegretol) may manage sensory symptoms, such as pain, numbness, burning, and tingling sensations. Selective serotonin reuptake inhibitors may also treat depression.
- Adaptive devices and physical therapy assist with motor dysfunction, such as problems with balance, strength, and muscle coordination.
- Beta-adrenergic blockers, sedatives, or diuretics may be used to alleviate tremors.
- Speech therapy may manage dysarthria.
- Antihistamines, vision therapy, or exercises may minimize vertigo.
- Vision therapy or adaptive lenses may manage visual problems.

Special considerations

Management considerations focus on educating the patient and family:

- Assist with physical therapy. Increase patient comfort with massages and relaxing baths. Make sure the bath water isn't too hot because it may temporarily intensify otherwise subtle symptoms. Assist with active, resistive, and stretching exercises to maintain muscle tone and joint mobility, decrease spasticity, improve coordination, and boost morale.
- Educate the patient and her family concerning the chronic course of MS. Emphasize the need to avoid stress, infections, and fatigue and to maintain independence by developing new ways of performing daily activities. Be sure to tell the patient to avoid exposure to infections.
- Stress the importance of eating a nutritious, well-balanced diet that contains sufficient roughage and adequate fluids to prevent constipation.
- Evaluate the need for bowel and bladder training during hospitalization. Encourage adequate fluid intake and regular urination. Eventually, the patient may require urinary drainage by self-catheterization (or, in men, condom drainage). Teach the correct use of suppositories to help establish a regular bowel schedule.
- Watch for adverse drug effects. For instance, dantrolene may cause muscle weakness and decreased muscle tone.
- Promote emotional stability. Help the patient establish a daily routine to maintain optimal functioning. Activity level is regulated by tolerance level. Encourage regular rest periods to prevent fatigue and daily physical exercise.
- Inform the patient that exacerbations are unpredictable, necessitating physical and emotional adjustments in lifestyle.
- For more information, refer the patient to the National Multiple Sclerosis Society.

Myasthenia gravis

Myasthenia gravis causes sporadic but progressive weakness and abnormal fatigability of striated (skeletal) muscles. Symptoms are exacerbated by exercise and repeated movement and relieved by anticholinesterase drugs. Usually, this disorder affects muscles innervated by the cranial nerves (face, lips, tongue, neck, and throat) but can affect any muscle group.

Myasthenia gravis follows an unpredictable course of periodic exacerbations and remissions. There's no known cure. Drug treatment has improved the prognosis and allows patients to lead relatively normal lives, except during exacerbations. When the disease involves the respiratory system, it may be life-threatening.

Myasthenia gravis affects 1 in 25,000 people at any age, but incidence peaks between ages 20 and 40. It's three times more common in women than in men in this age-group; however, after age 40, the incidence is similar in women and men.

About 20% of infants born to mothers with myasthenia gravis have transient (or occasionally persistent) myasthenia for 2 to 3 weeks. This disease may coexist with immune and thyroid disorders; 15% of patients with myasthenia gravis have thymomas. Remissions occur in about 25% of patients.

Causes

Myasthenia gravis causes a failure in transmission of nerve impulses at the neuromuscular junction. The site of action is the postsynaptic membrane. Theoretically, antireceptor antibodies block, weaken, or reduce the number of acetylcholine receptors available at each neuromuscular junction, impairing muscle depolarization necessary for movement. (See *Impaired transmission in myasthenia gravis.*)

The exact cause of myasthenia gravis is unknown. However, it's believed to be the result of:

- autoimmune response
- ineffective acetylcholine release
- inadequate muscle fiber response to acetylcholine.

In addition, certain medications, such as antibiotics, beta-adrenergic blockers, lithium, magnesium, Proscar, verapamil, and quinidine, can exacerbate the disease.

Signs and symptoms

Myasthenia gravis may occur gradually or suddenly. Signs and symptoms include:

- weak eye closure, ptosis, and diplopia from impaired neuromuscular transmission to the cranial nerves supplying the eye muscles (may be the only symptom present)
- skeletal muscle weakness and fatigue, increasing through the day but decreasing with rest (in the early stages, easy fatigability of certain muscles with or without other findings and, later, possibly severe enough to cause paralysis)
- progressive muscle weakness and accompanying loss of function, depending on the muscle group affected, that becomes more intense during menses and after emotional stress,

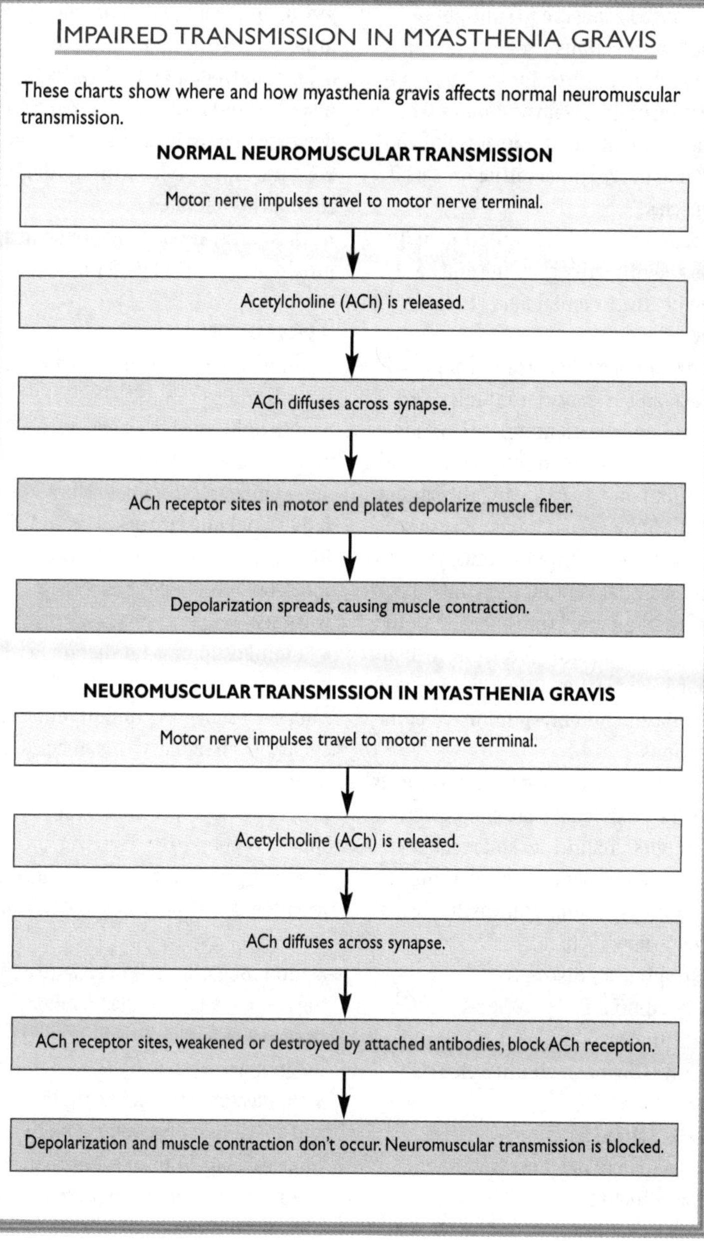

Impaired transmission in myasthenia gravis

These charts show where and how myasthenia gravis affects normal neuromuscular transmission.

prolonged exposure to sunlight or cold, or infections

- blank and expressionless facial appearance and nasal vocal tones secondary to impaired transmission of cranial nerves innervating the facial muscles
- frequent nasal regurgitation of fluids and difficulty chewing and swallowing from cranial nerve involvement
- drooping eyelids from weakness of facial and extraocular muscles
- weakened neck muscles that may become too weak to support the head without bobbing, causing the patient to tilt her head back to be able to see
- weakened respiratory muscles, decreased tidal volume and vital capacity from impaired transmission to the diaphragm making breathing difficult and predisposing the patient to pneumonia and other respiratory tract infections
- respiratory muscle weakness (myasthenic crisis) that's possibly severe enough to require an emergency airway and mechanical ventilation.

Complications of myasthenia gravis may include:

- respiratory distress
- pneumonia
- aspiration
- myasthenic or cholinergic crisis.

Diagnosis

Tests to help diagnose myasthenia gravis include:

- The tensilon test confirms diagnosis of myasthenia gravis, revealing temporarily improved muscle function within 30 to 60 seconds after I.V. injection of edrophonium or neostigmine and lasting up to 30 minutes.
- Electromyography with repeated neural stimulation shows progressive decrease in muscle fiber contraction.
- Serum antiacetylcholine antibody titer may be elevated.
- Chest X-ray reveals thymoma (in approximately 15% of patients).

Treatment

Treatment of myasthenia gravis may include:

- anticholinesterase drugs, such as neostigmine (Prostigmin) and pyridostigmine (Mestinon), to counteract fatigue and muscle weakness and allow about 80% of normal muscle function (less effective as disease worsens)
- immunosuppressant therapy with corticosteroids, azathioprine (Imuran), cyclosporine (Sandimmune) and cyclophosphamide (Cytoxan) used in a progressive fashion (moving on to next drug when previous drug response is poor) to decrease the immune response toward acetylcholine receptors at the neuromuscular junction
- immunoglobulin G (BayGam) during acute relapses or plasmapheresis in severe exacerbations to suppress the immune system
- thymectomy to remove thymomas and possibly induce remission in some cases of adult-onset myasthenia
- tracheotomy, positive-pressure ventilation, and vigorous suctioning to remove secretions for treatment of acute exacerbations that cause severe respiratory distress

- in myasthenic crisis, discontinuation of anticholinesterase drugs until respiratory function improves as well as immediate hospitalization and vigorous respiratory support.

Special considerations

Careful baseline assessment, early recognition and treatment of potential crises, supportive measures, and thorough patient teaching can minimize exacerbations and complications of myasthenia gravis. Continuity of care is essential. Care measures include:

- Establish an accurate neurologic and respiratory baseline. Thereafter, monitor tidal volume and vital capacity regularly. The patient may need a ventilator and frequent suctioning to remove accumulating secretions.
- Be alert for signs of an impending myasthenic crisis (increased muscle weakness, respiratory distress, and difficulty talking or chewing).
- Be alert for signs of impending cholinergic crisis (profound weakness, increased respiratory secretions, and respiratory failure).
- To prevent relapses, adhere closely to the ordered drug administration schedule. Be prepared to give atropine for anticholinesterase overdose or toxicity.
- Plan exercise, meals, patient care, and activities to make the most of energy peaks. For example, give medication 20 to 30 minutes before meals to facilitate chewing or swallowing. Allow the patient to participate in his care.
- When swallowing is difficult, give soft, solid foods instead of liquids to lessen the risk of choking.
- After a severe exacerbation, try to increase social activity as soon as possible.
- Patient teaching is essential because myasthenia gravis is usually a lifelong condition. Help the patient plan daily activities to coincide with energy peaks. Stress the need for frequent rest periods throughout the day. Emphasize that periodic remissions, exacerbations, and day-to-day fluctuations are common.
- Teach the patient how to recognize adverse effects and signs of anticholinesterase toxicity (headaches, weakness, sweating, abdominal cramps, nausea, vomiting, diarrhea, excessive salivation, and bronchospasm) and corticosteroid toxicity (euphoria, insomnia, edema, and increased appetite).
- Warn the patient to avoid strenuous exercise, stress, infection, and needless exposure to the sun or cold. All of these things may worsen signs and symptoms. Wearing an eye patch or glasses with one frosted lens may help the patient with diplopia.
- Encourage the patient to wear medical identification jewelry at all times.
- For more information and an opportunity to meet other myasthenia gravis patients who lead full, productive lives, refer the patient to the Myasthenia Gravis Foundation.

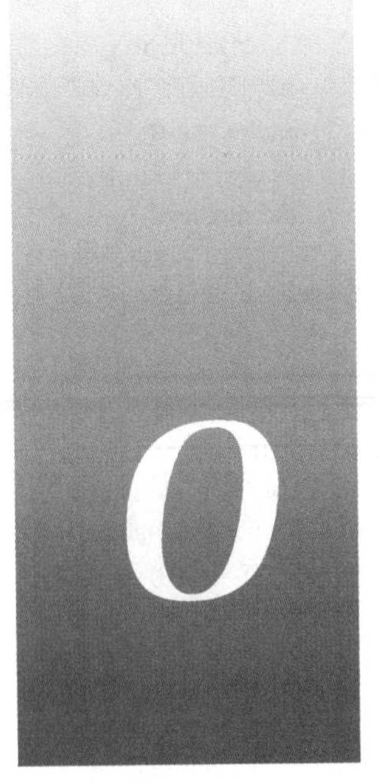

Obsessive-compulsive disorder

Obsessive thoughts and compulsive behaviors represent recurring efforts to control overwhelming anxiety, guilt, or unacceptable impulses that persistently enter the consciousness. The word *obsession* refers to a recurrent idea, thought, impulse, or image that's intrusive and inappropriate, causing marked anxiety or distress. A *compulsion* is a ritualistic, repetitive, and involuntary defensive behavior or action. Performing a compulsive behavior reduces the patient's anxiety and increases the probability that the behavior will recur. Compulsions are commonly associated with obsessions.

Patients with obsessive-compulsive disorder (OCD) are prone to abuse psychoactive substances, such as alcohol and anxiolytics, in an attempt to relieve their anxiety. In addition, other anxiety disorders, Tourette syndrome, attention deficient hyperactivity disorder (ADHD), and major depression commonly coexist with OCD. OCD is typically a chronic condition with remissions and flare-ups and is likely to begin during adolescence. Mild forms of the disorder are relatively common in the population at large. Although OCD tends to affect men and women equally, men typically have the disorder earlier in life than women, with most men being diagnosed between ages 6 and 15, whereas women are typically diagnosed in their 20s. Also, men are more likely to have chronic OCD whereas women are more likely to have acute, or episodic, OCD.

Causes

The cause of OCD is unknown. Research indicates that there are abnormalities in central nervous system serotonin transmission and in the paralimbic circuit. Some studies suggest the possibility of brain lesions, but the most useful research and clinical studies base an explanation on psychological theories. In addition, major depression, organic brain syndrome, and schizophrenia may contribute to the onset of OCD. Some authorities think OCD is closely related to certain eating disorders. Also, someone who has a blood relative with OCD is more likely to develop OCD than someone who doesn't. Even so, not everyone who has a relative with the disorder will necessarily develop it.

Signs and symptoms

The psychiatric history of a patient with this disorder may reveal the presence of obsessive thoughts, words, or mental images that persistently and involuntarily invade the consciousness. Some common obsessions include thoughts of violence (such as stabbing, shooting, maiming, or hitting), thoughts of contamination (images of dirt, germs, or feces), repetitive doubts and worries about a tragic event, and repeating or counting images, words, or objects in the environment. The patient recognizes that the obsessions are a product of her own mind and that they interfere with normal daily activities.

The patient's history may also reveal the presence of compulsions, which are irrational and recurring impulses to repeat a certain behavior. Common compulsions include repetitive touching, sometimes combined with counting; doing and undoing (for instance, opening and closing doors or rearranging things); washing (especially hands); and checking (to be sure no tragedy has occurred since the last time she checked). In many cases, the patient's anxiety is so strong that she'll avoid the situation or the object that evokes the impulse.

When the obsessive-compulsive phenomena are mental, observation may reveal no behavioral abnormalities. However, compulsive acts may be observed. Feelings of shame, nervousness, or embarrassment may prompt the patient to try limiting these acts to her own private time.

Diagnosis

For characteristic findings in patients with this condition, see *Diagnosing OCD*, page 374. Coexisting disorders, such as depression, ADHD, and eating, personality, or anxiety disorders, can make OCD more difficult to diagnose. Although there's no laboratory test that diagnoses OCD, the disorder usually causes severe distress and interferes with a person's normal routine,

Diagnosing OCD

The diagnosis of obsessive-compulsive disorder (OCD) is made when the patient's signs and symptoms meet the established criteria put forth in the *Diagnostic and Statistical Manual of Mental Disorders*, Fourth Edition, Text Revision. These signs and symptoms are outlined here.

Obsessions or compulsions

Obsessions are defined as all of the following:

- Recurrent and persistent thoughts, impulses, or images perceived to be intrusive and inappropriate by the patient, causing anxiety or distress at some point in time during the disturbance.
- The thoughts, impulses, or images aren't simply excessive worries about real-life problems.
- The person attempts to ignore or suppress such thoughts or impulses, or to neutralize them with some other thought or action.
- The person recognizes that the obsessions are the products of her mind and not externally imposed.

Compulsions are defined as all of the following:

- Repetitive behaviors or mental acts performed by the person, who feels driven to perform them in response to an obsession or according to rules that must be applied rigidly.
- The behavior or mental acts are aimed at preventing or reducing distress or preventing some dreaded event or situation. However, the activity is clearly excessive or unconnected in a realistic way with what it's designed to neutralize or prevent.
- The patient recognizes that her behavior is excessive or unreasonable (may not be true for young children or for patients whose obsessions have evolved into overvalued ideas).

Additional criteria

- At some point, the person recognizes that the obsessions or compulsions are excessive or unreasonable.
- The obsessions or compulsions cause marked distress, are time-consuming (take more than 1 hour per day), or significantly interfere with the person's normal routine, occupational functioning, or usual social activities or relationships.
- If another axis I disorder is present, the content of the obsession is unrelated to it; for example, the ideas, thoughts, or images aren't about food in the presence of an eating disorder, about drugs in the presence of a psychoactive substance abuse disorder, or about guilt in a major depressive disorder.
- The disturbance isn't due to the direct physiologic effects of a substance or a general medical condition.

work, social activities, and relationships.

Treatment

OCD is tenacious, but improvement occurs in 60% to 70% of patients who obtain treatment. Current treatment usually involves a combination of medication and cognitive behavioral therapy. Other types of psychotherapy may also be helpful.

The most effective medications are selective serotonin reuptake inhibitors, such as fluoxetine (Prozac), paroxetine (Paxil), sertraline (Zoloft), and fluvoxamine (Luvox); and tricyclic antidepressants such as clomipramine (Anafranil). These drugs help decrease the frequency and intensity of the obsessions and compulsions. Improvement usually takes three or more weeks and the patient will have to continue the medication indefinitely.

Behavioral therapies — aversion therapy, thought stopping, thought switching, flooding, implosion therapy, and exposure and response prevention — have also been effective. (See *Behavioral therapies*.)

Special considerations

- Approach the patient unhurriedly.
- Provide an accepting atmosphere; don't appear shocked, amused, or critical of the ritualistic behavior.
- Keep the patient's physical health in mind. For example, compulsive hand washing may cause skin breakdown; rituals or preoccupations may cause inadequate food and fluid intake and exhaustion. Provide for basic needs, such as rest, nutrition, and grooming, if the patient becomes involved in ritualistic thoughts and behaviors to the point of self-neglect.
- Let the patient know you're aware of her behavior. For example, you might say, "I noticed you've made your bed three times today; that must be very tiring for you." Help the patient explore feelings associated with the behavior. For example, ask her, "What do you think about while you're performing your chores?"
- Make reasonable demands and set reasonable limits, explaining their purpose clearly. Avoid creating situations that increase frustration and provoke anger, which may interfere

Behavioral therapies

These behavioral therapies are used to treat a patient with obsessive-compulsive disorder:

- *Aversion therapy* involves application of a painful stimulus to create an aversion to the obsession that leads to undesirable behavior (compulsion).
- *Thought stopping* breaks the habit of fear-inducing anticipatory thoughts. The patient learns to stop unwanted thoughts by saying the word "stop" and then focusing her attention on achieving calmness and muscle relaxation.
- *Thought switching* attempts to replace fear-inducing self-instructions with competent self-instructions. In doing so, the patient learns to replace negative thoughts with positive ones until the positive thoughts become strong enough to overcome the anxiety-provoking ones.
- *Flooding* is frequent, full-intensity exposure (through the use of imagery) to an object that triggers a symptom. It must be used with caution because it produces extreme discomfort.
- *Implosion therapy* is a form of desensitization that calls for repeated exposure to a highly feared object.
- *Response prevention* involves preventing compulsive behavior by distraction, persuasion, or redirection of activity. This treatment may require hospitalization or involvement of the family to be effective.

with treatment or may trigger an obsessive or compulsive thought.

- Explore patterns leading to the behavior or recurring problems.
- Engage the patient in activities to create positive accomplishments and to raise self-esteem and confidence.
- Encourage active diversionary activities, such as whistling or humming a tune, to divert attention from the unwanted thoughts and to promote a pleasurable experience.
- Help the patient develop new ways to solve problems, and cultivate more effective coping skills by setting limits on unacceptable behavior (for example, by limiting the number of times per day she may indulge in compulsive behavior). Gradually shorten the time allowed. Help her focus on other feelings or problems for the remainder of the time.
- Identify insight and improved behavior (reduced compulsive behavior and fewer obsessive thoughts). Evaluate behavioral changes by your own observations and the patient's reports.
- Identify disturbing topics of conversation that reflect underlying anxiety or terror.
- Help the patient identify progress and set realistic expectations of herself and others.
- Work with the patient and other treatment team members to establish behavioral goals and to help the patient tolerate anxiety in pursuing these goals.
- Provide support to family members and educate them on OCD to help them manage OCD and prevent its recurrence and complications.

Osteoarthritis

Osteoarthritis, commonly referred to as *degenerative joint disease*, is the most common joint disorder. It's a chronic condition causing the deterioration of joint cartilage and the formation of reactive new bone at the margins and subchondral areas of the joints. It usually affects weight-bearing joints (knees, feet, hips, lumbar vertebrae). Osteoarthritis is widespread (affecting more than 60 million persons in the United States) and is most common in women. Typically, its earliest symptoms manifest in middle age and progress from there.

Disability depends on the site and severity of involvement and can range from minor limitation of finger movement to severe disability in persons with hip or knee involvement. The rate of progression varies, and joints may remain stable for years in an early stage of deterioration.

SPECIAL NEEDS

In older women, the most common sites for osteoporosis are the hands and the knees.

Causes

Osteoarthritis occurs in synovial joints. The primary defect in both idiopathic and secondary osteoarthritis is loss of articular cartilage due to functional changes in chondrocytes (cells responsible for the formation of the proteoglycans, glycoproteins that act as cementing material in the cartilage, and collagen). New bone, called *osteophyte* (bone spur), then forms at joint margins as the articular cartilage erodes, causing gross alteration of the bony contours and enlargement of the joint.

Idiopathic osteoarthritis, a normal part of aging, results from many factors, including:

- metabolic factors (endocrine disorders such as hyperparathyroidism) and genetic factors (decreased collagen synthesis)
- chemical factors (drugs that stimulate the collagen-digesting enzymes in the synovial membrane such as steroids)
- mechanical factors (repeated stress on the joint).

Secondary osteoarthritis usually follows an identifiable predisposing event that leads to degenerative changes, such as:

- trauma (most common cause)
- congenital deformity
- hormonal changes (particulary low estrogen levels)
- obesity.

Signs and symptoms

Symptoms, which increase with poor posture, obesity, and occupational stress, include:

- deep, aching joint pain due to degradation of the cartilage, inflammation, and bone stress, particularly after exercise or weight bearing (the most common symptom, usually relieved by rest)
- stiffness in the morning and after exercise (relieved by rest)
- crepitus, or "grating" of the joint during motion due to cartilage damage
- Heberden's nodes (bony enlargements of the distal interphalangeal joints) due to repeated inflammation
- altered gait from contractures due to overcompensation of the muscles supporting the joint
- decreased range of motion (ROM) due to pain and stiffness
- joint enlargement due to stress on the bone and disordered bone growth
- localized headaches (may be a direct result of cervical spine arthritis).

Complications of osteoarthritis include:

- irreversible joint changes and node formation (with nodes eventually becoming red, swollen, and tender, causing numbness and loss of finger dexterity)
- subluxation of the joint
- decreased joint ROM
- joint contractures
- pain (can be debilitating in later stages)
- loss of independence in activities of daily living.

Diagnosis

Findings that help diagnose osteoarthritis include:

- absence of systemic symptoms (ruling out inflammatory joint disorder)
- arthroscopy showing bone spurs and narrowing of joint space
- increased erythrocyte sedimentation rate (with extensive synovitis).

X-rays of the affected joint help confirm the diagnosis but may be normal in the early stages. X-rays may require many views and typically show:

- narrowing of joint space or margin

Specific care for arthritic joints

Care for an arthritic joint depends on the affected joint:

- *Hand*—Apply hot soaks and paraffin dips to relieve pain as ordered.
- *Lumbar and sacral spine*—Recommend a firm mattress or bed board to decrease morning pain.
- *Cervical spine*—Check cervical collar for constriction; watch for redness with prolonged use.
- *Hip*—Use moist heat pads to relieve pain, and administer antispasmodic drugs as ordered. Assist with range-of-motion (ROM) and strengthening exercises, always making sure the patient gets the proper rest afterward. Check crutches, cane, braces, and walker for proper fit, and teach the patient to use them correctly. For example, the patient with unilateral joint involvement should use an orthopedic appliance (such as a cane or walker) on the unaffected side. Advise use of cushions when sitting and use of an elevated toilet seat.
- *Knee*—Assist with prescribed ROM exercises, exercises to maintain muscle tone, and progressive resistance exercises to increase muscle strength. Provide elastic supports or braces, if needed.

Minimizing long-term effects

To minimize the long-term effects of osteoarthritis, teach the patient to:

- plan for adequate rest during the day, after exertion, and at night
- take medication exactly as prescribed and report adverse effects immediately
- avoid overexertion, take care to stand and walk correctly, minimize weight-bearing activities, and be especially careful when stooping or picking up objects
- always wear well-fitting supportive shoes and avoid worn-down heels
- install safety devices at home such as guard rails in the bathroom
- perform ROM exercises as gently as possible
- maintain proper body weight to reduce strain on joints
- avoid percussive activities.

- cystlike bony deposits in joint space and margins as well as sclerosis of the subchondral space
- joint deformity due to degeneration or articular damage
- bony growths at weight-bearing areas
- joint fusion.

Treatment

The goal of treatment is to relieve pain, maintain or improve mobility, and minimize disability. Treatment may include:

- weight loss to reduce stress on the joint
- balance of rest and exercise, such as swimming
- medications, including aspirin, fenoprofen (Nalfon), ibuprofen (Motrin), indomethacin (Indocin), phenylbutazone, and other nonsteroidal anti-inflammatory drugs; propoxyphene (Darvon); COX-2 inhibitors, such as celecoxib (Celebrex); and analgesic creams such as capsaicin (Capsin) (see *Specific care for arthritic joints*)

- support or stabilization of joint with crutches, braces, cane, walker, cervical collar, or traction to reduce stress
- intra-articular injections of corticosteroids (every 4 to 6 months) to possibly delay node development in the hands (if used too frequently, may accelerate arthritic progression by depleting the normal ground substance of the cartilage).

Surgical treatment, reserved for patients with severe disability or uncontrollable pain, may include:

- arthroplasty (partial or total replacement of the deteriorated part of the joint with a prosthetic appliance)
- arthrodesis (surgical fusion of bones, primarily in the spine [laminectomy])
- osteoplasty (scraping and lavage of deteriorated bone from the joint)
- osteotomy (change in alignment of bone to relieve stress by excision of a wedge of bone or cutting of the bone).

Special considerations

- Promote adequate rest, particularly after activity. Plan rest periods during the day, and provide for adequate sleep at night. Moderation is the key — teach the patient to pace daily activities.
- Assist with physical therapy, and encourage the patient to perform gentle, isometric ROM exercises.
- If the patient needs surgery, provide appropriate preoperative and postoperative care.
- Provide emotional support and reassurance to help the patient cope with limited mobility. Explain that osteoarthritis isn't a systemic disease.

Osteoporosis

Osteoporosis is a metabolic bone disorder in which the rate of bone resorption accelerates while the rate of bone formation slows, causing a loss of bone mass. Bones affected by this disease lose calcium and phosphate salts and become porous, brittle, and abnormally vulnerable to fractures. Osteoporosis may be primary or secondary to an underlying disease, such as Cushing's syndrome or hyperthyroidism. It primarily affects the weight-bearing vertebrae. Only when the condition is advanced or severe, as in secondary disease, do similar changes occur in the skull, ribs, and long bones. Usually, the femoral heads and pelvic acetabula are selectively affected.

Of those affected by osteoporosis, 80% are women. Primary osteoporosis is often called *postmenopausal osteoporosis* because it most commonly develops in postmenopausal women. (See *What's osteoporosis?* pages 380 and 381.)

Causes

In normal bone, the rates of bone formation and resorption are constant; replacement follows resorption immediately, and the amount of bone replaced equals the amount of bone resorbed. Osteoporosis develops when the remodeling cycle is interrupted, and new bone formation falls behind resorption. When bone is resorbed

What's osteoporosis?

Osteoporosis is a metabolic disease of the skeleton that reduces the amount of bone tissue. Bones weaken as local cells resorb, or take up, bone tissue. Trabecular bone at the core becomes less dense, and cortical bone on the perimeter loses thickness.

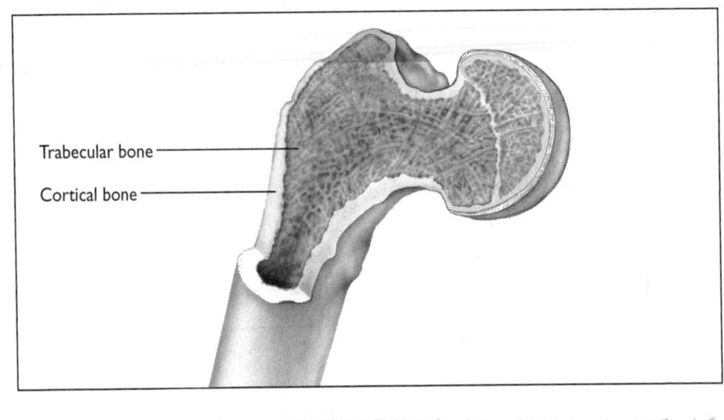

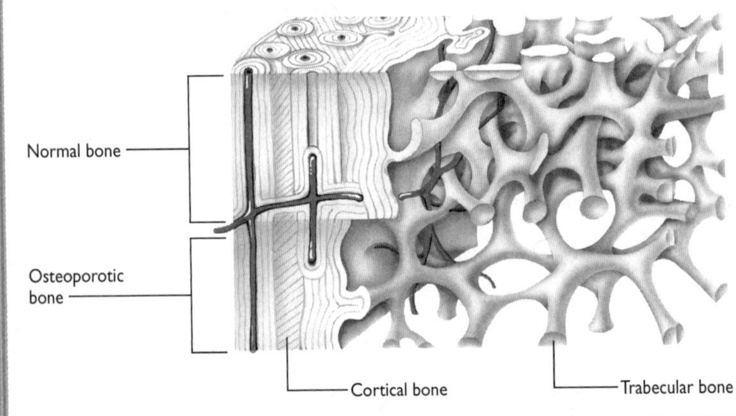

faster than it forms, the bone becomes less dense.

The cause of primary osteoporosis is unknown, but contributing factors include:

- mild but prolonged negative calcium balance due to inadequate dietary intake of calcium (possibly an important contributing factor)
- declining gonadal and adrenal function
- faulty protein metabolism due to relative or progressive estrogen deficiency (estrogen stimulates osteoblastic activity and limits the osteoclastic-stimulating effects of parathyroid hormones)
- sedentary lifestyle.

Bone formation and resorption

Bone consists of 30% organic and 70% mineral substances. The organic portion, called *osteoid,* acts as the matrix or framework for the mineral portion.

Bone cells called *osteoblasts* produce the osteoid matrix. The mineral portion, which consists of calcium and other minerals, hardens the osteoid matrix.

Large bone cells called *osteoclasts* reshape mature bone by resorbing the mineral and organic components. Bone formation and resorption are normal, continuous processes. However, in osteoporosis, osteoblasts continue to produce bone, but resorption by osteoclasts exceeds bone formation.

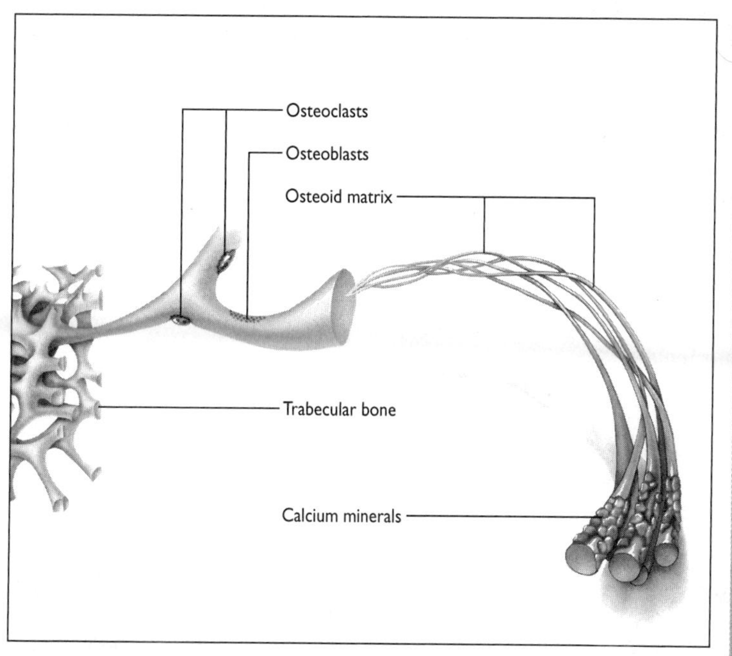

The many causes or risk factors of secondary osteoporosis include:

- prolonged therapy with steroids or heparin (heparin promotes bone resorption by inhibiting collagen synthesis or enhancing collagen breakdown)
- total immobilization or disuse of a bone (as in hemiplegia)
- alcoholism
- malnutrition
- malabsorption
- scurvy
- lactose intolerance
- endocrine disorders, such as hyperthyroidism, hyperparathyroidism, Cushing's syndrome, diabetes mellitus (plasma calcium and phosphate

concentrations are maintained by the endocrine system)

- osteogenesis imperfecta
- Sudeck's atrophy (localized to hands and feet, with recurring attacks)
- medications (aluminum-containing antacids, corticosteroids, anticonvulsants)
- cigarette smoking.

There are many other risk factors that have been identified, including:

- history of a fracture after age 50 or in a first-degree relative
- current low bone mass
- being female
- being thin or having a small frame
- advanced age
- family history of osteoporosis
- estrogen deficiency as a result of menopause, especially early or surgically induced
- abnormal absence of menstruation (amenorrhea)
- anorexia nervosa
- low testosterone levels in men

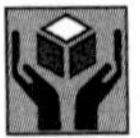

SPECIAL NEEDS

Caucasian or Asian women are at higher risk for osteoporosis, although Black and Hispanic women are at significant risk as well.

Signs and symptoms

Osteoporosis is typically discovered suddenly, such as:

- a postmenopausal woman bends to lift something, hears a snapping sound, then feels a sudden pain in her lower back
- vertebral collapse causes back pain that radiates around the trunk (most common presenting feature) and is aggravated by movement or jarring.

In another common pattern, osteoporosis can develop insidiously, showing:

- increasing deformity, kyphosis, loss of height, decreased exercise tolerance, and a markedly aged appearance
- spontaneous wedge fractures, pathologic fractures of the neck and femur, Colles' fractures of the distal radius after a minor fall, and hip fractures (common as bone is lost from the femoral neck).

Possible complications of osteoporosis include:

- spontaneous fractures as the bones lose volume and become brittle and weak
- shock, hemorrhage, or fat embolism (fatal complications of fractures).

Diagnosis

Differential diagnosis must exclude other causes of bone loss, especially those affecting the spine, such as metastatic cancer or advanced multiple myeloma. History is the key to identifying the specific cause of osteoporosis. Diagnosis may include:

- dual-energy X-ray absorptiometry (DEXA), the gold standard for measuring bone mass of the extremities, hips, and spine
- X-rays showing typical degeneration in the lower thoracic and lumbar vertebrae (vertebral bodies possibly appearing flattened and denser than normal, with bone mineral loss evident only in later stages)
- computed tomography scan to assess spinal bone loss

▪ normal serum calcium, phosphorus, and alkaline phosphatase levels and possibly elevated parathyroid hormone level
▪ bone biopsy showing bone that appears thin and porous but otherwise normal.

PREVENTION POINTER

In September of 2002, the U.S. Preventative Services Task Force panel recommended that all women age 65 and over should get bone density tests of the hip every 5 years and those women who are at higher risk for osteoporosis-related fractures should start screening at age 60. Medicare covers the cost of the test every 2 years for postmenopausal women if ordered by a physician.

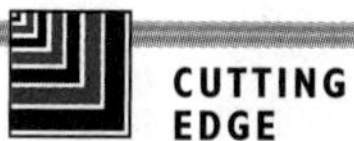

CUTTING EDGE

HRT AND OSTEOPOROSIS

In May 2002, the Women's Health Initiation Study reported an increased risk of breast cancer in postmenopausal women who took estrogen or hormone replacement therapy (ERT/HRT). In addition, no conclusive evidence was found to support the use of ERT or HRT for the treatment or prevention of osteoporosis. The American College of Obstetricians and Gynecologists stated after the May 2002 results that ERT and HRT for long-term prevention of osteoporosis should be used cautiously until more research on the subject becomes available.

Treatment

Treatment to control bone loss, prevent fractures, and control pain may include:
▪ physical therapy emphasizing gentle exercise and activity and regular, moderate weight-bearing exercise to slow bone loss and possibly reverse demineralization (the mechanical stress of exercise stimulates bone formation)
▪ supportive devices such as a back brace
▪ surgery, if indicated, for pathologic fractures
▪ selective estrogen receptor modulators (such as Evista) that have been approved by the Food and Drug Administration for postmenopausal women to increase bone density (see *HRT and osteoporosis*)
▪ analgesics and local heat to relieve pain.

In addition to selective estrogen receptor modulators, medications to treat osteoporosis include:
▪ calcium and vitamin D supplements to support normal bone metabolism, except when contraindicated, as with calcium supplements in patients with renal disease (see *Teriparatide,* page 384)
▪ calcitonin (Calcimar) to reduce bone resorption and slow the decline in bone mass
▪ bisphosphonates, such as etidronate (Didronel) or alendronate sodium (Fosamax) to increase bone density and restore lost bone (strict dosage precautions required; possible adverse effects, including gastric distress)

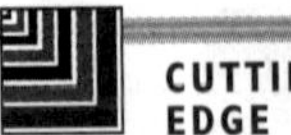

CUTTING EDGE

Teriparatide

Teriparatide, newly approved by the Food and Drug Administration, is derived from human parathyroid hormone, the main regulator of calcium and phosphate metabolism. In a study of 1,637 postmenopausal women with osteoporosis, researchers found that women who were treated with the new drug Forteo (teriparatide), along with calcium and vitamin D supplements had significant increases in bone mineral density compared to those who were taking a placebo along with the supplements.

Other studies have shown that teriparatide reduces the risk of fractures. However, the long-term effects of the drug are unknown, so using teriparatide for more than 2 years isn't recommended.

- vitamin C, calcium, and protein to support skeletal metabolism (through a balanced diet rich in nutrients).

Other measures include:

- early mobilization after surgery or trauma
- decreased alcohol and tobacco consumption
- careful observation for signs of malabsorption, (fatty stools, chronic diarrhea)
- prompt, effective treatment of the underlying disorder (to prevent secondary osteoporosis).

Special considerations

Your care plan should focus on the patient's fragility, stressing careful positioning, ambulation, and prescribed exercises.

- Check the patient's skin daily for redness, warmth, and new sites of pain, which may indicate new fractures. Encourage activity; help the patient walk several times daily. As appropriate, perform passive range-of-motion exercises or encourage the patient to perform active exercises. Make sure the patient regularly attends scheduled physical therapy sessions.
- Impose safety and fall precautions. Keep the bed's side-rails in the raised position. Move the patient gently and carefully at all times. Encourage her to wear comfortable, flat shoes with rubber soles to prevent slipping and falling. Explain to her family and ancillary health care personnel how easily an osteoporotic patient's bones can fracture.
- Make sure the patient and her family clearly understand the prescribed drug regimen. Tell them how to recognize significant adverse effects and to report them immediately. The patient should also report any new pain sites immediately, especially after trauma, no matter how slight. Advise her to sleep on a firm mattress and avoid excessive bed rest. Make sure she knows how to wear her back brace.
- Teach the patient good body mechanics — to stoop before lifting anything and to avoid twisting movements and prolonged bending.
- Instruct the female patient taking estrogen about the proper technique for breast self-examination. Tell her to perform this examination at least

once per month and to report any lumps immediately. Emphasize the need for regular gynecologic examinations. Tell her to report abnormal bleeding promptly.

PREVENTION POINTER

Remind the woman that, even at an early age, adequate daily intake of calcium and vitamin D as well as performing regular weight-bearing and resistance exercises remains the foundation of osteoporosis prevention and treatment.

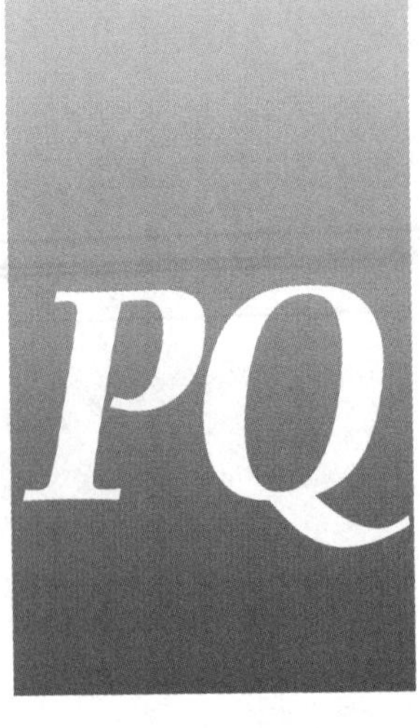

Panic disorder

Panic disorder represents anxiety in its most severe form. It's an anxiety disorder characterized by unexpected and recurrent episodes of intense apprehension, terror, and impending doom, usually accompanied by physical symptoms that mimic a heart attack or other serious medical condition. Initially unpredictable, panic attacks may later become associated with specific situations, places, or tasks. As the attacks become more frequent, the person commonly develops agoraphobia, also known as *phobic avoidance* — the avoidance of those situations, places, or tasks that trigger the attacks, rendering the person unable to leave a known, safe surrounding such as her home because of intense fear and anxiety. Panic disorder may also coexist with other disorders, such as depression and substance abuse.

Panic disorder typically has an onset in late adolescence or early adulthood, commonly in response to a sudden loss. It may also be triggered by severe separation anxiety experienced during early childhood. Panic disorder is twice as common in women as men and even higher for panic disorder with agoraphobia. In addition, women who experience more severe symptoms are more likely to have recurrences after wellness and experience the illness for a longer period. Without treatment, panic disorder can persist for years with alternating exacerbations and remissions.

Causes

Although the exact cause of panic disorder isn't known, many investigators theorize that, as in other anxiety disorders, panic disorder may stem from a combination of physical, psychological, and biological factors, including heredity. For example, some studies emphasize the role of stressful events or unconscious conflicts that occur early in childhood. Another study found that children of parents with panic disorder were (themselves) more likely to suffer from panic attacks.

Recent evidence indicates that alterations in brain biochemistry, especially in norepinephrine, serotonin, and gamma-aminobutyric acid activity, may also contribute to panic disorder. Another area of research for the treatment of panic disorder focuses on the amygdala, a very small and complicated structure inside the brain that controls the body's response to fear. Recent research suggests that the abnormal activation of the amygdala is associated with anxiety disorders.

Signs and symptoms

The patient with panic disorder typically complains of repeated episodes of unexpected apprehension, fear or, in rare cases, intense discomfort. These panic attacks may last for minutes or hours and leave the patient shaken, fearful, and exhausted. They may occur several times per week — sometimes even daily. Because the attacks may initially occur spontaneously without exposure to a known anxiety-producing situation, place, or task, the patient generally worries between attacks about when the next episode will occur.

Physical examination of the patient during a panic attack may reveal signs of intense anxiety, such as hyperventilation, tachycardia, palpitations, dizziness, trembling, and profuse sweating. She may also complain of difficulty breathing, digestive disturbances, and chest pain.

Diagnosis

For specific *Diagnosis and Statistical Manual of Mental Disorders*, Fourth Edition, Text Revision *(DSM-IV-TR)* findings in patients with panic disorder, see *Diagnosing panic disorder*, page 388. Because many medical conditions can mimic panic disorder, additional tests may be ordered to rule out an organic basis for symptoms. For example, an electrocardiogram (ECG) can rule out a myocardial infarction; tests for serum glucose levels rule out hypoglycemia; studies of urine catecholamines and vanillylmandelic acid rule out pheochromocytoma; and thyroid function tests rule out hyperthyroidism. Urine and serum toxicology tests may reveal the presence of psychoactive substances that can precipitate panic attacks, including barbiturates, caffeine, and amphetamines.

Diagnosing panic disorder

The diagnosis of panic disorder is confirmed when the patient meets the criteria put forth in the *Diagnostic and Statistical Manual of Mental Disorders,* Fourth Edition, Text Revision, for panic attack or panic disorder with or without agoraphobia. These criteria are outlined below.

Panic attack

A discrete period of intense fear or discomfort in which at least four of the following symptoms develop abruptly and reach a peak within 10 minutes:

- palpitations, pounding heart, or tachycardia
- sweating
- trembling or shaking
- shortness of breath or smothering sensations
- feeling of choking
- chest pain or discomfort
- nausea or abdominal distress
- dizziness or faintness
- depersonalization or derealization
- fear of losing control or going crazy
- fear of dying
- numbness or tingling sensations (paresthesia)
- hot flashes or chills.

Panic disorder with agoraphobia

- The person experiences recurrent unexpected panic attacks and at least one of the attacks has been followed by 1 month (or more) of one (or more) of the following:
  - persistent concern about having additional attacks
  - worry about the implications of the attack or its consequences
  - significant change in behavior related to the attacks.
- The person exhibits agoraphobia.
- The panic attacks aren't due to the direct physiologic effects of a substance or a general medical condition.
- The panic attacks aren't better accounted for by another mental disorder, such as social phobia, specific phobia, obsessive-compulsive disorder, posttraumatic stress disorder, or separation anxiety disorder.

Panic disorder without agoraphobia

- The person experiences recurrent unexpected panic attacks and at least one of the attacks has been followed by 1 month (or more) of one (or more) of the following:
  - persistent concern about having additional attacks
  - worry about the implications of the attack or its consequences
  - significant change in behavior related to the attacks.
- The panic attacks aren't due to the direct physiologic effects of a substance or a general medical condition.
- The panic attacks aren't better accounted for by another mental disorder, such as social phobia, specific phobia, obsessive-compulsive disorder, posttraumatic stress disorder, or separation anxiety disorder.

Treatment

Panic disorder may respond to behavioral-cognitive therapy, supportive psychotherapy, or drug therapy, or a combination of these treatments. Behavioral-cognitive therapy works best when agoraphobia accompanies panic disorder because identifying the anxiety-inducing situation is easier.

Supportive psychotherapy commonly uses cognitive techniques to enable the patient to view anxiety-provoking situations more realistically and to recognize panic symptoms as a misinterpretation of essentially harmless physical sensations.

Drug therapy includes antianxiety drugs, such as diazepam, alprazolam, and clonazepam, and beta-adrenergic blockers such as propranolol to provide symptomatic relief. Antidepressants, including tricyclic antidepressants, selective serotonin reuptake inhibitors (specifically paroxetine and sertraline) and monoamine oxidase (MAO) inhibitors, are also effective.

Special considerations

- If the patient is experiencing an acute panic attack, stay with the patient until the attack subsides. If left alone, she may become even more anxious.
- Maintain a calm, serene approach. Statements such as, "I won't let anything here hurt you," and, "I'll stay with you," can assure the patient that you're in control of the immediate situation. Avoid giving her insincere expressions of reassurance.
- The patient's perceptual field may be narrowed; excessive stimuli may cause her to feel overwhelmed. Dim or brighten lights as necessary.
- If the patient loses control, move her to a smaller, quieter space.
- The patient may be so overwhelmed that she can't follow lengthy or complicated instructions. Speak in short, simple sentences and slowly give one direction at a time. Avoid giving lengthy explanations and asking too many questions.
- Allow the patient to pace around the room (if she isn't in danger of hurting herself or anyone else) to help expend energy. Show her how to take slow, deep breaths if she's hyperventilating.
- Avoid touching the patient until you've established rapport. Unless she trusts you, she may be too stimulated or frightened to find touch reassuring.
- Administer appropriate medication as prescribed.
- During and after a panic attack, encourage the patient to express her feelings. Discuss her fears and help her identify situations or events that trigger the attacks.
- Teach the patient relaxation techniques and how she can use them to relieve stress or avoid a panic attack.
- Review with the patient the adverse effects of the drugs she'll be taking. Caution her to notify the physician before discontinuing the medication because abrupt withdrawal could cause severe symptoms.
- Encourage the patient and her family to use community resources, such as support groups and meetings, and refer them to the Anxiety Disorders Association of America.

Pelvic inflammatory disease

According to the National Institutes of Health, pelvic inflammatory disease (PID) is "the most common and serious complication of sexually transmitted diseases (STDs) among women," aside from acquired immunodeficiency syndrome (AIDS). PID is any acute, subacute, recurrent, or chronic infection of the upper genital tract. It can affect the uterus, oviducts, ovaries, and other related reproductive structures with adjacent tissue involvement. It includes inflammation of the fallopian tubes (salpingitis) and ovaries (oophoritis), which can extend to the connective tissue lying between the broad ligaments (parametritis). Early diagnosis and treatment prevent damage to the reproductive system.

PID affects more than 1 million women each year, with the highest incidence among teenagers. PID causes infertility in more than 100,000 women each year. It's also the major cause of ectopic pregnancies.

Causes

PID can result from infection with aerobic or anaerobic organisms that travel from the urethra and cervix into the upper genital tract. Although many different organisms can cause PID, *Neisseria gonorrhoeae* and *Chlamydia trachomatis* are two of the most common because they most readily penetrate the bacteriostatic barrier of cervical mucus.

Normally, cervical secretions have protective and defensive functions. Conditions or procedures that alter or destroy the cervical mucus impair these bacteriostatic mechanisms and allow bacteria present in the cervix or vagina to ascend into the uterine cavity; such procedures include conization or cauterization of the cervix.

Uterine infection can also follow the transfer of contaminated cervical mucus into the endometrial cavity by instrumentation. Consequently, PID can follow insertion of an intrauterine device, use of a biopsy curet or an irrigation catheter, or tubal insufflation. Other predisposing factors include abortion, pelvic surgery, and infection during or after pregnancy. Bacteria may also enter the uterine cavity through the bloodstream or from drainage from a chronically infected fallopian tube, a pelvic abscess, a ruptured appendix, diverticulitis of the sigmoid colon, or other infectious foci. Common bacteria found in cervical mucus are staphylococci, streptococci, diphtheroids, chlamydiae, and coliforms, including *Pseudomonas* and *Escherichia coli*. Uterine infection can result from one or several of these organisms or may follow the multiplication of normally nonpathogenic bacteria in an altered endometrial environment.

Risk factors for PID include:

- women with STDs
- prior episode of PID
- sexually active teenager
- increased number of sexual partners
- lack of consistent condom use
- lack of contraceptive use (including hormonal contraceptives that, while protecting against or reducing the severity of the symptoms of PID, don't protect against contracting STDs)
- douching.

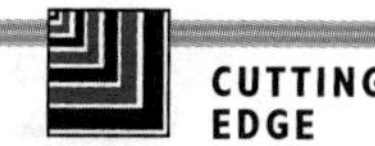

Guidelines for diagnosing PID

In 2002, the Centers for Disease Control and Prevention (CDC) modified its criteria for diagnosing pelvic inflammatory disease (PID). The original criteria required all three findings of lower abdominal tenderness, adnexal tenderness, and cervical motion tenderness to be present. However, they found this requirement to be too narrow, causing too many cases of PID to go undiagnosed and untreated. The CDC now recommends that PID should be diagnosed in any sexually active female with at least one of the findings that has no other cause: adnexal tenderness, uterine tenderness, or cervical motion tenderness.

Additional findings that may support the diagnosis of PID, to be considered along with the women's risk factors and history of STDs or PID, include:

- fever greater than 101° F (38.3° C)
- cervical mucopurulent discharge
- white blood cells in vaginal secretions
- increased erythrocyte sedimentation rate
- increased C-reactive protein
- confirmation of *Neisseria gonorrhoeae* or *Chlamydia trachomatis*.

Signs and symptoms

Clinical features of PID vary with the affected area but generally include a profuse, purulent vaginal discharge, sometimes accompanied by low-grade fever and malaise (particularly if gonorrhea is the cause). The patient also experiences lower abdominal pain; movement of the cervix or palpation of the adnexa may be extremely painful. Other symptoms may include right upper abdominal pain, painful sexual intercourse, and irregular menstrual bleeding. PID caused by a chlamydial infection, however, may produce only mild symptoms.

If left untreated, PID may cause infertility, tubal pregnancy, chronic pelvic pain, and may lead to potentially fatal septicemia and shock.

Diagnosis

For the most up-to-date guidelines for diagnosing PID from the Centers for Disease Control and Prevention (CDC), see *Guidelines for diagnosing PID*.

Some diagnostic tests that are likely to be ordered are:

- urine pregnancy test
- urine or cervical testing for *N. gonorrhea* and *C. trachomatis*
- wet preparation of vaginal secretions for the presence of WBCs and clue cells that, along with findings of increased pH and a positive whiff test, indicates bacterial vaginosis, which is associated with PID
- urinalysis or urine dipstick and urine culture
- syphilis and HIV screening
- CBC, ESR, and C-reactive protein.

Differential diagnosis includes:

- ectopic pregnancy

- appendicitis
- urinary tract infection or pyelonephritis
- constipation
- gastroenteritis
- rupture, bleeding, or torsion of an ovarian cyst
- mittelschmerz pain
- irritable bowel syndrome
- renal colic.

Treatment

To prevent progression of PID, antibiotic therapy begins immediately after culture specimens are obtained. Such therapy can be reevaluated as soon as laboratory results are available (usually after 24 to 48 hours). Infection may become chronic if treated inadequately.

Usually, because PID is caused by multiple organisms, the patient is prescribed at least two antibiotics. The CDC guidelines for outpatient treatment include ofloxacin (Floxin) and metronidazole (Flagyl) for 14 days or ceftriaxone (Rocephin) or another third-generation cephalosporin with doxycycline (Vibramycin) for 14 days.

For those women that must be hospitalized due to increased severity of the illness or other complications, such as pregnancy, AIDS, or inability to take oral forms of antibiotics, the CDC guidelines for inpatient treatment include doxycycline with cefoxitin (Mefoxin) or cefotetan (Cefotan) or a combination of clindamycin (Cleocin) and gentamicin (Garamycin). Alternative investigational inpatient regimens include ofloxacin and metronidazole, ampicillin and sulbactam (Unasyn) and doxycycline, and ciprofloxacin (Cipro) with mebendazole (Vermox) and doxycycline.

Development of a pelvic abscess necessitates adequate drainage. A ruptured abscess is life-threatening. If this complication develops, the patient may need a total abdominal hysterectomy with bilateral salpingo-oophorectomy to avoid shock and sepsis. Alternatively, laparoscopic drainage with preservation of the ovaries and uterus appears to hold promise.

Special considerations

- After establishing that the patient has no drug allergies, administer appropriate antibiotics and analgesics.
- Check for fever. If it persists, carefully monitor fluid intake and output for signs of dehydration.
- Watch for abdominal rigidity and distention, which are possible signs of developing peritonitis. Provide frequent perineal care if vaginal drainage occurs.
- To prevent a recurrence, explain the nature and seriousness of PID, and encourage the patient to comply with the treatment regimen.
- Because PID may cause painful intercourse, advise the patient to consult with her primary health care provider about sexual activity.

PREVENTION POINTER

- If the patient is having sex, encourage her to use a condom to prevent the transmission of STDs.

▪ Stress the need for the patient's sexual partner to be examined for STDs and, if the partner tests positive, be treated for infection at the same time as the patient even if the partner is asymptomatic to prevent reinfection.
▪ Warn patient that signs of discharge with odor or bleeding between menses may be a sign of infection. Treating an infection early can prevent PID from developing.
▪ To prevent infection after minor gynecologic procedures, such as dilatation and curettage, tell the patient to immediately report fever, increased vaginal discharge, or pain. After such procedures, instruct her to avoid douching and sexual intercourse for at least 7 days.

Pelvic pain and pelvic masses

Pelvic pain and pelvic masses are common symptoms experienced by women and can be due to several causes. Both can be described as acute or chronic, cyclic or noncyclic, localized or generalized, or a combination. Specific characteristics vary with the cause. It's important to note that sudden, severe pain with mass indicates a serious disorder such as an ectopic pregnancy, and requires immediate evaluation and treatment. Chronic pelvic pain is defined as pelvic pain that lasts for more than 6 months.

Ten percent of all outpatient visits to a gynecologist are for pelvic pain, and in the United States, chronic pelvic pain has a prevalence of 3% (approximately 9.2 million women). It affects women of reproductive age and older.

Causes

Many gynecologic conditions cause pelvic pain and pelvic masses:

▪ Several types of infections can lead to pelvic pain, such as vaginitis, urinary tract infection, and pelvic inflammatory disease (PID). Bacteria enter via the genitourinary tract and cause inflammation.
▪ Pelvic pain may occur early in pregnancy, especially in the right lower quadrant, due to the dextrorotation of the uterus as it grows. It's sometimes referred to as *round ligament pain.*
▪ Spontaneous abortion, whether missed, threatened, incomplete, or complete, can induce pelvic pain.
▪ Ectopic pregnancy, the implantation of the fertilized ovum in a place other than the uterus (most commonly one of the fallopian tubes), can produce lower abdominal pain (commonly unilateral) with a tender mass.
▪ Endometriosis, the presence of endometrial tissue outside of the endometrium, may cause pelvic pain with dyspareunia (difficult or painful sexual intercourse). Uterosacral nodules may be felt during physical examination.
▪ An endometrial polyp is a mass of tissue holding on to the surface of the endometrium by a pedicle. It isn't commonly associated with pain.
▪ Fibroids are masses of smooth muscle and fibrous connective tissue in the uterus.
▪ One symptom of premenstrual syndrome (PMS) is described as pelvic

heaviness or pressure and is most commonly felt 7 to 10 days before menses.
- Mittelschmerz can cause pain in the middle of the menstrual cycle due to ovulation.
- Dysmenorrhea is pain that occurs during menses.
- Ovarian cysts are masses, which are usually benign sacs that contain fluid or semisolid material. They may cause unilateral adnexal pain. Severe pain occurs with rupture or torsion.
- Adhesions from prior surgeries can cause pain as well as masses.
- Pelvic malignancy can present as a mass but isn't commonly associated with pelvic pain.

Pelvic pain may also be caused by nongynecologic conditions, such as:
- GI disorders, such as appendicitis, irritable bowel syndrome, spastic colon, chronic constipation, diverticulitis, and inflammatory bowel disease
- musculoskeletal problems
- prior physical or sexual abuse.

Signs and symptoms

Pelvic pain may be described in many ways, such as cramping, bloating, discomfort, pressure, stabbing, or aching. Pelvic masses can be small, large, localized to a single mass, or consist of multiple masses. Pelvic masses themselves may cause pain. Many associated signs and symptoms may occur with pelvic pain and masses, including:
- dyspareunia, or pain with deep thrusting during sexual intercourse
- cervical motion tenderness
- vaginal fornix pain
- adnexal tenderness
- enlarged, bulky uterus
- uterosacral nodules
- nausea and vomiting
- severe pain with rupture of ovarian cysts, adnexal torsion, or hemorrhage
- fever
- leukocytosis (increased white blood cell count)
- cervical discharge
- adnexal enlargement
- back pain
- leg pain.

Diagnosis

Diagnostic tests used to identify the cause of pelvic pain or masses depend on the suspected cause. Tests may include:
- specimen cultures
- serum or urine pregnancy test
- complete blood count to rule out anemia if bleeding is present
- erythrocyte sedimentation rate or C-reactive protein, to identify inflammatory or infectious process
- ultrasonography
- X-rays
- computed tomography scan
- magnetic resonance imaging
- laparoscopy, if the client is in severe pain and the diagnosis is unclear, pathology is suspected, or there's minimal or no response to therapy
- laparoscopic pain mapping
- ultrasound, sigmoidoscopy, colonoscopy, or barium enema if a GI problem is suspected

- urinalysis, cystourethroscopy, or urodynamic studies if infection of the urinary tract is suspected.

When evaluating for chronic pelvic pain, it's absolutely necessary to perform laparoscopy and cystoscopy because chronic pelvic pain can be caused by endometriosis, interstitial cystitis, or both.

Treatment

Treatment of pelvic pain and masses should be directed to the cause of the pain. However, a cause isn't always identified, and although treatment of symptoms is commonly attempted, pain isn't always relieved. In fact, it may worsen with treatment. Treatments may include:

- antibiotics
- nonsteroidal anti-inflammatory drugs
- gonadotropin-releasing hormone agonists
- hormonal contraceptives
- embolization of fibroids
- surgical removal of fibroids, cysts, or endometrial growths
- laparoscopic laser surgery
- uterosacral nerve ablation for central pelvic pain or dysmenorrhea unresponsive to medical therapy
- presacral neurectomy
- hysterectomy
- nerve block or transection
- antidepressants.

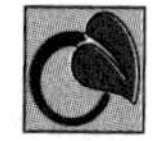

ALTERNATIVE THERAPIES

Relaxation exercises, hypnosis, biofeedback, and physical therapy have been used as adjuncts in the treatment of pelvic pain. Acupuncture may also offer relief. Psychotherapy may be needed to help the woman deal with the stress of having chronic pain.

Special considerations

- Encourage the woman to keep a "diary" of the pain, which may help the client and clinician identify possible causes.
- Provide nutritional counseling to the client with a GI problem, such as constipation, that may contribute to pelvic pain.
- Educate the client about diagnostic procedures and treatment.
- Encourage good hygiene practices if an infectious cause is suspected or determined.
- Make appropriate referrals for counseling, surgery, or other specialists.
- Supportive care is crucial in caring for these clients. Many women suffering chronic pelvic pain are frustrated by the lack of a diagnosis, lack of relief, or both.

Polycystic ovary syndrome

Polycystic ovary syndrome (PCOS) is also known as *hyperandrogenic anovulation* and *Stein-Leventhal syndrome*. It's a metabolic disorder characterized by a chronic hyperandrogenic state and multiple ovarian cysts. It's the most common endocrine disorder in women. About 5% to 10% of women in their reproductive years are affected. It's also the leading cause of infertility in women. Among those women who seek treatment for infertility, more than 75% have some degree of PCOS, usually manifested by anovulation alone. Other implications of PCOS include obesity, amenorrhea, oligomenorrhea, diabetes, cardiovascular disease, endometrial cancer, and excessive body hair (hirsutism).

Causes

The precise cause of PCOS is unknown. However, it has been associated with many factors, including:

- obesity
- enlarged ovaries
- abnormal uterine bleeding
- irregular or absent menstruation
- oily skin
- acne.

Some theories about the cause of PCOS include:

- abnormal enzyme activity triggering excess androgen secretion from the ovaries and adrenal glands
- endocrine abnormalities (such as increased insulin production, which also increases male hormone levels), which cause or worsen all of the signs and symptoms of PCOS
- heredity.

Signs and symptoms

PCOS tends to begin soon after the onset of menarche. A general feature of all anovulation syndromes is a lack of pulsatile release of gonadotropin-releasing hormone. Initial ovarian follicle development is normal. Many small follicles begin to accumulate because there's no selection of a dominant follicle. These follicles may respond abnormally to hormonal stimulation, such as by forming cysts instead of releasing an egg each month. These cysts eventually fill up the ovaries.

Signs and symptoms of classic PCOS include:

- mild pelvic discomfort that lasts longer than 6 months
- abdominal pain or bloating
- lower back pain
- dyspareunia
- abnormal uterine bleeding secondary to irregular menstrual cycle (usually menstrual cycle greater than 35 days or less than 8 cycles per year to complete absence of menses (amenorrhea)
- polycystic ovaries (not definitively diagnostic of PCOS, although seen in 67% to 86% of patients with PCOS)
- elevated luteinizing hormone
- cervical discharge
- obesity (usually centered around the midsection)
- increased androgen levels, such as testosterone
- increased insulin levels (diabetes)
- hirsutism (excess hair on the face and body)
- increased blood pressure, cholesterol, or lipid levels
- acne
- male-pattern hair loss.

Certain complications occur in patients with PCOS. (See *Complications of PCOS.*)

Diagnosis

Diagnosis of PCOS includes:

- history and physical examination showing bilaterally enlarged polycys-

tic ovaries and menstrual irregularities, usually dating back to menarche
- visualization of the ovary through ultrasound, laparoscopy, or surgery, commonly for another condition (may confirm ovarian cysts)
- slightly elevated urinary 17-ketosteroid levels and anovulation (shown by basal body temperature graphs and endometrial biopsy)
- elevated ratio of luteinizing hormone to follicle-stimulating hormone (usually 3:1 or greater) and elevated levels of testosterone and androstenedione (androgen)
- unopposed estrogen action during the menstrual cycle due to anovulation
- direct visualization by laparoscopy to rule out paraovarian cysts of the broad ligament, salpingitis, endometriosis, and neoplastic cysts
- absence of any other underlying causative disorders, such as ovarian cancer and tumor of the adrenal gland.

Treatment

There's no cure for PCOS, so the focus of treatment is to prevent further problems and control symptoms. Treatment of PCOS includes monitoring the patient's weight to maintain a normal body mass index in order to reduce risks associated with insulin resistance, which may cause spontaneous ovulation in some women. Treatment also depends on the patient's lipid and glucose levels.

Complications of PCOS

Possible complications of polycystic ovary syndrome (PCOS) include:
- increased risk of endometrial cancer due to sustained estrogenic stimulation of the endometrium
- increased risk of cardiovascular disease, such as hyperlipidemia and myocardial infarction
- increased risk of developing type 2 diabetes mellitus due to insulin resistance
- obesity
- hirsutism
- secondary amenorrhea
- oligomenorrhea
- infertility
- increased risk of miscarriage if pregnancy occurs.

Prognosis is good for ovulation and fertility with appropriate treatment. With proper screening, many of these long-term complications can be avoided.

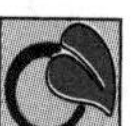

ALTERNATIVE THERAPIES

Because obesity increases insulin levels, weight loss, diet, and exercise may be sufficient treatment for PCOS.

Treatment of PCOS may include the administration of such drugs as:
- metformin (Glucophage) to decrease insulin levels, which will increase ovulation
- clomiphene (Clomid) to induce ovulation
- medroxyprogesterone (Provera) for 10 days each month for a patient who wants to become pregnant

- low-dose hormonal contraceptives to treat abnormal bleeding for the patient who requires reliable contraception; also to regulate the menstrual cycle, reduce androgen levels, and help clear acne
- progestin to protect the endometrium from estrogen exposure, although no contraceptive protection is provided (usually prescribed to women who aren't candidates for hormonal contraceptives due to smoking, hypertension, or other contraindications)
- topical creams or antiandrogens (spironolactone) to decrease hair production

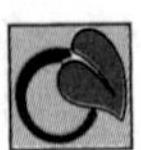

ALTERNATIVE THERAPIES

For treatment of excess body hair, waxing, electrolysis, or laser therapy may be helpful.

Special considerations

- Preoperatively, watch for signs of cyst rupture, such as increasing abdominal pain, distention, and rigidity. Monitor vital signs for fever, tachypnea, or hypotension (possibly indicating peritonitis or intraperitoneal hemorrhage).
- Provide emotional support, offering appropriate reassurance if the patient fears cancer or infertility.
- Assure the patient that unwanted excess hair may be removed by a variety of methods and can even be removed permanently.
- For those women who are infertile but still wish to conceive, provide them with information on alternative options such as in vitro fertilization.

Pregnancy-induced hypertension

Pregnancy-induced hypertension (PIH), also known — although incorrectly — as *toxemia of pregnancy*, is a potentially life-threatening disorder that usually develops late in the second trimester or in the third trimester. *Preeclampsia*, the nonconvulsive form of PIH, develops in about 7% of pregnancies. Preeclampsia may be mild or severe, and the incidence is significantly higher in low socioeconomic groups. *Eclampsia* is the convulsive form of PIH. About 5% of females with preeclampsia develop eclampsia; of these, about 15% die from PIH itself or its complications. Fetal mortality is high due to the increased incidence of premature delivery and uteroplacental insufficiency.

Causes

The cause of PIH is unknown; however, geographic, ethnic, racial, nutritional, immunologic, and familial factors as well as preexisting cardiovascular disease (such as diabetes mellitus, hypertension, and hyperlipidemia) may contribute to its development. Age is also a risk factor for PIH. Primiparas over age 35 and those women with large placentas from multiple pregnancies are at higher risk for preeclampsia.

Signs and symptoms

Mild preeclampsia generally produces:

- hypertension
- proteinuria (less than 5 g/24 hours)
- generalized edema

- sudden weight gain of more than 3 lb (1.4 kg) per week during the 2nd trimester or more than 1 lb (0.5 kg) per week during the third trimester.

Severe preeclampsia is marked by increased hypertension and proteinuria, eventually leading to the development of oliguria. HELLP syndrome (hemolysis, elevated liver enzymes, and low platelets) is a severe variant of preeclampsia. Other symptoms that may indicate worsening preeclampsia include blurred vision due to retinal arteriolar spasms, epigastric pain or heartburn, and severe frontal headache.

In eclampsia, all the clinical manifestations of preeclampsia are magnified and are associated with seizures and, possibly, coma, premature labor, stillbirth, renal failure, and hepatic damage.

Diagnosis

The following findings suggest mild preeclampsia:

- *elevated blood pressure reading* — 140 systolic, or a rise of 30 mm Hg or greater above the patient's normal systolic pressure, measured on two occasions, 6 hours apart; 90 diastolic, or a rise of 15 mm Hg or greater above the patient's normal diastolic pressure, measured on two occasions, 6 hours apart
- *proteinuria* — more than 300 mg/24 hours.

The following findings suggest severe preeclampsia:

- *higher blood pressure readings* — 160/110 mm Hg or higher on two occasions, 6 hours apart, on bed rest
- *increased proteinuria* — 5 g/24 hours or more
- *oliguria* — urine output less than or equal to 400 ml/24 hours
- *deep tendon reflexes* — possibly hyperactive as central nervous system (CNS) irritability increases.

Typical clinical features — especially seizures — with typical findings for severe preeclampsia strongly suggest eclampsia. Ophthalmoscopic examination may reveal vascular spasm, papilledema, retinal edema or detachment, and arteriovenous nicking or hemorrhage.

Real-time ultrasonography, stress and nonstress tests, and biophysical profiles evaluate fetal status. In the stress test, oxytocin is administered to stimulate contractions and then fetal heart tones are monitored electronically. In the nonstress test, fetal heart tones are monitored electronically during periods of fetal activity without oxytocin stimulation. Electronic monitoring reveals stable or increased fetal heart tones during periods of fetal activity.

Ultrasonography aids evaluation of fetal health by assessing fetal breathing movements, gross body movements, fetal tone, reactive fetal heart rate, and qualitative amniotic fluid volume.

Treatment

Therapy for preeclampsia is designed to halt the disorder's progress — specifically, the early effects of eclampsia, such as seizures, residual hypertension, and renal shutdown — and ensure fetal survival. Some physicians advocate the prompt induction of labor, especially if the patient is near term; others may take a more conservative approach. Therapy may include anticonvulsants (such as magnesium sulfate), along with complete bed rest, to relieve anxiety, reduce hypertension, and evaluate response to therapy. Antihypertensive therapy doesn't alter the potential for developing eclampsia. Diuretics aren't appropriate during pregnancy.

If the patient's blood pressure fails to respond to bed rest and sedation and persistently rises above 160/100 mm Hg, or if CNS irritability increases, magnesium sulfate may produce general sedation, promote diuresis, and prevent seizures. Cesarean birth or oxytocin induction may be required to terminate the pregnancy.

Emergency treatment of eclamptic seizures consists of immediate administration of magnesium sulfate I.V., oxygen administration, and continuous electronic fetal monitoring. After the seizures subside and the patient's condition stabilizes, delivery should proceed with induction of labor or cesarean birth, depending on the circumstances.

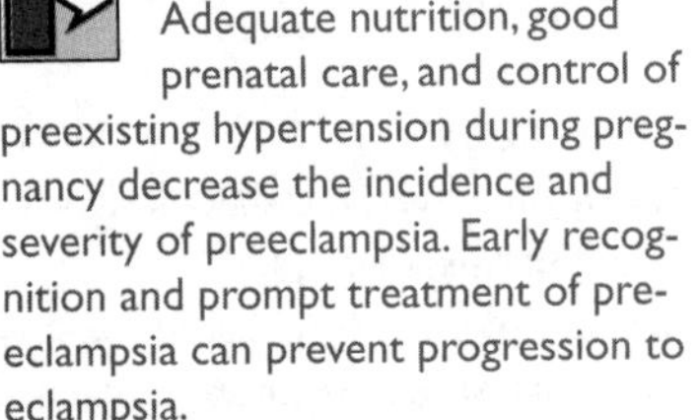

PREVENTION POINTER

Adequate nutrition, good prenatal care, and control of preexisting hypertension during pregnancy decrease the incidence and severity of preeclampsia. Early recognition and prompt treatment of preeclampsia can prevent progression to eclampsia.

Special considerations

- Monitor the patient regularly for changes in blood pressure, pulse rate, respiration, fetal heart tones, vision, level of consciousness, deep tendon reflexes, and for headache unrelieved by medication. Report changes immediately. Assess these signs before administering medications. Absence of patellar reflexes may indicate magnesium sulfate toxicity.
- Assess fluid balance by measuring intake and output and by checking daily weight.
- Observe for signs of fetal hypoxemia by closely monitoring the results of stress and nonstress tests.
- Instruct the patient to lie in a left lateral position to increase venous return, cardiac output, and renal blood flow.
- Keep emergency resuscitative equipment and drugs available in case of seizures and cardiac or respiratory arrest. Also keep calcium gluconate readily available at the bedside because it counteracts the toxic effects of magnesium sulfate.
- To protect the patient from injury, maintain seizure precautions. Don't leave an unstable patient unattended.
- Assist with emergency medical treatment for the convulsive patient. Provide a quiet, darkened room until the patient's condition stabilizes and enforce absolute bed rest. Carefully monitor administration of magnesium sulfate and give oxygen, as ordered. Don't administer anything by mouth. Insert an indwelling urinary catheter for accurate measurement of intake and output.

- Inform the patient about tests that evaluate fetal status because the baby's welfare is of prime concern.
- Provide emotional support for the patient and family. If the patient's condition necessitates premature delivery, point out that infants of mothers with PIH are usually small for gestational age but sometimes fare better than other premature babies of the same weight, possibly because they have developed adaptive responses to stress in utero.

Premenstrual syndrome

Premenstrual syndrome (PMS) is defined as a recurrent, cyclical set of varying physical and behavioral symptoms that appear 7 to 14 days before menses and usually subside with onset. Depending on the symptoms and their severity, they usually interfere with some aspect of a woman's life. The effects of PMS range from minimal discomfort to severe, disruptive symptoms and can include nervousness, irritability, depression, and multiple somatic complaints.

Researchers believe that 70% to 90% of women experience PMS at some time during their childbearing years, usually between ages 25 and 45. According to the *DSM-IV-TR*, a more severe form of PMS is referred to as premenstrual dysphoric disorder (PMDD). PMDD includes the psychological manifestations of PMS. (See *About PMDD*, page 402.)

Causes

The list of biological theories offered to explain the cause of PMS is impressive. It includes such conditions as progesterone deficiency in the luteal phase of the menstrual cycle and vitamin deficiencies. Although there's no evidence that PMS is hormonally mediated, failure to identify a specific disorder with a specific mechanism suggests that PMS represents a variety of manifestations triggered by normal physiologic hormonal changes.

Signs and symptoms

Clinical effects vary widely among patients and may include behavioral symptoms, somatic symptoms, or both. These symptoms include:

- *behavioral* — mild to severe personality changes, mood changes, anxiety, nervousness, hostility, irritability, agitation, sleep disturbances (either insomnia or hypersomnia), fatigue, lethargy, and depression as well as overeating, food cravings, and increased appetite
- *somatic* — breast tenderness or swelling, abdominal tenderness or bloating, weight gain, joint pain, headache, edema, diarrhea or constipation, and exacerbations of skin problems (such as acne or rashes), respiratory problems (such as asthma), or neurologic problems (such as seizures).

Diagnosis

The patient history shows typical symptoms related to the menstrual cycle. To help ensure an accurate history, the patient may be asked to record

About PMDD

Premenstrual dysphoric disorder (PMDD) is a cyclical occurrence of psychiatric symptoms that starts after ovulation (usually the week before the onset of menstruation) and ends within the first day or two of menses. PMDD is a severe form of premenstrual syndrome (PMS). Similar to PMS, its underlying cause or causes and pathophysiology remain unclear. Researchers theorize that normal cyclic changes in the body cause abnormal responses to neurotransmitters such as serotonin, resulting in physical and behavioral symptoms. It affects as many as 1 in 20 American women who have regular menstrual periods. It's unclear why some women are affected and not others.

How PMDD and PMS differ

PMDD is characterized by severe monthly mood swings and physical symptoms that interfere with everyday life and interactions. PMDD symptoms are abnormal and unmanageable as compared to PMS. Physically, the symptoms are similar. Behaviorally and emotionally, however, PMDD symptoms are more serious. Although depression, anxiety, and sadness are common with PMS, in PMDD, these symptoms are extreme. Some women may feel the urge to hurt or kill themselves or others.

PMDD criteria

The Diagnostic and Statistical Manual, Fourth Edition, Text Revision, sets these criteria for diagnosing PMDD:

- functional impairment
- predominant mood symptoms, with one being affective
- symptoms beginning 1 week before the onset of menstruation
- symptoms that aren't due to any underlying primary mood disorder.

In addition, at least five of the following symptoms must be present:

- "low mood"
- tension
- mood swings
- irritability
- decreased interests
- difficulty concentrating
- fatigue
- appetite changes
- insomnia or hypersomnia
- physical symptoms
- feelings of being overwhelmed.

menstrual symptoms and body temperature on a calendar for 2 to 3 months prior to diagnosis. Estrogen and progesterone blood levels may be evaluated to help rule out hormonal imbalance. A psychological evaluation is also recommended to rule out or detect any underlying psychiatric disorders.

Treatment

Educating and reassuring patients that PMS is a real physiologic syndrome are important parts of treatment. Because treatment is predominantly symptomatic, each patient must learn to cope with her own individual set of symptoms. Treatment may include antidepressants, vitamins such as B_6 (pyridoxine), hormonal contraceptives, selective serotonin reuptake inhibitors, prostaglandin inhibitors, diuretics, and nonsteroidal anti-inflammatory drugs.

Herbal remedies for PMS

The following chart includes herbs used to remedy the symptoms of PMS along with indications for each. Check with your physician before taking any herbal remedies because they may have severe interactions or interfere with the effectiveness of a prescribed medication.

Herb	Indications
St. John's wort	▪ Treats moodiness and sadness
Kava kava	▪ Treats anxiety ▪ Improves mood
Chaste berry	▪ Reduces anger, headache, and breast fullness ▪ Regulates monthly periods and treats amenorrhea and dysmenorrhea
Dong quai (angelica)	▪ Treats irregular, painful, or meek menses
Taurine	▪ Treats anxiety and hyperactivity
Gamma-linolenic acid (GLA) (Evening primrose oil)	▪ Improves brain function ▪ Treats breast tenderness, depression, irritability, swelling, and bloating
Buchu	▪ Treats bloating and excess water weight

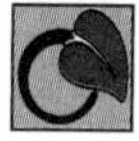

ALTERNATIVE THERAPIES

Other therapies that have been effective for some women include:

- diet low in simple sugars, caffeine, alcohol, and salt starting three days before usual onset of symptoms
- frequent exercise and yoga
- calcium carbonate intake to reduce cramping and moodiness
- magnesium oxide to reduce headache, fluid retention, and moodiness
- various herbal remedies. (See *Herbal remedies for PMS.*)

Special considerations

- Inform the patient that self-help groups exist for women with PMS; if appropriate, help her contact such a group.
- Obtain a complete patient history to help identify any emotional problems that may contribute to PMS. If necessary, refer the patient for psychological counseling.

PREVENTION POINTER

Discuss ways in which the patient can modify her lifestyle, such as regular exercise, changes to her diet, and avoidance of salt, refined sugars, and such stimulants as caffeine and alcohol. These actions may decrease PMS symptoms.

- Suggest that the patient seek further medical consultation if symptoms are severe and interfere with her normal lifestyle.

Psoriasis

Psoriasis is a chronic, recurrent disease marked by epidermal proliferation and characterized by recurring partial remissions and exacerbations. Flare-ups are commonly related to specific systemic and environmental factors but may be unpredictable. Widespread involvement is called *exfoliative* or *erythrodermic psoriasis.*

Psoriasis affects about 21% of the population in the United States. Although this disorder usually affects young adults, it may occur at any age, including infancy. Genetic factors predetermine the incidence of psoriasis; researchers have discovered a significantly greater incidence of certain human leukocyte antigens (HLAs) in families with psoriasis. Although some studies found that psoriasis is equally prevalent between men and women, other studies have found that psoriasis was slightly more prevalent in women.

Flare-ups can usually be controlled with therapy. Appropriate treatment depends on the type of psoriasis, extent of the disease, the patient's response, and the effect of the disease on the patient's lifestyle. No permanent cure exists and all methods of treatment are palliative.

Causes

Causes of psoriasis include:

- genetically determined tendency to develop psoriasis
- possible immune disorder, as shown in the HLA type in families
- environmental factors
- isomorphic effect or Koebner's phenomenon, in which lesions develop at sites of injury due to trauma
- flare-up of guttate (drop-shaped) lesions due to infections, especially beta-hemolytic streptococci.

Other contributing factors include:

- pregnancy
- endocrine changes
- climate (cold weather tends to exacerbate psoriasis)
- emotional stress.

Signs and symptoms

Possible signs and symptoms include:

- itching and occasional pain from dry, cracked, encrusted lesions (most common)
- erythematous and, usually, well-defined plaques, sometimes covering large areas of the body (psoriatic lesions)
- lesions most commonly on the scalp, chest, elbows, knees, back, and buttocks
- plaques with characteristic silver scales that either flake off easily or thicken, covering the lesion; scale removal can produce fine bleeding
- occasional small guttate lesions (usually thin and erythematous, with few scales), either alone or with plaques.

Rarely, psoriasis becomes pustular, taking one of two forms:

- localized pustular psoriasis, with pustules on the palms and soles that remain sterile until opened

- generalized pustular (von Zumbusch) psoriasis, typically occurring with fever, leukocytosis, and malaise, with groups of pustules coalescing to form lakes of pus on red skin (also remain sterile until opened), commonly involving the tongue and oral mucosa
- erythrodermic psoriasis (least common form), which is an inflammatory form of the disorder characterized by periodic fiery erythema and exfoliation of the skin with severe itching and pain.

Possible complications of psoriasis include spread to fingernails, producing small indentations or pits and yellow or brown discoloration (about 60% of patients); accumulation of thick, crumbly debris under the nail, causing it to separate from the nail bed (onycholysis); infection, secondary to itching; and arthritic symptoms, usually in one or more joints of the fingers or toes, the larger joints, or sometimes the sacroiliac joints, which may progress to spondylitis, and morning stiffness (in some patients).

Diagnosis

Diagnosis is based on:

- patient history, appearance of the lesions and, if needed, the results of skin biopsy
- serum uric acid level (usually elevated in severe cases due to accelerated nucleic acid degradation) without indications of gout
- human leukocyte antigens (HLA)-Cw6, -B13, -B27 and -B57 (may be present in early-onset familial psoriasis).

Treatment

Treatment for psoriasis may include:

- aspirin and local heat to help alleviate the pain of psoriatic arthritis; NSAIDs in severe cases
- ultraviolet B (UVB) or natural sunlight exposure to retard rapid cell production to the point of minimal erythema
- tar preparations or crude coal tar applications to the affected areas about 15 minutes before exposure to UVB, or left on overnight and wiped off the next morning
- gradually increasing exposure to UVB (outpatient treatment or day treatment avoids long hospitalizations and prolongs remission)
- steroid creams and ointments applied twice daily, preferably after bathing to facilitate absorption, and overnight use of occlusive dressings to control symptoms, if necessary.
- intralesional steroid injection for small, stubborn plaques
- anthralin ointment (Anthra-Derm) or paste mixture for well-defined plaques (not applied to unaffected areas due to injury and staining of normal skin) with application of petroleum jelly around affected skin before applying anthralin
- anthralin (Anthra-Derm) and steroids (anthralin application at night and steroid use during the day)
- calcipotriene ointment (Dovonex), a vitamin D analogue (best when alternated with a topical steroid)
- Goeckerman regimen (combines tar baths and UVB treatments) to help achieve remission and clear the skin

in 3 to 5 weeks (severe chronic psoriasis)
- Ingram technique (variation of the Goeckerman regimen) using anthralin (Anthra-Derm) instead of tar
- administration of psoralens (plant extracts that accelerate exfoliation) with exposure to high intensity ultraviolet A (UVA); also called *psoralen plus UVA (PUVA) therapy*
- cytotoxin, usually methotrexate (Mexate) (last-resort treatment for refractory psoriasis)
- acitretin (Soriatane), a retinoid compound (for extensive psoriasis)
- cyclosporine (Neoral), an immunosuppressant (in resistant cases)
- tar shampoo followed by a steroid lotion (psoriasis of the scalp).

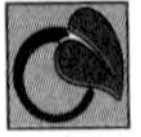

ALTERNATIVE THERAPIES

Low-dose antihistamines, oatmeal baths, emollients, and open wet dressings may help relieve pruritus.

Special considerations

Design your patient's care plan to include patient teaching and careful monitoring for adverse effects of therapy:

- Make sure the patient understands the prescribed therapy; provide written instructions to avoid confusion. Teach correct application of prescribed ointments, creams, and lotions. A steroid cream, for example, should be applied in a thin film and rubbed gently into the skin until the cream disappears. All topical medications, especially those containing anthralin and tar, should be applied with a downward motion to avoid rubbing them into the follicles. Gloves must be worn because anthralin stains and injures the skin. After application, the patient may dust herself with powder to prevent anthralin from rubbing off on her clothes. Warn the patient never to put an occlusive dressing over anthralin. Suggest use of mineral oil, then soap and water, to remove anthralin. Caution the patient to avoid scrubbing her skin vigorously to prevent Koebner's phenomenon. If a medication has been applied to the scales to soften them, suggest the patient use a soft brush to remove them.
- Watch for adverse effects, especially allergic reactions to anthralin, atrophy and acne from steroids, and burning, itching, nausea, and squamous cell epitheliomas from PUVA.
- For patients on methotrexate therapy, initially monitor the patient and his CBC (red blood cell, white blood cell, and platelet counts) weekly, then monthly, because cytotoxins may cause hepatic or bone marrow toxicity. Liver biopsy may be done to assess the effects of methotrexate. Patients taking methotrexate shouldn't drink alcohol due to the increased risk of hepatotoxicity.
- Caution the patient receiving PUVA therapy to stay out of the sun on the day of treatment, and to protect her eyes with sunglasses that block out UVA rays for 24 hours after treatment. Tell her to wear goggles during exposure to this light.
- Know that there's no effective topical treatment for psoriasis of the nails.

■ Be aware that psoriasis can cause psychological problems. Assure the patient that psoriasis isn't contagious and, although exacerbations and remissions occur, they're controllable with treatment. However, be sure she understands that there's no cure. Also, because stressful situations tend to exacerbate psoriasis, help the patient learn effective stress management techniques and coping mechanisms. Explain the relationship between psoriasis and arthritis, but point out that psoriasis causes no other systemic disturbances. Refer all patients to the National Psoriasis Foundation, which provides information and directs patients to local chapters. (See *Psoriasis: What you can do.*)

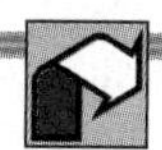

PREVENTION POINTER

Psoriasis: What you can do

■ Avoid scratching or rubbing psoriasis patches.
■ Bathe once or twice daily in warm water.
■ Avoid hot water.
■ Avoid harsh soaps and detergents.
■ Pat yourself dry; never rub.
■ Apply a heavy, oil-based moisturizer twice daily after each bath.
■ Avoid creams, lotions, or oils that contain alcohol.
■ Avoid unprotected or prolonged exposure to sunlight.
■ Avoid applying irritants, such as heavily scented perfumes and cosmetics.
■ Wear loose-fitting, comfortable, breathable clothing, such as cotton.

Pyelonephritis, acute

Acute pyelonephritis, also known as *acute infective tubulointerstitial nephritis*, is a sudden inflammation caused by bacteria that primarily affects the interstitial area and the renal pelvis or, less commonly, the renal tubules. It's one of the most common renal diseases. With treatment and continued follow-up care, prognosis is good and extensive permanent damage is rare. It's more common in females than in males. It can also cause pregnant women to have premature labor.

Causes

Acute pyelonephritis results from bacterial infection of the kidneys. Infecting bacteria are usually normal intestinal and fecal flora that grow readily in urine. The most common causative organism is *Escherichia coli*, but *Proteus*, *Pseudomonas*, *Staphylococcus aureus*, and *Enterococcus faecalis* (formerly *Streptococcus faecalis*) may also cause this infection.

Typically, the infection spreads from the bladder to the ureters, then to the kidneys, as in vesicoureteral reflux. Vesicoureteral reflux may result from congenital weakness at the junction of the ureter and the bladder. Bacteria refluxed to intrarenal tissues may create colonies of infection within 24 to 48 hours. Infection may also result from instrumentation (such as catheterization, cystoscopy, or urologic surgery), hematogenic infection (as in septicemia or endocarditis) or, possibly, lymphatic infection.

Pyelonephritis may also result from an inability to empty the bladder (for example, in patients with neurogenic bladder), urinary stasis, or urinary obstruction due to tumors, strictures, or benign prostatic hyperplasia.

Pyelonephritis occurs more commonly in females, probably because of a shorter urethra and the proximity of the urinary meatus to the vagina and the rectum, which allow bacteria to reach the bladder more easily, and a lack of the antibacterial prostatic secretions produced in the male. Incidence increases with age and is higher in the following groups:

- *sexually active women.* Intercourse increases the risk of bacterial contamination.
- *pregnant women.* About 5% develop asymptomatic bacteriuria; if untreated, about 40% develop pyelonephritis.
- *diabetics.* Neurogenic bladder causes incomplete emptying and urinary stasis; glycosuria may support bacterial growth in the urine.
- *persons with other renal diseases.* Compromised renal function aggravates susceptibility.

Signs and symptoms

Typical clinical features include urgency, frequency, burning during urination, dysuria, nocturia, and hematuria (usually microscopic but may be gross). Urine may appear cloudy and have an ammonia-like or fishy odor. Other common symptoms include a temperature of 102° F (38.9° C) or higher, shaking chills, flank pain, anorexia, and general fatigue.

These symptoms characteristically develop rapidly over a few hours or a few days. Although these symptoms may disappear within days, even without treatment, residual bacterial infection is likely and may cause symptoms to recur later.

SPECIAL NEEDS

Elderly patients may exhibit GI or pulmonary symptoms rather than the usual febrile responses to pyelonephritis. In children younger than age 2, fever, vomiting, nonspecific abdominal complaints, or failure to thrive may be the only signs of acute pyelonephritis.

Diagnosis

Diagnosis requires urinalysis and culture. Typical findings include:

- *pyuria (pus in urine).* Urine sediment reveals the presence of leukocytes singly, in clumps, and in casts and, possibly, a few red blood cells.
- *significant bacteriuria.* Urine culture reveals more than 100,000 organisms/mm^3 of urine.
- *low-specific gravity and osmolality.* These findings result from a temporarily decreased ability to concentrate urine.
- *slightly alkaline urine pH.* Alkaline urine pH results from the production of urease from the bacteria or organism, which breaks down the urea.
- *proteinuria, glycosuria, and ketonuria.* These findings usually occur in patients with diabetes who are at

increased risk for infections including pyelonephritis.

Computed tomography scan also helps in the evaluation of acute pyelonephritis. CT scan of the kidneys, ureters, and bladder may reveal calculi, tumors, or cysts in the kidneys and the urinary tract. Excretory urography may show asymmetrical kidneys.

Treatment

Treatment focuses on antibiotic therapy appropriate to the specific infecting organism after identification by urine culture and sensitivity studies. For example, *Enterococcus* requires treatment with ampicillin, penicillin G, or vancomycin. *Staphylococcus* requires penicillin G or, if resistance develops, semisynthetic penicillin, such as nafcillin, or a cephalosporin. *E. coli* may be treated with sulfisoxazole, nalidixic acid, and nitrofurantoin. *Proteus* may be treated with ampicillin, sulfisoxazole, nalidixic acid, and a cephalosporin. *Pseudomonas* requires gentamicin, tobramycin, or carbenicillin. When the infecting organism can't be identified, therapy usually consists of a broad-spectrum antibiotic, such as ampicillin or cephalexin. If the patient is pregnant, antibiotics must be prescribed cautiously. Urinary analgesics such as phenazopyridine are also appropriate.

Symptoms may disappear after several days of antibiotic therapy. Although urine usually becomes sterile within 48 to 72 hours, the full course of such therapy is 10 to 14 days. Follow-up treatment includes reculturing urine 1 week after drug therapy stops and then periodically for the next year to detect residual or recurring infection. Most patients with uncomplicated infections respond well to therapy and don't suffer reinfection.

If infection results from obstruction or vesicoureteral reflux, antibiotics may be less effective; treatment may then necessitate surgery to relieve the obstruction or correct the anomaly. Patients at high risk for recurring urinary tract and kidney infections, such as those with prolonged use of an indwelling catheter or maintenance antibiotic therapy, require long-term follow-up. Recurrent episodes of acute pyelonephritis can eventually result in chronic pyelonephritis. (See *Chronic pyelonephritis*, page 410.)

Special considerations

Patient care is supportive during antibiotic treatment of underlying infection:

- Administer antipyretics for fever.
- Force fluids to achieve urine output of more than 2,000 ml/day to help empty the bladder of contaminated urine. Don't encourage intake of more than 2 to 3 qt (2 to 3 L) because this may decrease the effectiveness of the antibiotics.
- Provide an acid-ash diet to prevent stone formation.
- Teach proper technique for collecting a clean-catch urine specimen. Be sure to refrigerate or culture a urine specimen within 30 minutes of collection to prevent overgrowth of bacteria.

Chronic pyelonephritis

Chronic pyelonephritis is a persistent kidney inflammation that can scar the kidneys and may lead to chronic renal failure. Its etiology may be bacterial, metastatic, or urogenous. This disease is most common in patients who are predisposed to recurrent acute pyelonephritis, such as those with urinary obstructions or vesicoureteral reflux.

Patients with chronic pyelonephritis may have a childhood history of unexplained fevers or bedwetting. Clinical effects may include flank pain, anemia, low urine specific gravity, proteinuria, leukocytes in urine and, especially in late stages, hypertension. Uremia rarely develops from chronic pyelonephritis unless structural abnormalities exist in the excretory system. Bacteriuria may be intermittent. When no bacteria are found in the urine, diagnosis depends on excretory urography (renal pelvis that may appear small and flattened) and renal biopsy.

Effective treatment of chronic pyelonephritis requires control of hypertension, elimination of the existing obstruction (when possible), and long-term antibiotic therapy.

- Stress the need to complete prescribed antibiotic therapy, even after symptoms subside. Encourage long-term follow-up care for high-risk patients.

PREVENTION POINTER

- To prevent further infection, observe strict sterile technique during catheter insertion and care.
- Instruct females to prevent bacterial contamination by wiping the perineum from front to back after defecation.
- Advise routine checkups for patients with a history of urinary tract infections. Teach them to recognize signs of infection, such as cloudy urine, burning on urination, urgency, and frequency, especially when accompanied by a low-grade fever.
- Tell patients with a history of urinary tract infections to drink plenty of fluid and to void frequently.
- Advise females to void after sexual intercourse to help flush out bacteria in the bladder.

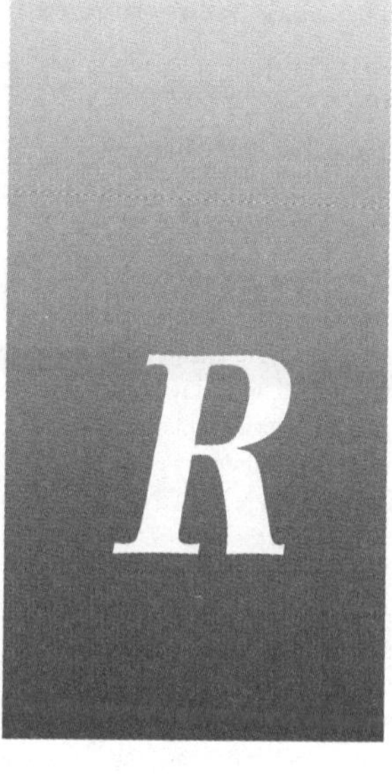

Rape-trauma syndrome

The term *rape* refers to illicit sexual intercourse without consent. It's a violent assault in which sex is used as a weapon to inflict varying degrees of physical, emotional, and psychological trauma. Rape-trauma syndrome is a form, or subcategory, of posttraumatic stress disorder (PTSD) that affects almost all rape survivors. Rape-trauma syndrome occurs during the period following a rape or attempted rape and refers to the victim's acute short-term and long-term reactions and the methods she uses to cope with the trauma.

In the United States, 1.3 adult women are raped every minute, which amounts to over 680,000 women each year. The incidence of reported rapes is highest in large cities and continues to rise. However, many rapes — possibly even most — are never reported. Known victims of rape range from ages 2 months to 97 years. The age-group most affected is 10- to 19-year-old females; the average victim's age is 13½. About one in seven reported rapes involves a prepubertal child; most of these cases involve manual, oral, or genital contact with the child's genitals by a member of the child's family. Over 50% of rapes oc-

Examining the rape victim

When a rape victim arrives in the emergency department, assess her physical injuries. If she isn't seriously injured, allow her to remain clothed and take her to a private room, where she can talk with you or a counselor before the necessary physical examination.

Interviewing the rape victim

Remember, immediate reactions to rape differ and include crying, laughing, hostility, confusion, withdrawal, or outward calm; anger and rage may not surface until later. During the attack, the victim may have felt demeaned, helpless, and afraid for her life; afterward, she may feel ashamed, guilty, shocked, and vulnerable and have a sense of disbelief and lowered self-esteem. Offer support and reassurance. Help her explore her feelings; listen, convey trust and respect, and remain nonjudgmental. Don't leave her alone unless she asks you to.

Obtaining an accurate history

Being careful to upset the victim as little as possible, obtain an accurate history of the rape, pertinent to physical assessment. (Remember, your notes may be used as evidence if the rapist is tried.) Follow these guidelines:

- Record the victim's statements in the first person, using quotation marks, and document objective information provided by others. Never speculate as to what may have happened or record subjective impressions or thoughts.
- Include the time the victim arrived at the hospital, the date and time of the alleged rape, and the time that the victim was examined.
- Ask the victim if she's allergic to penicillin or other drugs, if she has had recent illnesses (especially venereal disease), and if she was pregnant before the attack.
- Find out the date of her last menstrual period and details of her obstetric and gynecologic history.

Conducting the physical examination

Thoroughly explain the examination to the woman and tell her it's necessary to rule out internal injuries and obtain a specimen for venereal disease testing and, if semen is present, for DNA testing. Obtain her informed consent for treatment and for the police report. Allow her some control, if possible; for instance, ask her if she's ready to be examined or if she would rather wait a bit. Follow these additional guidelines:

- Before the examination, ask the victim whether she douched, bathed, or washed before coming to the hospital. Note this on her chart.
- Ask her to change into a hospital gown. Place her clothing in paper bags and label each bag and its contents. (Never use plastic bags because secretions and seminal stains will mold, destroying valuable evidence.)
- Tell the victim she may urinate but warn her not to wipe or otherwise clean the perineal area. Stay with her or ask a counselor to stay with her throughout the examination.
- During the examination, assist in specimen collection, including those for semen and gonorrhea. Carefully label all specimens with the patient's name, the physician's name, and the location from which the specimen was obtained. List all specimens in your notes. Specimens will be used for evidence, so accuracy is essential. Most emergency departments have "rape kits" that include containers for specimens.
- Carefully collect and label fingernail scrapings and foreign material obtained

EXAMINING THE RAPE VICTIM *(continued)*

by combing the victim's pubic hair, which also provide valuable evidence. Note to whom you give these specimens.

- Even if the victim wasn't beaten, the physical examination (including a pelvic examination by a gynecologist) will probably show signs of physical trauma, especially if the attack was prolonged. Depending on specific body areas attacked, a patient may have a sore throat, mouth irritation, difficulty swallowing, ecchymoses, or rectal pain and bleeding. As ordered, obtain a pharyngeal specimen for a gonorrhea culture and rectal aspirate for acid phosphatase or sperm analysis.
- If additional physical violence accompanied the rape, the victim may have hematomas, lacerations, bleeding, severe internal injuries, and hemorrhage. X-rays may reveal fractures. If severe injuries require hospitalization, introduce the victim to her primary nurse if possible.
- If the rape occurred outdoors, the woman may suffer from exposure.
- Before the victim's pelvic area is examined, take vital signs; if she is wearing a tampon, remove it, wrap it, and label it as evidence.
- The pelvic examination is typically very distressing for the victim. Reassure her and allow her as much control as possible.
- Assist in photographing the patient's injuries (this may be delayed for a day or repeated when bruises and ecchymoses are more apparent).

cur in the home; about one-third of these involve a male intruder who forces his way into a home. In about 50% of the cases, the victim has some casual acquaintance with the attacker. Most rapists are men ages 15 to 24 and have planned the attack. (See *Examining the rape victim.*)

In most cases, the rapist is a man and the victim is a woman or a male or female child. However, rapes do occur between persons of the same sex, especially in prisons, schools, hospitals, and other institutions. In rare instances, a man or child is sexually abused by a woman.

The prognosis for rape-trauma syndrome is good if the rape victim receives physical (treatment of injuries and for diseases) and emotional support and counseling to help her deal with her feelings. Victims who articulate their feelings are able to cope with fears, interact with others, and return to normal routines faster than those who don't. (See *Child rape victim,* page 414.)

Causes

Some of the cultural, sociologic, and psychological factors that contribute to rape include increasing exposure to sex, permissiveness, cynicism about relationships, feelings of anger, and powerlessness amid social pressures. Many rapists feel violence or hatred toward women or have sexual problems, such as impotence or premature ejaculation. They may feel socially isolated and be unable to form warm,

Child rape victim

If the rape victim is a child, carefully interview her to assess how well she'll be able to deal with the situation after going home. Interview the child alone, away from her parents. Tell the parents that this is being done for the child's comfort, not to keep secrets from them. Ask them what words the child is comfortable with when referring to parts of the anatomy.

History and examination

A young child will place only as much importance on an experience as others do unless there's physical pain. A good question to ask is, "Did someone touch you when you didn't want to be touched?" As with other rape victims, record information in the child's own words. A complete pelvic examination is necessary only if penetration has occurred; such an examination requires parental consent and an analgesic or a local anesthetic.

Need for counseling

The child and the parents will need counseling to minimize possible emotional disturbances. Encourage the child to talk about the experience, and try to alleviate any confusion. After a rape, a young child may regress; an older child may become fearful about being left alone. The child's behavior may change at school or at home.

Help the parents understand that it's normal for them to feel angry and guilty, but warn them against displacing or projecting these feelings onto the child. Instruct them to assure the child that they aren't angry with her or him; that the child is good and didn't cause the incident; that they're sorry it happened, but glad the child is all right; and that the family will work problems out together.

loving relationships. Some rapists may be psychopaths who need to commit violence to achieve physical pleasure; others rape to satisfy a need for power. Some may have been physically and sexually abused as children.

Signs and symptoms

Rape survivors respond differently to their experience. Some may experience severe symptoms of rape trauma syndrome, while others may experience some or no symptoms at all. However, rape survivors that experience symptoms have consistently described certain symptoms that, when clustered together, fall into two distinct stages that define rape-trauma syndrome — the acute phase (immediate reaction) and the reorganization phase.

Acute phase

During the acute phase, the most common feeling is an intense sense of fear, such as an intense fear that the rapist will return, fear of men in general, fear of being alone, fear of going outside, fear of sleeping, or other fears. Physical effects include shock, pain, loss of appetite, somnolence or insomnia, and wound healing; emotional reactions typically include shaking, crying, sadness, numbness, dissociation or detachment, vivid dreams or recurrent nightmares, and mood swings. Flashbacks and feelings of grief, anger, fear, guilt, self-blame, humiliation, shame, embarrassment, or revenge may color the victim's social interactions. Counseling helps the victim identify her coping mechanisms. She may relate more easily to a counselor of the same sex.

Reorganization phase

During the reorganization phase, which usually begins 1 to 3 weeks after the rape and may last months or years, the victim is concerned with restructuring her life. Commonly, she initially has nightmares in which she's powerless; later dreams show her gradually gaining more control. When she's alone, she may also suffer from "daymares" — frightening thoughts about the rape. She may have reduced sexual desire or may develop fear of intercourse or mistrust of men. As the reorganization phase progresses, the survivor begins to show coping skills and begins to integrate the rape into her life. Slowly, the incident won't be such a central and daily focus of her life. She'll be able to carry on daily activities without constant reminders or fears related to the assault.

Complications of rape and rape-trauma syndrome are:

- sexually transmitted diseases
- emotional trauma that may last years
- pelvic injury
- pregnancy (rare).

Diagnosis

The previous description of the stages that characterizes a rape survivor's symptoms is to assist in understanding what they experience rather than for diagnostic purposes. Because rape-trauma syndrome is a subcategory of PTSD, its diagnosis falls under the *DSM-IV-TR* criteria for PTSD. (See *Diagnosing PTSD,* pages 416 and 417.)

Treatment

Immediate treatment of the rape victim consists of supportive measures and protection against venereal disease, human immunodeficiency virus (HIV) testing and, if the patient wishes, testing for pregnancy:

- Give antibiotics, as ordered, to prevent venereal disease.
- Because cultures can't detect gonorrhea or syphilis for 5 to 6 days after the rape, stress the importance of returning for follow-up venereal disease testing.
- To prevent pregnancy as a result of the rape, the patient may be given 2 tablets of Norgestrel and ethinylestradiol (Ovral) orally immediately, plus 2 tablets 12 hours later. If so, explain the possible adverse effects of Ovral. The victim may wait 3 to 4 weeks and undergo dilatation and curettage or vacuum aspiration to abort a pregnancy.
- If the patient has vulvar lacerations, the physician will clean the area and repair the lacerations after all the evidence is obtained. Topical use of ice packs may reduce vulvar swelling.

Diagnosing PTSD

The American Psychiatric Association criteria for a diagnosis of posttraumatic stress disorder (PTSD), which is outlined in the *Diagnostic and Statistical Manual,* Fourth Edition, Text Revision, includes:

A. The person has been exposed to a traumatic event in which both of the following were present:

1. The person experienced, witnessed, or was confronted with an event or events that involved actual or threatened death or serious injury, or a threat to the physical integrity of self or others.

2. The person's response involved intense fear, helplessness, or horror. (*Note:* In children, this may be expressed instead by disorganized or agitated behavior.)

B. The traumatic event is persistently reexperienced in one (or more) of the following ways:

1. recurrent and intrusive distressing recollections of the event, including images, thoughts, or perceptions (*Note:* In young children, repetitive play may occur in which themes or aspects of the trauma are expressed.)

2. recurrent distressing dreams of the event (*Note:* In children, there may be frightening dreams without recognizable content.)

3. acting or feeling as if the traumatic event were recurring (includes a sense of reliving the experience, illusions, hallucinations, and dissociative flashback episodes, including those that occur on awakening or when intoxicated) (*Note:* In young children, trauma-specific reenactment may occur.)

4. intense psychological distress at exposure to internal or external cues that symbolize or resemble an aspect of the traumatic event

5. physiologic reactivity on exposure to internal or external cues that symbolize or resemble an aspect of the traumatic event.

C. Persistent avoidance of stimuli associated with the trauma and numbing of general responsiveness (not present before the trauma), as indicated by three (or more) of the following:

1. efforts to avoid thoughts, feelings, or conversations associated with the trauma

2. efforts to avoid activities, places, or people that arouse recollections of the trauma

3. inability to recall an important aspect of the trauma

4. markedly diminished interest or participation in significant activities

5. feeling of detachment or estrangement from others

6. restricted range of affect (e.g., unable to have loving feelings)

7. sense of a foreshortened future (e.g., doesn't expect to have a career, marriage, children, or a normal life span).

D. Persistent symptoms of increased arousal (not present before the trauma), as indicated by two (or more) of the following:

1. difficulty falling or staying asleep

2. irritability or outburst of anger

3. difficulty concentrating

4. hypervigilance

5. exaggerated startle response.

- Duration of the disturbance (symptoms in criteria B, C, and D) is more than 1 month.
- The disturbance causes clinically significant distress or impairment in social,

(continued)

Diagnosing PTSD *(continued)*

occupational, or other important areas of functioning.

Specify if:

- *acute*—if duration of symptoms is less than 3 months
- *chronic*—if duration of symptoms is 3 months or more.

Specify if:

- *with delayed onset*—if onset of symptoms is at least 6 months after the stressor.

- Offer all rape victims testing for HIV infection as well as medical counseling and follow-up.
- Give sedatives or tranquilizers for a short time to decrease anxiety.

There's no definitive treatment for rape-trauma syndrome or PTSD. Treatment of the rape survivor experiencing rape-trauma syndrome will vary with each individual and may include:

- exposure therapy, which involves gradually facing a feared situation or memory to reduce its associated anxiety and distress
- cognitive therapy, which focuses on how the person views the world after the life-shattering event and attempts to restructure the survivor's feelings of safety, trust, power, and control and consists of offering emotional support in a calm and nonjudgmental manner
- SSRIs, which are the first medications to be approved for treating PTSD
- medications to treat specific symptoms, such as severe anxiety and insomnia
- suicide precautions if the rape survivor considers suicide.

In addition, the rape survivor will need to be treated for a variety of complications that may arise from the rape, such as physical injuries, chronic pain, bereavement, and depression or anger.

Special considerations

- Most states require hospitals to report rapes even if the patient doesn't press charges or assist the police. If the police interview the patient in the hospital, be supportive and encourage her to recall details of the rape. Your kindness and empathy are invaluable. The patient may also want you to call her family. Help her to verbalize anticipation of her family's response.
- Refer the patient for psychological counseling, if needed, to cope with the aftereffects of the attack.
- If the patient is engaged in legal proceedings during this time, she'll be forced to relive the trauma, which may leave her feeling lonely and isolated, perhaps even temporarily halting her emotional recovery. To help her cope, encourage her to write her thoughts, feelings, and reactions in a

daily diary, and refer her to organizations such as Women Organized Against Rape or a local rape crisis center for empathy, advice, and support groups. (See *Legal tips for rape examination.*)

- Remember that the assault affects every aspect of the rape survivor's life, including social interactions, intimacy, other relationships, job, home, and health.

Legal tips for rape examination

If your hospital observes a protocol for emergency care of rape victims, it may include a rape evidence kit. If it does, follow the kit's instructions carefully. Include only medically relevant information in your notes.

If you're called as a witness during a trial, try to provide the judge and jury with pertinent facts while maintaining your own credibility.

Courtroom tips

- Go to court tastefully dressed and well-groomed.
- Keep your posture erect and look confident.
- Look the prosecuting and defense attorneys in the eye when answering their questions but avoid long eye contact with the victim—this may cause you to appear biased.
- Don't offer speculations about the rape or volunteer information. Just answer questions that you're asked. If you don't know an answer, don't be afraid to say so.

Raynaud's disease

Raynaud's disease is one of several primary (idiopathic) arteriospastic disorders characterized by episodic vasospasm and, therefore, decreased blood circulation in the small peripheral arteries and arterioles. It occurs bilaterally, usually affecting the hands or, less commonly, the feet and is precipitated by exposure to cold or stress. Raynaud's disease is most prevalent in females, particularly those between puberty and age 40. Women are five times more likely than men to develop it. It's usually a benign condition, requiring no specific treatment and causing no serious sequelae. However, approximately 30% of cases progress after diagnosis, while 15% improve.

Raynaud's phenomenon, however, is a secondary condition that's usually associated with several connective disorders, such as scleroderma, systemic lupus erythematosus (SLE), or polymyositis. Raynaud's phenomenon is more complicated and severe than Raynaud's disease, and it has a progressive course, leading to ischemia, gangrene, and possible amputation. Distinguishing between the two disorders is difficult because some patients who experience mild symptoms of Raynaud's disease for several years may later develop overt connective tissue disease, especially scleroderma.

Causes

Although family history is a risk factor, the exact cause of Raynaud's disease is unknown. Raynaud's phenomenon, however, may develop secondary to:

- connective tissue disorders, such as scleroderma, rheumatoid arthritis, SLE, or polymyositis
- pulmonary hypertension
- thoracic outlet syndrome
- arterio-occlusive disease
- myxedema
- trauma
- serum sickness
- exposure to heavy metals
- previous damage from cold exposure
- long-term exposure to cold, vibrating machinery (such as operating a jackhammer), or pressure to the fingertips (such as in typists and pianists).

Although the cause is unknown, several theories account for reduced digital blood flow, including:

- intrinsic vascular wall hyperactivity to cold
- increased vasomotor tone due to sympathetic stimulation
- antigen-antibody immune response (the most likely theory because abnormal immunologic test results accompany Raynaud's phenomenon).

Signs and symptoms

Signs and symptoms of Raynaud's disease may include:

- blanching of the fingers bilaterally after exposure to cold or stress as vasoconstriction or vasospasm reduces blood flow (followed by cyanosis due to increased oxygen extraction resulting from sluggish blood flow and then, as the spasm resolves, the fingers turning red as blood rushes back into the arterioles)
- cold and numbness, possibly occurring during the vasoconstrictive phase because of ischemia
- throbbing, aching pain; swelling; and tingling, possibly occurring during the hyperemic phase
- trophic changes, such as sclerodactyly, ulcerations, or chronic paronychia, possibly occurring as a result of ischemia in long-standing disease
- possible cutaneous gangrene as a result of prolonged ischemia, necessitating amputation of one or more digits (extremely rare).

Diagnosis

Tests that help diagnose Raynaud's disease include:

- Clinical criteria include skin color changes induced by cold or stress; bilateral involvement; absence of gangrene or, if present, minimal cutaneous gangrene; normal arterial pulses; and patient history of symptoms for at least 2 years.
- Antinuclear antibody (ANA) titer is used to identify autoimmune diseases, such as a connective tissue disease, as an underlying cause of Raynaud's phenomenon. Further tests, such as the erythrocyte sedimentation rate (ESR) and the nailfold capillary study, must be performed if ANA titer is positive.
- Arteriography rules out arterial occlusive disease.
- Doppler ultrasonography may show reduced blood flow if symptoms result from arterial occlusive disease.
- Cold stimulation test where the temperature of the hand or foot is tak-

en at rest and then again every 5 minutes after the hand or foot is submerged in ice water for 20 seconds. Raynaud's disease is suspected if the temperature of the hand or foot doesn't reach the at-rest temperature in 20 minutes or less.

Treatment

Treatment of Raynaud's disease typically involves:

- teaching the patient to avoid triggers, such as cold and mechanical or chemical injury
- encouraging the patient to stop smoking and avoid decongestants and caffeine to reduce vasoconstriction
- keeping fingers and toes warm to reduce vasoconstriction
- calcium channel blockers, such as nifedipine, diltiazem, and nicardipine, or nitroglycerine paste to produce vasodilation and prevent vasospasm
- adrenergic blockers, such as phenoxybenzamine or reserpine, which may improve blood flow to fingers or toes
- sympathectomy to prevent ischemic ulcers by promoting vasodilation (necessary in less than 25% of patients)
- treatment of the co-existing condition if the patient has secondary Raynaud's phenomenon, including corticosteroids if it's a connective tissue disorder
- amputation, if ischemia causes ulceration and gangrene.

ALTERNATIVE THERAPIES

Certain herbs (not regulated by the U.S. Food and Drug Administration), including vitamin E, magnesium, fish oils, peony, dong quai, cayenne, ginger, and prickly ash, are believed to decrease the vessel spasms of Raynaud's disease to improve circulation to the extremities.

Additionally, hypnosis, biofeedback training, relaxation exercises, and visualization are believed to reduce stress and anxiety and improve temperature control of the extremities.

Special considerations

- Warn the patient against exposure to the cold. Tell her to wear mittens or gloves in cold weather or when handling cold items or defrosting the freezer.
- Advise the patient to avoid stressful situations and to stop smoking.
- Instruct the patient to inspect her skin frequently and to seek immediate care for signs of skin breakdown or infection.
- Teach the patient about drugs, their use, and their adverse effects.
- Provide psychological support and reassurance to allay the patient's fear of amputation and disfigurement.

Rheumatoid arthritis

Rheumatoid arthritis (RA) is the most common form of arthritis. It's a chronic, systemic inflammatory disease that primarily attacks peripheral joints and the surrounding muscles, tendons, ligaments, and blood vessels. Partial remissions and unpredictable exacerbations mark the course of this potentially crippling disease. RA is three times more common in women than men. RA occurs worldwide, affecting more than 2.1 million people in the United States alone, 1.5 million of which are women. RA affects all races and ethnicities. Although it usually begins in middle age, RA may occur at any age including childhood and adolescence.

RA usually requires lifelong treatment and, sometimes, surgery. In most patients, it follows an intermittent course and allows normal activity between flare-ups. However, in 10% of affected people, total disability from severe joint deformity, associated extra-articular symptoms such as vasculitis, or both, occur. The prognosis worsens with the development of nodules, vasculitis, and high titers of rheumatoid factor (RF).

Causes

The cause of the chronic inflammation characteristic of RA isn't known. Possible theories include:

- abnormal immune activation (occurring in a genetically susceptible individual) leading to inflammation, complement activation, and cell proliferation within joints and tendon sheaths
- possible infection (viral or bacterial), hormone action, or lifestyle factors influencing onset
- development of an immunoglobulin (Ig) M antibody against the body's own IgG, or *rheumatoid factor* (RF), which aggregates into complexes and generates inflammation, causing eventual cartilage damage and triggering other immune responses.

If not arrested, the inflammatory process in the joints occurs in four stages:

- Synovitis develops from congestion and edema of the synovial membrane and joint capsule. Infiltration by lymphocytes, macrophages, and neutrophils continues the local inflammatory response. These cells and fibroblast-like synovial cells produce enzymes that help to degrade bone and cartilage.
- Pannus (thickened layers of granulation tissue) covers and invades cartilage and eventually destroys the joint capsule and bone.
- Fibrous ankylosis (fibrous invasion of the pannus and scar formation) occludes the joint space. Bone atrophy and misalignment cause visible deformities and disrupt the articulation of opposing bones, which causes muscle atrophy, imbalance and, possibly, partial dislocations (subluxations).
- Fibrous tissue calcifies, resulting in bony ankylosis and total immobility.

Signs and symptoms

RA usually develops insidiously and initially causes nonspecific signs and symptoms, most likely related to the initial inflammatory reactions before the inflammation of the synovium, including:

- fatigue
- malaise
- anorexia and weight loss
- persistent, low-grade fever
- lymphadenopathy
- vague articular symptoms.

As the disease progresses, signs and symptoms may include:

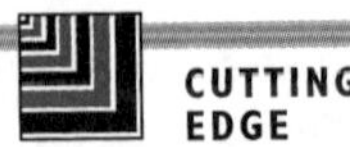

CUTTING EDGE

RA AND HEART ATTACK

In February of 2003, *Circulation: Journal of the American Heart Association* published results of a study in which researchers concluded that women with rheumatoid arthritis (RA) had a higher risk of heart attacks compared to women without RA. In fact, the risk increased twofold. In addition, women who had RA for 10 or more years were three times more likely to have a heart attack compared to women without RA.

The association of RA and heart attack is linked to fatty build-up in blood vessels (a known cause of heart attack) as a consequence of inflammation from RA. Another possible link between RA and heart attack is decreased physical activity due to pain and discomfort from RA and adverse effects of some of its drug therapies.

Researchers are still trying to determine whether early treatment of RA will also reduce the risk of a heart attack. Even so, they believe these findings show that RA should be a recognized risk factor for increased risk of heart attack, especially in women, and that health care providers should consider more aggressive cardiac prevention measures in these patients.

- specific localized, bilateral, symmetrical articular symptoms, commonly in the fingers at the proximal interphalangeal, metacarpophalangeal, and metatarsophalangeal joints and possibly extending to the wrists, knees, elbows, and ankles from inflammation of the synovium
- stiffening of affected joints after inactivity, especially on arising in the morning, due to progressive synovial inflammation and destruction
- spindle-shaped fingers from marked edema and congestion in the joints
- joint pain and tenderness — at first only with movement but eventually even at rest — due to prostaglandin release, edema, and synovial inflammation and destruction
- feeling of warmth at joint from inflammation
- diminished joint function and deformities as synovial destruction continues
- flexion deformities or hyperextension of metacarpophalangeal joints, subluxation of the wrist, and stretching of tendons pulling the fingers to the ulnar side (ulnar drift), or characteristic swan-neck or boutonnière deformity from joint swelling and loss of joint space
- carpal tunnel syndrome from synovial pressure on the median nerve causing paresthesia in the fingers.

Extra-articular findings may include:

- gradual appearance of rheumatoid nodules (subcutaneous, round or oval, nontender masses found in 20% of RF-positive patients), usually on elbows, hands, or Achilles tendon from destruction of the synovium
- vasculitis possibly leading to skin lesions, leg ulcers, and multiple systemic complications from infiltration

of immune complexes and subsequent tissue damage and necrosis in the vasculature

- pericarditis, pulmonary nodules or fibrosis, pleuritis, or inflammation of the sclera and overlying tissues of the eye from immune complex invasion and subsequent tissue damage and necrosis
- peripheral neuropathy with numbness or tingling in the feet or weakness and loss of sensation in the fingers from infiltration of the nerve fibers
- stiff, weak, or painful muscles secondary to limited mobility and decreased use.

With RA, the patient may also experience complications including myocardial infarction. (See *RA and heart attack*, and *Complications of RA*.)

Complications of RA

Complications of rheumatoid arthritis (RA) include:

- fibrosis and ankylosis
- soft tissue contractures
- pain
- joint deformities
- Sjögren's syndrome
- destruction of second cervical vertebra
- spinal cord compression
- temporomandibular joint disease
- infection
- osteoporosis
- myositis (inflammation of voluntary muscles)
- cardiopulmonary lesions
- lymphadenopathy
- peripheral neuritis
- myocardial infarction.

Diagnosis

Test results indicating RA include:

- X-rays showing bone demineralization and soft-tissue swelling (early stages), cartilage loss and narrowed joint spaces and, ultimately, cartilage and bone destruction and erosion, subluxations, and deformities (later stages)
- RF titer positive in 75% to 80% of patients (titer of 1:160 or higher)
- synovial fluid analysis showing increased volume and turbidity but decreased viscosity and elevated white blood cell counts (usually greater than 10,000/mm^3)
- serum protein electrophoresis possibly showing elevated serum globulin levels
- erythrocyte sedimentation rate and C-reactive protein levels showing elevations in 85% to 90% of patients (may be useful to monitor response to therapy because elevation commonly parallels disease activity)
- complete blood count usually showing moderate anemia, slight leukocytosis, and slight thrombocytosis.

Treatment

Treatment for RA involves drug therapy and supportive measures. (See *Drug therapy for RA*, pages 424 and 425.) These treatments include:

- salicylates, particularly aspirin (mainstay of therapy), to decrease inflammation and relieve joint pain

(Text continues on page 426.)

Drug therapy for RA

The following flowchart identifies the major pathophysiologic events in rheumatoid arthritis (RA) and shows where in this chain of events the major drug therapies act to control the disease.

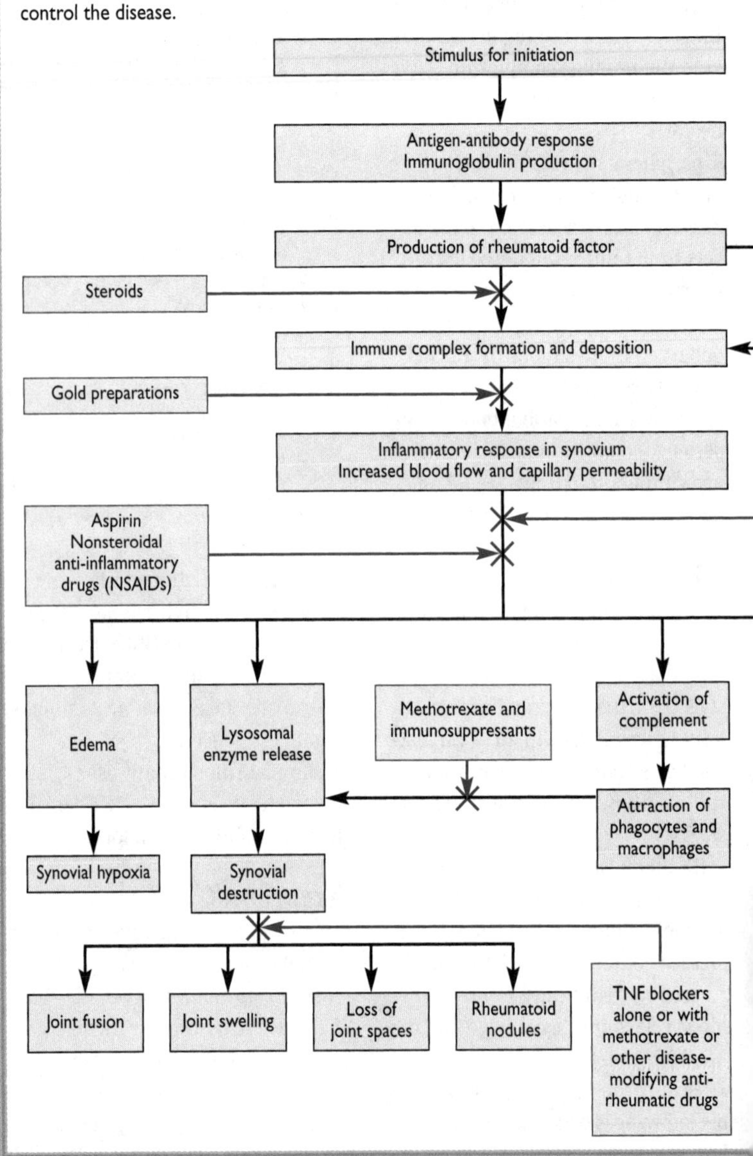

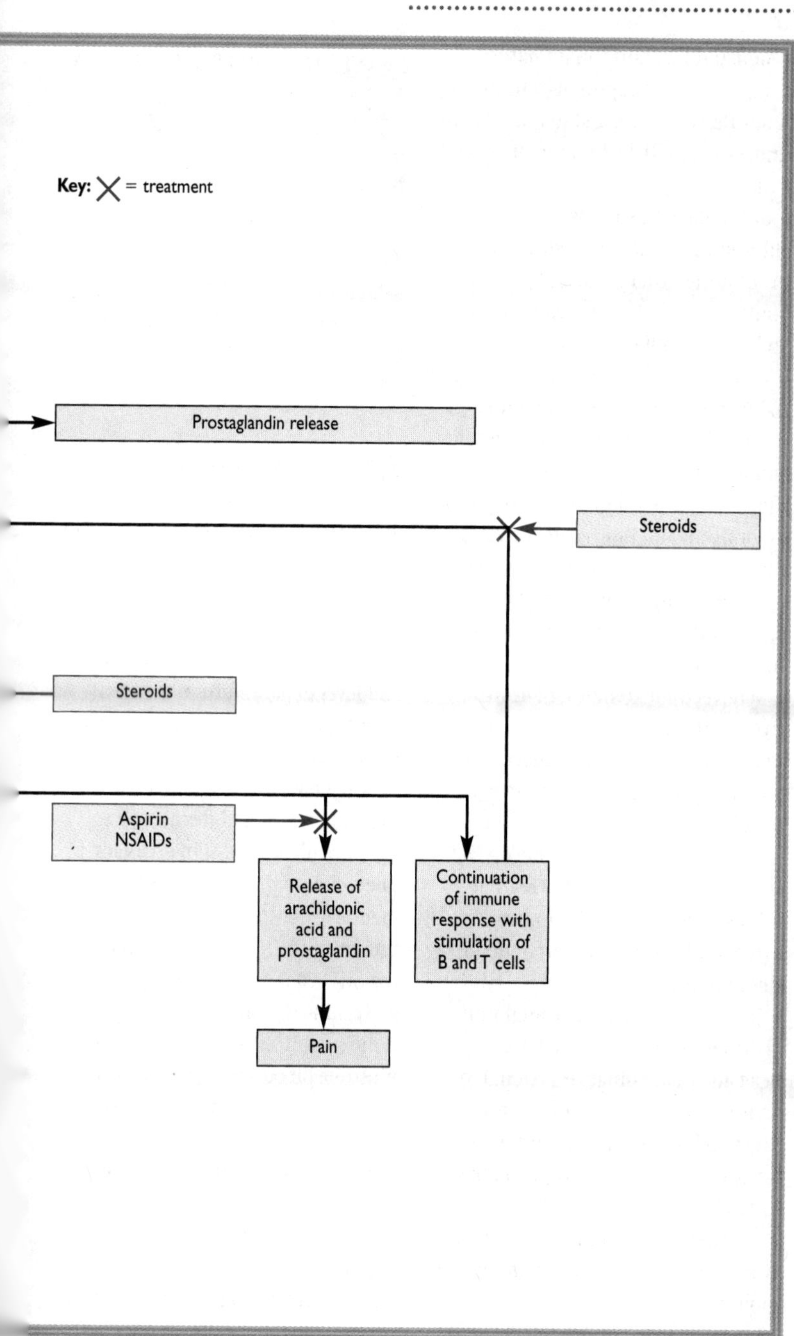
Key: = treatment
Prostaglandin release
Steroids
Steroids
Aspirin
NSAIDs
Release of arachidonic acid and prostaglandin
Continuation of immune response with stimulation of B and T cells
Pain

- nonsteroidal anti inflammatory drugs, such as fenoprofen (Nalfon), ibuprofen (Motrin), and indomethacin (Indocin), to relieve inflammation and pain
- antimalarials, such as hydroxychloroquine (Plaquenil), sulfasalazine (Azulfidine), gold salts, and penicillamine (Cuprimine), to reduce acute and chronic inflammation
- corticosteroids such as prednisone in low doses for anti-inflammatory effects and in higher doses for immunosuppressive effect on T cells
- azathioprine (Imuran), cyclosporine (Neoral), and methotrexate (Folex) in early disease for immunosuppression by suppressing T and B lymphocyte proliferation that's causing destruction of the synovium
- synovectomy (removal of destructive, proliferating synovium, usually in the wrists, knees, and fingers) to possibly halt or delay the course of the disease
- osteotomy (cutting of bone or excision of a wedge of bone) to realign joint surfaces and redistribute stress
- tendon transfers to prevent deformities or relieve contractures
- joint reconstruction or total joint arthroplasty, including metatarsal head and distal ulnar resectional arthroplasty, insertion of a Silastic prosthesis between metacarpophalangeal and proximal interphalangeal joints (severe disease)
- arthrodesis (joint fusion) for stability and relief from pain (sacrifices joint mobility)

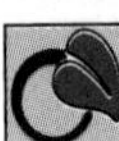

ALTERNATIVE THERAPIES

Acupuncture, which may be effective in treating some forms of arthritis (according to the National Institutes of Health, although other experts, such as the American College of Rheumatology, disagree) and exercise, such as range-of-motion, strengthening, and aerobic (biking or swimming) exercise have been effective in decreasing RA symptoms.

Special considerations

- Assess all joints carefully. Look for deformities, contractures, immobility, and inability to perform everyday activities.
- Monitor vital signs, and note weight changes, sensory disturbances, and level of pain. Administer analgesics, as ordered, and watch for adverse effects.
- Provide meticulous skin care. Check for rheumatoid nodules as well as pressure ulcers and skin breakdown due to immobility, vascular impairment, corticosteroid treatment, or improper splinting. Use lotion or cleansing oil — not soap — for dry skin.
- Explain all diagnostic tests and procedures. Tell the patient to expect multiple blood samples to confirm diagnosis and enable accurate therapy.
- Monitor the duration — not the intensity — of morning stiffness because duration more accurately reflects the severity of the disease. Encourage the patient to take hot showers or baths at bedtime or in the morning to reduce the need for pain medication.

- Apply splints carefully and correctly. Observe for pressure ulcers if the patient is in traction or wearing splints.
- Explain the nature of the disease. Make sure the patient and her family understand that RA is a chronic disease that requires major changes in lifestyle. Emphasize that there are no miracle cures, despite claims to the contrary.
- Encourage a balanced diet but make sure the patient understands that special diets won't cure RA. Stress the need for weight control because obesity adds further stress to joints.
- Urge the patient to perform activities of daily living, such as dressing and feeding herself (supply easy-to-open cartons, lightweight cups, and unpackaged silverware). Allow the patient enough time to calmly perform these tasks.
- Provide emotional support. Remember that the patient with chronic illness easily becomes depressed, discouraged, and irritable. Encourage the patient to discuss her fears concerning dependency, sexuality, body image, and self-esteem. Refer her to an appropriate social service agency as needed.
- Discuss sexual aids, alternative positions, pain medication, and moist heat to increase mobility.
- Before discharge, make sure the patient knows how and when to take prescribed medication and how to recognize possible adverse effects.
- Teach the patient how to stand, walk, and sit correctly. Tell her to sit in chairs with high seats and armrests; she'll find it easier to get up from a chair if her knees are lower than her hips. If she doesn't own a chair with a high seat, recommend putting blocks of wood under the legs of a favorite chair. Suggest an elevated toilet seat.
- Instruct the patient to pace daily activities, resting for 5 to 10 minutes out of each hour and alternating sitting and standing tasks. Adequate sleep is important and so is correct sleeping posture. She should sleep on her back on a firm mattress and should avoid placing a pillow under her knees, which encourages flexion deformity.
- Teach her to avoid putting undue stress on joints by using the largest joint available for a given task, avoiding positions of flexion and promoting positions of extension, holding objects parallel to the knuckles as briefly as possible, always using her hands toward the center of her body, sliding — not lifting — objects whenever possible, and supporting weak or painful joints as much as possible. Enlist the aid of the occupational therapist to teach her how to simplify activities and protect arthritic joints. Stress the importance of shoes with proper support.
- Suggest dressing aids (long-handled shoehorn, reacher, elastic shoelaces, zipper-pull, and buttonhook) and helpful household items (easy-to-open drawers, handheld shower nozzle, handrails, and grab bars). The patient who has trouble maneuvering fingers into gloves should wear mittens. Tell her to dress while in a sitting position as often as possible.

- Refer the patient to the Arthritis Foundation for more information on coping with the disease.

Rosacea

A chronic skin eruption, rosacea produces flushing and dilation of the small blood vessels in the face, especially the nose and cheeks. Papules and pustules may also occur but without the characteristic comedones of acne vulgaris. Rosacea is most common in white women between ages 30 and 50. When it occurs in men, however, it's usually more severe and commonly associated with rhinophyma, which is characterized by dilated follicles and reddened, thickened, and bulbous skin on the nose. Ocular involvement may result in blepharitis, conjunctivitis, uveitis, or keratitis. Rosacea usually spreads slowly and rarely subsides spontaneously.

Causes

Although the cause of rosacea is unknown, stress, infection, vitamin deficiency, menopause, and endocrine abnormalities can aggravate it. Anything that produces flushing — for example, hot beverages, such as tea or coffee; tobacco; alcohol; spicy foods; physical activity; sunlight; and extreme heat or cold — can also aggravate rosacea.

Signs and symptoms

Rosacea generally begins with periodic flushing across the central oval of the face, accompanied later by telangiectasia, papules, pustules, and nodules. Rhinophyma is commonly associated with severe rosacea but may occur alone. Rhinophyma usually appears first on the lower half of the nose, and produces red, thickened skin and follicular enlargement. It's found almost exclusively in men over age 40. Related ocular lesions are uncommon.

Diagnosis

Typical vascular and acneiform lesions — without the comedones characteristically associated with acne vulgaris — and rhinophyma in severe cases confirm rosacea.

Treatment

Treatment of the acneiform component of rosacea consists of oral tetracycline (Sumycin) or erythromycin (Erythocin) in gradually decreasing doses as symptoms subside. Resistant cases can be treated with oral metronidazole (Flagyl). Isotretinoin (Accutane) is also effective. Topical metronidazole gel (MetroGel) helps resolve papules, pustules, and erythema. Combination acne products, including over-the-counter and prescription products (such as Sulfacet-R Lotion and Clearasil) are available in flesh tones, control pustules, and hide redness. They can be used alone or with oral antibiotics. Topical application of 1% hydrocortisone cream reduces erythema and inflammation. Other treatments include electrolysis to destroy large, dilated blood vessels and removal of excess tissue in patients with rhinophyma. (See *Preventing rosacea flare-ups*.)

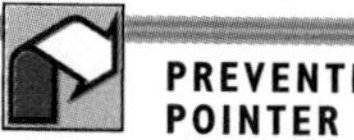

PREVENTION POINTER

PREVENTING ROSACEA FLARE-UPS

Some women find that certain stimuli will cause them to flush and cause a flare-up. Common stimuli that will trigger such a flare-up include sun exposure, stress, heat, physical or strenuous activity, spicy foods, hot drinks such as tea, hot baths, extreme temperatures (hot and cold), windy weather, and skin products that are harsh (such as those products that contain alcohol). To prevent flare-ups, tell her to:

- avoid direct sun exposure
- if outside, wear sunscreen and a hat that will shield her face from the sun
- stay in air-conditioned rooms when it's hot and humid outside
- avoid going outside in extremely cold or windy weather, if possible
- avoid spicy foods
- avoid drinking hot beverages; rather, drink them at room temperature
- avoid hot baths
- use noncomedogenic and nonalcoholic skin products
- avoid alcohol
- avoid facials or facial massages
- avoid high-intensity workouts
- take prescription medication as directed.

Special considerations

- Instruct the patient to avoid hot beverages, alcohol, extended sun exposure, and other possible causes of flushing.
- Assess the effect of rosacea on body image. Because it's always apparent on the face, your support is essential.
- Refer your patient to a dermatologist, as necessary.

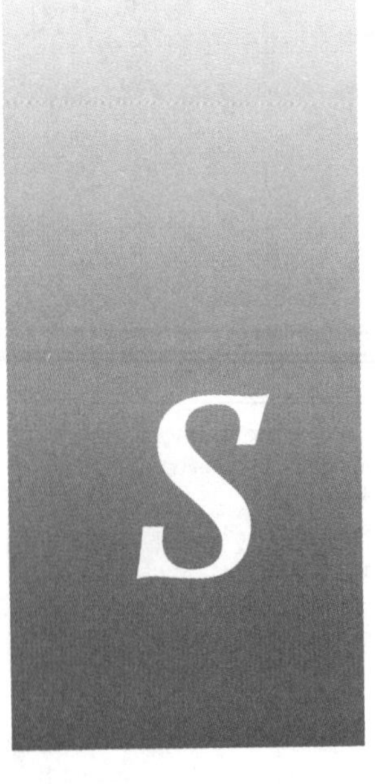

Sarcoidosis

Sarcoidosis is a multisystem, granulomatous disorder that characteristically produces lymphadenopathy, pulmonary infiltration, and skeletal, liver, eye, or skin lesions. It occurs most commonly in young adults (ages 20 to 40). In the United States, sarcoidosis occurs predominantly among blacks, and affects twice as many women as men. Acute sarcoidosis usually resolves within 2 years. Chronic, progressive sarcoidosis, which is uncommon, is associated with pulmonary fibrosis and progressive pulmonary disability.

Causes

The cause of sarcoidosis is unknown, but the following factors may play a role:

- hypersensitivity response (possibly from T-cell imbalance) to such agents as atypical mycobacteria, fungi, and pine pollen
- genetic predisposition (suggested by a slightly higher incidence of sarcoidosis within the same family)
- chemicals, such as zirconium and beryllium, that can lead to illnesses resembling sarcoidosis, suggesting an extrinsic cause for this disease.

Signs and symptoms

Initial symptoms of sarcoidosis include arthralgia (in the wrists, ankles, and elbows), fatigue, malaise, and weight loss. Other clinical features vary according to the extent and location of the fibrosis:

- *respiratory* — breathlessness, cough (usually nonproductive), substernal pain; pulmonary hypertension and cor pulmonale (complications in advanced pulmonary disease)
- *cutaneous* — erythema nodosum, subcutaneous skin nodules with maculopapular eruptions, and extensive nasal mucosal lesions
- *ophthalmic* — anterior uveitis (common), glaucoma, and blindness (rare)
- *lymphatic* — bilateral hilar and right paratracheal lymphadenopathy and splenomegaly
- *musculoskeletal* — muscle weakness, polyarthralgia, pain, and punched-out lesions on phalanges
- *hepatic* — granulomatous hepatitis, which usually produces no symptoms
- *genitourinary* — hypercalciuria
- *cardiovascular* — arrhythmias (premature beats, bundle-branch or complete heart block) and, rarely, cardiomyopathy
- *central nervous system (CNS)* — cranial or peripheral nerve palsies, basilar meningitis, seizures, and pituitary and hypothalamic lesions producing diabetes insipidus.

Diagnosis

Diagnosis of sarcoidosis is one of exclusion. Once differential diagnoses are excluded, other tests may be ordered. Typical clinical features with appropriate laboratory data and X-ray findings suggest sarcoidosis. A positive Kveim skin test supports the diagnosis. In this test, the patient receives an intradermal injection of an antigen prepared from human sarcoidal spleen or lymph nodes from patients with sarcoidosis. If the patient has active sarcoidosis, granuloma develops at the injection site in 2 to 6 weeks. This reaction is considered positive when a biopsy of the skin at the injection site shows discrete epithelioid cell granuloma.

Other relevant findings include:

- *chest X-ray* — bilateral hilar and right paratracheal adenopathy with or without diffuse interstitial infiltrates and, occasionally, large nodular lesions present in lung parenchyma
- *lymph node, skin, or lung biopsy* — noncaseating granulomas with negative cultures for mycobacteria and fungi
- *other laboratory data* — rarely, increased serum calcium, mild anemia, leukocytosis, and hyperglobulinemia
- *pulmonary function tests* — decreased total lung capacity and compliance and decreased diffusing capacity
- *arterial blood gas (ABG) analysis* — decreased arterial oxygen saturation.

Negative tuberculin skin test, fungal serologies, and sputum cultures for mycobacteria and fungi as well as negative biopsy cultures help rule out infection.

Treatment

Asymptomatic sarcoidosis requires no treatment. However, sarcoidosis that causes ocular, respiratory, CNS, cardiac, or systemic symptoms (such as fever and weight loss) requires treatment with systemic or topical steroids as does sarcoidosis that produces hypercalcemia or destructive skin lesions. Such therapy is usually continued for 1 to 2 years, but some patients may need lifelong therapy. Other measures include a low-calcium diet and avoidance of direct exposure to sunlight in patients with hypercalcemia.

Special considerations

- Watch for and report complications. Be aware of any abnormal laboratory results (anemia, for example) that could alter patient care.
- For the patient with arthralgia, administer analgesics as ordered. Record signs of progressive muscle weakness.
- Provide a nutritious, high-calorie diet and plenty of fluids. If the patient has hypercalcemia, suggest a low-calcium diet. Weigh the patient regularly to detect weight loss.
- Monitor respiratory function. Check chest X-rays for the extent of lung involvement; note and record any bloody sputum or increase in sputum. If the patient has pulmonary hypertension or end-stage cor pulmonale, check ABG levels, observe for arrhythmias, and administer oxygen as needed.
- Because steroids may induce or worsen diabetes mellitus, perform fingerstick glucose tests at least every 12 hours at the beginning of steroid therapy. Also, watch for other steroid adverse effects, such as fluid retention, electrolyte imbalance (especially hypokalemia), moon face, hypertension, and personality change. Remember that the patient on long-term or high-dose steroid therapy is vulnerable to infection.
- During or after steroid withdrawal (particularly in association with infection or other types of stress), watch for and report vomiting, orthostatic hypotension, hypoglycemia, restlessness, anorexia, malaise, and fatigue.
- When preparing the patient for discharge, stress the need for compliance with prescribed steroid therapy and regular, careful follow-up examinations and treatment. Refer the patient with failing vision to community support and resource groups and the American Foundation for the Blind, if necessary.

Scleroderma

Scleroderma literally means "hard skin." It's an uncommon disorder of diffuse connective tissue disease characterized by inflammatory and then degenerative and fibrotic changes (hardening and scarring) in the skin, blood vessels, synovial membranes, skeletal muscles, and internal organs (especially the esophagus, intestinal tract, thyroid, heart, lungs, and kidneys). There are two major types of scleroderma — localized and systemic — and each type has many subtypes.

Localized scleroderma usually affects only the skin. It has three main subtypes: morphea, generalized morphea, and linear. Systemic scleroderma affects multiple systems, including blood vessels, internal organs, muscles, joints, and the intestines. It's divided into two subtypes: systemic-limited scleroderma (also known as *CREST*) and systemic-diffuse. There's also a type called *scleroderma sine sclerosis*, which affects the internal organs but doesn't have the characteristic skin ulcers of systemic scleroderma.

Scleroderma occurs in 3 to 4 times as many women as men, especially those between ages 30 and 50. The peak incidence of occurrence is in women ages 50 to 60. Scleroderma usually progresses slowly. When the condition is limited to the skin, the prognosis is usually favorable. However, approximately 30% of patients with systemic scleroderma die within 5 years of onset. Death is usually caused by infection or renal or heart failure.

Causes

The cause of scleroderma is unknown, but some possible causes include:

- systemic exposure to silica dust or polyvinyl chloride
- anticancer agents, such as bleomycin (Blenoxane), or nonopioid analgesics such as pentazocine (Talwin)
- fibrosis due to an abnormal immune system response
- underlying vascular cause with tissue changes initiated by a persistent perfusion. For example, in some patients, muscles and joints become fibrotic.

Signs and symptoms

Scleroderma is characterized by diffuse fibrosis, degenerative changes, and vascular changes in the skin, articular structures, and internal organs. It usually begins in the fingers and extends proximally to the upper arms, shoulders, neck, and face. The skin atrophies, edema and infiltrates containing CD4+ T cells surround the blood vessels, and inflamed collagen fibers become edematous, losing strength and elasticity. The dermis becomes tightly bound to the underlying structures, resulting in atrophy of the affected dermal appendages and destruction of the distal phalanges by osteoporosis. As the disease progresses, this atrophy can affect other areas.

Possible signs and symptoms of scleroderma include:

- skin thickening, commonly limited to the distal extremities and face but possibly involving internal organs (systemic-limited scleroderma)
- CREST syndrome (calcinosis, Raynaud's phenomenon, esophageal dysfunction, sclerodactyly, and telangiectasia), a benign subtype of systemic-limited scleroderma
- generalized skin thickening and involvement of internal organs (systemic-diffuse scleroderma)
- patchy skin changes with a teardrop shape known as *morphea* (localized scleroderma)
- band of thickened skin on the face or extremities that severely damages underlying tissues, causing atrophy and deformity (localized linear scleroderma)

- atrophy and deformity (most common in childhood)
- Raynaud's phenomenon (blanching, cyanosis, and erythema of the fingers and toes when exposed to cold or stress) and progressive phalangeal resorption, which may shorten the fingers (early symptoms)
- pain, stiffness, and swelling of fingers and joints (later symptoms)
- Sclerodactyly (taut, shiny skin over the entire hand and forearm due to skin thickening)
- tight and inelastic facial skin causing a masklike appearance and "pinching" of the mouth; contractures with progressive tightening
- thickened skin over proximal limbs and trunk (systemic-diffuse scleroderma)
- painful ulcers (systemic-limited and systemic-diffuse scleroderma)
- frequent reflux, heartburn, dysphagia, and bloating after meals due to GI dysfunction
- abdominal distention, diarrhea, constipation, and malodorous floating stool.

Complications of scleroderma include compromised circulation due to abnormal thickening of the arterial intima, possibly causing slowly healing ulcerations on fingertips or toes leading to gangrene; decreased food intake and weight loss due to GI symptoms; and arrhythmias and dyspnea due to cardiac and pulmonary fibrosis and renal crisis (malignant hypertension due to renal involvement), which may be fatal if untreated (advanced disease).

Diagnosis

Tests to aid diagnosis of scleroderma may include:

- typical cutaneous changes (the first clue to diagnosis)
- slightly elevated erythrocyte sedimentation rate, positive rheumatoid factor in 25% to 35% of patients, and positive antinuclear antibody test results
- urinalysis showing proteinuria, microscopic hematuria, and casts (with renal involvement)
- hand X-rays showing terminal phalangeal tuft resorption, subcutaneous calcification, and joint space narrowing and erosion
- chest X-rays showing bilateral basilar pulmonary fibrosis
- GI X-rays showing distal esophageal hypomotility and stricture, duodenal loop dilation, small-bowel malabsorption pattern, and large diverticula
- pulmonary function studies showing decreased diffusion and vital capacity
- electrocardiogram showing nonspecific abnormalities related to myocardial fibrosis
- skin biopsy showing changes consistent with disease progression, such as marked thickening of the dermis and occlusive vessel changes.

Treatment

There's no cure for scleroderma. Treatment aims to preserve normal body functions, minimize complications, and may include:

- immunosuppressants, including such common palliative drugs as cyclosporine (Neoral) and chlorambucil (Leukeran)

- vasodilators and antihypertensives, such as nifedipine (Adalat), prazosin (Minipress), or topical nitroglycerin (Nitro-Bid); digital sympathectomy; or, rarely, cervical sympathetic blockade to treat Raynaud's phenomenon
- digital plaster cast to immobilize the area, minimize trauma, and maintain cleanliness; possible surgical debridement for chronic digital ulceration
- antacids to reduce total acid level in GI tract; omeprazole (Prilosec), a proton-pump inhibitor to block the formation of gastric acid, periodic dilation, and a soft, bland diet for esophagitis with stricture
- broad-spectrum antibiotics to treat small-bowel involvement with erythromycin or tetracycline (preferred drugs) to counteract the bacterial overgrowth in the duodenum and jejunum related to hypomotility
- short-term benefit from vasodilators, such as nifedipine (Adalat) and hydralazine (Apresoline), to decrease contractility and oxygen demand and cause vasodilation (for pulmonary hypertension)
- angiotensin-converting enzyme (ACE) inhibitor to preserve renal function (early intervention in renal crisis)
- physical therapy to maintain function and promote muscle strength, heat therapy to relieve joint stiffness, and occupational therapy to help performance of daily activities easier (for hand debilitation).

Special considerations

- Assess motion restrictions, pain, vital signs, intake and output, respiratory function, and daily weight.
- Because of compromised circulation, warn against fingerstick blood tests.
- Remember that air conditioning may aggravate Raynaud's phenomenon.
- Help the patient and her family adjust to the patient's new body image and the limitations and dependence that these changes cause.
- Teach the patient to avoid fatigue by pacing activities and organizing schedules to include necessary rest.
- The patient and family need to accept the fact that this condition is incurable. Encourage them to express their feelings and help them cope with their fears and frustrations by offering information about the disease, its treatment, and relevant diagnostic tests.
- Whenever possible, let the patient participate in treatment by measuring her own intake and output, planning her own diet, giving herself heat therapy, and performing prescribed exercises independently.
- Refer the patient to support groups, which can be found in every state. Instruct the patient to call 1-800-872-HOPE or go to *www.scleroderma.org* to determine the closest location.

Sjögren's syndrome

The second most common autoimmune rheumatic disorder after rheumatoid arthritis (RA), Sjögren's syndrome is characterized by diminished lacrimal and salivary gland secretion (sicca complex). This syndrome occurs mainly in women (90% of patients); mean age of onset is 50. Sjögren's syndrome may be a primary disorder, or it may be associated with connective tissue disorders, such as RA, scleroderma, systemic lupus erythematosus, and polymyositis. In some patients, the disorder is limited to the exocrine glands (glandular Sjögren's syndrome); in others, it also involves other organs, such as the lungs and kidneys (extraglandular Sjögren's syndrome).

Causes

The cause of Sjögren's syndrome is unknown, but genetic and environmental factors probably contribute to its development. Viral or bacterial infection or, perhaps, exposure to pollen may trigger Sjögren's syndrome in a genetically susceptible individual. Tissue damage results from infiltration by lymphocytes or from the deposition of immune complexes. Lymphocytic infiltration may be classified as benign, malignant, or pseudolymphoma (nonmalignant but tumorlike aggregates of lymphoid cells).

Signs and symptoms

About 50% of patients with Sjögren's syndrome have confirmed RA and a history of slowly developing sicca complex. However, some seek medical help for rapidly progressive and severe oral and ocular dryness, in many cases accompanied by periodic parotid gland enlargement. Ocular dryness (xerophthalmia) leads to foreign body sensation (gritty, sandy eye), redness, burning, photosensitivity, eye fatigue, itching, and mucoid discharge. The patient may also complain of a film across his field of vision.

Oral dryness (xerostomia) leads to difficulty swallowing and talking; abnormal taste or smell sensation or both; thirst; ulcers of the tongue, buccal mucosa, and lips (especially at the corners of the mouth); and severe dental caries. Dryness of the respiratory tract leads to epistaxis, hoarseness, chronic nonproductive cough, recurrent otitis media, and increased incidence of respiratory infections.

Other effects may include dyspareunia and pruritus (associated with vaginal dryness), generalized itching, fatigue, recurrent low-grade fever, and arthralgia or myalgia. Lymph node enlargement may be the first sign of malignant lymphoma or pseudolymphoma.

Specific extraglandular findings in Sjögren's syndrome include interstitial pneumonitis; interstitial nephritis, which results in renal tubular acidosis in 25% of patients; Raynaud's phenomenon (20%); and vasculitis, usually limited to the skin and characterized by palpable purpura on the legs (20%). About 50% of patients show evidence of hypothyroidism related to autoimmune thyroid disease. A few patients develop systemic necrotizing vasculitis.

Diagnosis

Diagnosis of Sjögren's syndrome rests on the detection of two of the following three conditions: xerophthalmia, xerostomia (with salivary gland biopsy showing lymphocytic infiltration), and an associated autoimmune or lymphoproliferative disorder. Diagnosis must rule out other causes of oral and ocular dryness, including sarcoidosis, endocrine disorders, anxiety or depression, and effects of therapy, such as radiation to the head and neck. Over 200 commonly used drugs also produce dry mouth as an adverse effect. In patients with salivary gland enlargement and severe lymphoid infiltration, diagnosis must rule out cancer.

Laboratory values include elevated erythrocyte sedimentation rate in most patients, mild anemia and leukopenia in 30%, and hypergammaglobulinemia in 50%. Autoantibodies are also common, including anti-Sjögren's syndrome-A (anti-Ro) and anti-Sjögren's syndrome-B (anti-La), which are antinuclear and antisalivary duct antibodies. Between 75% and 90% of patients test positive for rheumatoid factor; 90%, for antinuclear antibodies.

Other tests help support this diagnosis. Schirmer's tearing test and slit-lamp examination with rose bengal dye are used to measure eye involvement. Salivary gland involvement is evaluated by measuring the volume of parotid saliva as well as secretory sialography and salivary scintigraphy. Lower-lip biopsy shows salivary gland infiltration by lymphocytes.

Treatment

Treatment is usually symptomatic and includes conservative measures to relieve ocular or oral dryness. Mouth dryness can be relieved by using a methylcellulose swab or spray and by drinking plenty of fluids, especially at mealtime. Meticulous oral hygiene is essential, including regular flossing, brushing, at-home fluoride treatment, and frequent dental checkups. Advise the patient to avoid drugs that decrease saliva production, such as atropine derivatives, antihistamines, anticholinergics, and antidepressants. If mouth lesions make eating painful, suggest high-protein, high-calorie liquid supplements to prevent malnutrition. Advise the patient to avoid sugar, which contributes to dental caries. Tobacco, alcohol, and spicy, salty, or highly acidic foods, which cause mouth irritation, should also be avoided.

Instill artificial tears as often as every half hour to prevent eye damage (corneal ulcerations and corneal opacifications) from insufficient tear secretions. Some patients may also benefit from instillation of an eye ointment at bedtime or twice-a-day use of sustained-release cellulose capsules (Lacrisert). Suggest the use of sunglasses to protect the patient's eyes from dust, wind, and strong light. Moisture chamber spectacles may also be helpful. Because dry eyes are more susceptible to infection, advise the patient to keep his face clean and avoid rubbing his eyes. If infection develops, antibiotics should be given immediately; topical steroids should be avoided.

To help relieve respiratory dryness, stress the need to humidify home and work environments. Suggest normal saline solution drops or aerosolized spray for nasal dryness. Advise the patient to avoid prolonged hot showers and baths and use moisturizing lotions to help ease dry skin. Suggest K-Y lubricating jelly as a vaginal lubricant.

Other treatment measures vary with associated extraglandular findings. Parotid gland enlargement requires local heat and analgesics. Pulmonary and renal interstitial disease necessitates the use of corticosteroids. Accompanying lymphoma is treated with a combination of chemotherapy, surgery, or radiation.

Special considerations

- Refer the patient to the Sjögren's Syndrome Foundation for additional information and support.
- Because Sjögren's syndrome may commonly coexist with other disorders, such as RA, systemic lupus erythematosus, scleroderma, or polymyositis and dermatomyositis, remember to treat the coexisting disorders.
- Refer the patient to a rheumatologist.

Squamous cell carcinoma

Squamous cell carcinoma (SCC) of the skin is an invasive tumor that arises from keratinizing epidermal cells and has a high metastatic potential to distant parts of the body. It's the second most common skin cancer, the third most common cancer in men, and the fourth most common cancer in women. It usually occurs in fair-skinned white males over age 60. Outdoor employment and residence in a sunny, warm climate (southwestern United States and Australia, for example) greatly increase the risk of developing SCC. However, the incidence of SCC affecting the skin and oral cavities in women is rising as more women are frequenting tanning salons, drinking alcohol, and smoking.

Causes

Predisposing factors associated with SCC include overexposure to the sun's ultraviolet rays, the presence of premalignant lesions (such as actinic keratosis or Bowen's disease), X-ray therapy, ingestion of herbicides containing arsenic, chronic skin irritation and inflammation, exposure to local carcinogens (such as tar and oil), and hereditary diseases (such as xeroderma pigmentosum and albinism). Women who use tanning lamps and tanning beds were also found to be at increased risk for SCC — 2½ times the risk of women who didn't use them. Smoking has recently been linked to skin cancer and may increase the risk of developing skin cancer threefold, independent of age, gender, sun exposure, and other predisposing factors that are listed above. Rarely, SCC may develop on the site of smallpox vaccination, psoriasis, or chronic discoid lupus erythematosus. (See *Premalignant skin lesions.*)

PREMALIGNANT SKIN LESIONS

This chart lists common diseases that result in premalignant skin lesions along with their cause, lesion characteristics, and treatment.

Disease	Cause	Lesion	Treatment
Actinic keratosis	Solar radiation	Reddish-brown lesions 1 mm to 1 cm in size (may enlarge if untreated) on face, ears, lower lip, bald scalp, dorsa of hands and forearms	Topical 5-fluorouracil, cryosurgery using liquid nitrogen, or curettage by electrodesiccation
Bowen's disease	Unknown	Brown to reddish-brown lesions, with scaly surface on exposed and unexposed areas	Surgical excision, topical 5-fluorouracil
Erythroplasia of Queyrat	Bowen's disease of the mucous membranes	Red lesions, with a glistening or granular appearance on mucous membranes, particularly the glans penis in uncircumcised males	Surgical excision
Leukoplakia	Smoking, alcohol, chronic cheek-biting, ill-fitting dentures, misaligned teeth	Lesions on oral, anal, and genital mucous membranes that vary in appearance from smooth and white to rough and gray	Elimination of irritating factors, surgical excision, or curettage by electrodesiccation (if lesion is still premalignant)

Signs and symptoms

SCC begins in the upper part of the epidermis and commonly develops on sun-exposed areas of the body, such as the face, ears, dorsa of the hands and forearms, and other sun-damaged areas. Lesions on sun-damaged skin tend to be less invasive and less likely to metastasize than lesions on unexposed skin. Squamous cell lesions may also begin within scars and skin ulcers that aren't necessarily in sun-exposed areas. Notable exceptions to this tendency are squamous cell lesions on the lower lip and the ears. These are almost invariably markedly invasive metastatic lesions with a generally poor prognosis.

Transformation from a premalignant lesion to SCC may begin with induration and inflammation of the preexisting lesion. When SCC arises from normal skin, the nodule grows slowly on a firm, indurated base. If untreated, this nodule eventually ulcerates and invades underlying tissues. Metastasis can occur to the regional lymph nodes, producing characteristic sys-

Staging SCC

The American Joint Committee on Cancer uses the following TNM (tumor, node, metastasis) system for staging squamous cell carcinoma (SCC).

Primary tumor
TX—primary tumor can't be assessed
T0—no evidence of primary tumor
Tis—carcinoma in situ
T1—tumor 2 cm or less in greatest dimension
T2—tumor between 2 and 5 cm in greatest dimension
T3—tumor more than 5 cm in greatest dimension
T4—tumor invades deep extradermal structures (such as cartilage, skeletal muscle, or bone)

Regional lymph nodes
NX—regional lymph nodes can't be assessed
N0—no evidence of regional lymph node involvement
N1—regional lymph node involvement

Distant metastasis
MX—distant metastasis can't be assessed
M0—no known distant metastasis
M1—distant metastasis

Staging categories
Squamous cell carcinoma progresses from mild to severe as follows:
Stage 0—Tis, N0, M0
Stage I—T1, N0, M0
Stage II—T2, N0, M0; T3, N0, M0
Stage III—T4, N0, M0; any T, N1, M0
Stage IV—any T, any N, M1.

temic symptoms of pain, malaise, fatigue, weakness, and anorexia. (See *Staging SCC*.)

Diagnosis

An excisional biopsy provides definitive diagnosis of SCC. Other appropriate laboratory tests depend on systemic symptoms.

Treatment

The size, shape, location, and invasiveness of a squamous cell tumor and the condition of the underlying tissue determine the treatment method used; a deeply invasive tumor may require a combination of techniques. All major treatment methods have excellent cure rates. In general, the prognosis is better with a well-differentiated lesion than with a poorly differentiated one in an unusual location. Depending on the lesion, treatment may consist of:

- wide surgical excision
- electrodesiccation and curettage (offers good cosmetic results for small lesions)
- cryosurgery (not for large invasive tumors or those tumors on certain parts of the body, such as the nose, eyes, ears, head, or legs)
- Mohs surgery (has the highest cure rate for tumors greater than 2 cm, recurring tumors, or certain cancers found along the nerves under the skin, face, or genital areas)

- radiation therapy (generally for older or debilitated patients and for those areas where surgery is difficult, such as the eyes, ears, nose, and throat)
- lymph node removal (for very large and deeply invasive tumors)
- chemosurgery (reserved for resistant or recurrent lesions)
- systemic chemotherapy (when the cancer has spread to lymph nodes or distant organs).

Special considerations

The care plan for patients with SCC should emphasize meticulous wound care, emotional support, and thorough patient instruction:

- Coordinate a consistent plan of care for changing the patient's dressings. Establishing a standard routine helps the patient and family learn how to care for the wound.
- Keep the wound dry and clean.
- Try to control odor with balsam of Peru, yogurt flakes, oil of cloves, or other odor-masking substances, although they're commonly ineffective for long-term use. Topical or systemic antibiotics also temporarily control odor and eventually alter the lesion's bacterial flora.
- Be prepared for other problems that accompany a metastatic disease (pain, fatigue, weakness, anorexia).
- Help the patient and family set realistic goals and expectations.
- Disfiguring lesions are distressing to both the patient and you. Try to accept the patient as she is to increase her self-esteem and strengthen a caring relationship.

PREVENTION POINTER

Preventing SCC

Teach patients to prevent squamous cell carcinoma (SCC) by:

- avoiding excessive sun exposure
- wearing protective clothing (hats, long sleeves)
- periodically examining the skin for precancerous lesions and having any removed promptly
- using strong sunscreening agents (at least sun protection factor 15) containing para-aminobenzoic acid, benzophenone, titanium dioxide, and zinc oxide; applying these agents 30 to 60 minutes before sun exposure; and reapplying throughout the duration of sun exposure
- using sunscreen to protect lips from sun damage
- wearing sunglasses to protect eyelids from UV damage and prevent eyes from getting cataracts.

- Teach the patient ways to avoid increasing her risk for future incidence of SCC. (See *Preventing SCC.*)

Stroke

A stroke, also known as a *cerebrovascular accident* or a *brain attack*, is a sudden impairment or disruption of cerebral circulation in one or more blood vessels. A stroke interrupts or diminishes blood supply and, therefore, the oxygen supply to or within the brain and commonly causes serious damage or necrosis in brain tissues. Chances for a complete recovery depend on how soon circulation returns to normal after a stroke. However, about one-half of the patients who survive a stroke remain permanently disabled and experience a recurrence within weeks, months, or years after the initial stroke. It's the leading serious neurologic disorder in the United States and the major cause of long-term disabilities in Americans.

Stroke is the third most common cause of death in the United States. It strikes over 500,000 persons per year and is fatal in approximately one-half of these persons. Although strokes may occur in younger persons, most patients experiencing strokes are over age 65. In fact, the risk of stroke doubles with each passing decade after age 55. Strokes are more common in men; however, more women die from strokes. In addition, women are at increased risk for strokes because of the use of hormonal contraceptives and pregnancy.

SPECIAL NEEDS

The incidence of stroke is also higher in Blacks. Blacks have a 60% higher risk of stroke than Whites or Hispanics of the same age. This increased risk is believed to be the result of an increased prevalence of hypertension in Blacks. In addition, strokes in Blacks usually result from disease in the small cerebral vessels, while strokes in Whites are typically the result of disease in the large carotid arteries. The mortality rate for Blacks from stroke is twice the rate for Whites.

Causes

Stroke typically results from one of three causes:

- thrombosis of the cerebral arteries supplying the brain or the intracranial vessels occluding blood flow (see *Types of stroke*)
- embolism from thrombus outside the brain, such as in the heart, aorta, or common carotid artery
- hemorrhage from an intracranial artery or vein, such as from hypertension, ruptured aneurysm, arteriovenous malformations, trauma, hemorrhagic disorder, or septic embolism.

Risk factors that have been identified as predisposing a patient to stroke include:

- hypertension
- heredity (family history of stroke)
- prior history of stroke
- advancing age (60% to 75% of all strokes occur in persons over age 65)
- history of transient ischemic attacks (TIAs) (see *Understanding TIAs*, page 444)
- cardiac disease, including arrhythmias, coronary artery disease, acute myocardial infarction, dilated cardiomyopathy, and valvular disease
- diabetes mellitus
- race (blacks more than whites)
- familial hyperlipidemia
- cigarette smoking
- increased alcohol intake
- obesity, sedentary lifestyle
- use of hormonal contraceptives, especially in women over age 35 and in women who smoke cigarettes
- premenopausal women with migraines.

Types of stroke

Strokes are typically classified as ischemic or hemorrhagic depending on the underlying cause. This chart describes the major types of stroke.

Type of stroke	Description
Ischemic: Thrombotic	▪ Thrombotic stroke is the most common type of stroke. ▪ Commonly the result of atherosclerosis, this type is also associated with hypertension, smoking, and diabetes. ▪ A thrombus in an extracranial or intracranial vessel blocks blood flow to the cerebral cortex. ▪ Carotid artery is the most commonly affected extracranial vessel. ▪ Common intracranial sites include bifurcation of carotid arteries, distal intracranial portion of vertebral arteries, and proximal basilar arteries. ▪ This type of stroke may occur during sleep or shortly after awakening, during surgery, or after a myocardial infarction.
Ischemic: Embolic	▪ Embolic stroke is the second most common type of stroke. ▪ An embolus from the heart or extracranial arteries floats into the cerebral bloodstream and lodges in the middle cerebral artery or branches. ▪ Embolus commonly originates during atrial fibrillation. ▪ This type of stroke typically occurs during activity and develops rapidly.
Ischemic: Lacunar	▪ Lacunar stroke is a subtype of thrombotic stroke. ▪ Hypertension creates cavities deep in the white matter of the brain, affecting the internal capsule, basal ganglia, thalamus, and pons. ▪ The lipid coating lining of the small penetrating arteries thickens and weakens its walls, causing microaneurysms and dissections.
Hemorrhagic	▪ Hemorrhagic stroke is the third most common type of stroke. ▪ Typically, hypertension or rupture of aneurysm is the cause. ▪ The ruptured artery causes diminished blood supply to an area and compression by accumulated blood.

Regardless of the cause of stroke, the underlying event is deprivation of oxygen and nutrients to the brain. Normally, if the arteries become blocked, autoregulatory mechanisms help maintain cerebral circulation until collateral circulation develops to deliver blood to the affected area. If the compensatory mechanisms become overworked or cerebral blood flow remains impaired for more than a few minutes, oxygen deprivation leads to infarction of brain tissue. The brain cells cease to function because they can neither store glucose or glycogen for use nor engage in anaerobic metabolism.

A thrombotic or embolic stroke causes ischemia. Some of the neurons served by the occluded vessel die from

Understanding TIAs

A transient ischemic attack (TIA) is an episode of neurologic deficit resulting from cerebral ischemia. The recurrent attacks may last from seconds to an hour. It's usually considered a warning sign for stroke. In 14% of patients who experience a TIA, another TIA or a full stroke will occur within 1 year.

In a TIA, microemboli released from a thrombus may temporarily interrupt blood flow, especially in the small distal branches of the brain's arterial tree. Small spasms in those arterioles may impair blood flow and also precede a TIA.

The most distinctive features of TIAs are transient focal deficits with complete return of function. The deficits usually involve some degree of motor or sensory dysfunction. They may also involve loss of consciousness and loss of motor or sensory function, but only for a brief time. Commonly the patient experiences weakness in the lower part of the face and arms, hands, fingers, and legs on the side opposite the affected region. Other manifestations may include transient dysphagia, numbness or tingling of the face and lips, double vision, slurred speech, and dizziness.

lack of oxygen and nutrients. This results in cerebral infarction, in which tissue injury triggers an inflammatory response that in turn increases intracranial pressure (ICP). Injury to the surrounding cells disrupts metabolism and leads to changes in ionic transport, localized acidosis, and free radical formation. Calcium, sodium, and water accumulate in the injured cells, and excitatory neurotransmitters are released. Consequently, continued cellular injury and swelling set up a vicious cycle of further damage.

When hemorrhage is the cause, impaired cerebral perfusion causes infarction, and the blood itself acts as a space-occupying mass, exerting pressure on the brain tissues. The brain's regulatory mechanisms attempt to maintain equilibrium by increasing blood pressure to maintain cerebral perfusion pressure. The increased ICP forces cerebrospinal fluid (CSF) out, thus restoring balance. If the hemorrhage is small, this correction may be enough to keep the patient alive with only minimal neurologic deficits. However, if bleeding is heavy, ICP increases rapidly and perfusion stops. Even if the pressure returns to normal, many brain cells die.

Initially, the ruptured cerebral blood vessels may constrict to limit blood loss. This vasospasm further compromises blood flow, leading to more ischemia and cellular damage. If a clot forms in the vessel, decreased blood flow also promotes ischemia. If the blood enters the subarachnoid space, meningeal irritation occurs. The blood cells that pass through the vessel wall into the surrounding tissue may also break down and block the arachnoid villi, causing hydrocephalus.

Signs and symptoms

The clinical features of stroke vary according to the affected artery and the

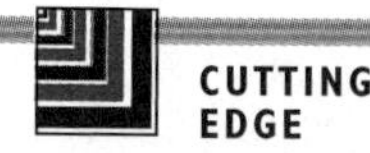

CUTTING EDGE

Different symptoms for women

In November 2002, the *Annals of Emergency Medicine* published findings of a study concluding that more than 60% of women who suffered a stroke had reported "nontraditional" stroke symptoms, meaning symptoms other than those that men usually experience.

The study further concluded that the higher mortality rate in women suffering stroke may be linked to the more nonspecific, non-neurologic symptoms women report, rather than the "typical" stroke symptoms men report. Although this finding will require further study, emergency health care professionals should be aware of these potential differences so that appropriate and proper stroke treatment is not delayed. The symptoms are outlined here.

Men

- Imbalance
- Sudden numbness or paralysis of the arms, face, or leg, especially on one side of the body
- Trouble with talking or understanding
- Trouble walking
- Sudden, severe headaches

Women

- Pain
- Changes in consciousness
- Disorientation
- Headaches
- Chest pains
- Shortness of breath

region of the brain it supplies, the severity of the damage, and the extent of collateral circulation developed. A stroke in one hemisphere causes signs and symptoms on the opposite side of the body; a stroke that damages cranial nerves affects structures on the same side as the infarction. In addition, symptoms of stroke in women may differ from those in men. (See *Different symptoms for women.*)

General symptoms of a stroke include:

- unilateral limb weakness
- speech difficulties
- numbness on one side
- headache
- vision disturbances (diplopia, hemianopsia, ptosis)
- dizziness
- anxiety
- altered level of consciousness (LOC).

Additionally, the artery affected usually classifies symptoms. Signs and symptoms associated with middle cerebral artery involvement include:

- aphasia
- dysphasia
- visual field deficits
- hemiparesis of affected side (more severe in the face and arm than in the leg).

Symptoms associated with carotid artery involvement include:

- weakness
- paralysis
- numbness

- sensory changes
- vision disturbances on the affected side
- altered LOC
- bruits
- headaches
- aphasia
- ptosis.

Symptoms associated with vertebrobasilar artery involvement include:

- weakness on the affected side
- numbness around lips and mouth
- visual field deficits
- diplopia
- poor coordination
- dysphagia
- slurred speech
- dizziness
- nystagmus
- amnesia
- ataxia.

Signs and symptoms associated with anterior cerebral artery involvement include:

- confusion
- weakness
- numbness, especially in the legs on the affected side
- incontinence
- loss of coordination
- impaired motor and sensory functions
- personality changes.

Signs and symptoms associated with posterior cerebral artery involvement include:

- visual field deficits (homonymous hemianopsia)
- sensory impairment
- dyslexia
- perseveration (abnormally persistent replies to questions)
- coma
- cortical blindness
- absence of paralysis (usually).

Complications vary with the severity and type of stroke but may include unstable blood pressure (from loss of vasomotor control), cerebral edema, fluid imbalances, sensory impairment, infections such as pneumonia, altered LOC, aspiration, contractures, pulmonary embolism, and death.

Diagnosis

- Computed tomography scan identifies an ischemic stroke within the first 72 hours of symptom onset and evidence of a hemorrhagic stroke (lesions larger than 1 cm) immediately.
- Magnetic resonance imaging assists in identifying areas of ischemia or infarction and cerebral swelling.
- Cerebral angiography reveals disruption or displacement of the cerebral circulation by occlusion, as in stenosis and acute thrombus, or hemorrhage.
- Digital subtraction angiography shows evidence of occlusion of cerebral vessels, lesions, or vascular abnormalities.
- Carotid duplex scan identifies the degree of stenosis.
- Brain scan shows ischemic areas but may not be conclusive for up to 2 weeks after a stroke.
- Single photon emission computed tomography and positron emission tomography scans identify areas of altered metabolism surrounding lesions

not yet distinguishable with other diagnostic tests.

- Transesophageal echocardiogram reveals cardiac disorders, such as atrial thrombi, atrial septal defect, or patent foramen ovale, as causes of thrombotic stroke.
- Lumbar puncture (performed if there are no signs of increased ICP) reveals bloody CSF when stroke is hemorrhagic.
- Ophthalmoscopy may identify signs of hypertension and atherosclerotic changes in retinal arteries.
- EEG helps identify damaged areas of the brain.

Treatment

Treatment is supportive to minimize and prevent further cerebral damage. Measures include:

- ICP management with monitoring, hyperventilation to decrease partial pressure of arterial carbon dioxide ($Paco_2$) to lower ICP, osmotic diuretics (mannitol) to reduce cerebral edema, and corticosteroids (dexamethasone) to reduce inflammation and cerebral edema
- stool softeners to prevent straining, which increases ICP
- anticonvulsants to treat or prevent seizures
- surgery for large cerebellar infarction to remove infarcted tissue and decompress remaining live tissue
- aneurysm repair to prevent further hemorrhage
- percutaneous transluminal angioplasty or stent insertion to open occluded vessels.

For ischemic stroke:

- thrombolytic therapy (tPA, alteplase [Activase]) within the first 3 hours after the onset of symptoms to dissolve the clot, remove occlusion, and restore blood flow, thus minimizing cerebral damage (see *Treating ischemic stroke*, page 448)
- anticoagulant therapy (heparin, warfarin) to maintain vessel patency and prevent further clot formation in cases of high-grade carotid stenosis or newly diagnosed cardiovascular disease.

For TIAs:

- antiplatelet agents (aspirin, ticlopidine, clopidogrel, Aggrenox) to reduce the risk of platelet aggregation and subsequent clot formation
- carotid endarterectomy to open partially occluded (greater than 70%) carotid arteries.

For hemorrhagic stroke:

- analgesics such as acetaminophen to relieve headache associated with hemorrhagic stroke.

Special considerations

During the acute phase, efforts focus on survival needs and the prevention of further complications. Effective care emphasizes continuing neurologic assessment, respiratory support, continuous monitoring of vital signs, careful positioning to prevent aspiration and contractures, management of GI problems, and careful monitoring of fluid, electrolyte, and nutritional status. Patient care must also include measures to prevent complications, such as infection:

Treating ischemic stroke

In an ischemic stroke, a thrombus occludes a cerebral vessel or one of its branches and blocks blood flow to the brain. The thrombus may have formed in that vessel or lodged there after traveling through the circulation from another site such as the heart. Prompt treatment with thrombolytic agents or anticoagulants helps minimize the effects of the occlusion. This flowchart shows how these drugs disrupt an ischemic stroke, thus minimizing the effects of cerebral ischemia and infarction. Keep in mind that thrombolytic agents should be used within 3 hours after onset of the patient's symptoms.

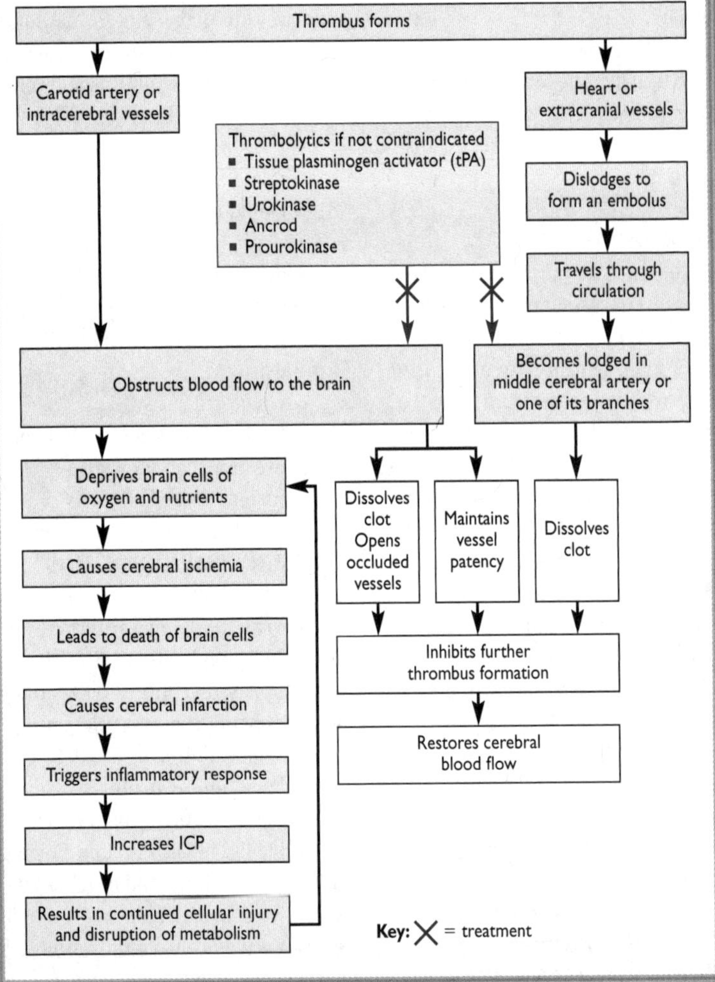

■ Maintain patent airway and oxygenation. Loosen constrictive clothing. Watch for ballooning of the cheek with respiration. The side that balloons is the side affected by the stroke. If the patient is unconscious, she could aspirate saliva, so keep her in a lateral position to allow secretions to drain naturally or suction secretions, as needed. Insert an artificial airway, and start mechanical ventilation or supplemental oxygen, if necessary.

■ Check vital signs and neurologic status, record observations, and report any significant changes to the physician. Monitor blood pressure, LOC, pupillary changes, motor function (voluntary and involuntary movements), sensory function, speech, skin color, temperature, signs of increased ICP, and nuchal rigidity or flaccidity. Remember, if a stroke is impending, blood pressure rises suddenly, the pulse is rapid and bounding, and the patient may complain of a headache. Also, watch for signs of pulmonary emboli, such as chest pains, shortness of breath, dusky color, tachycardia, fever, and changed sensorium. If the patient is unresponsive, monitor her blood gases often and alert the physician to increased $Paco_2$ or decreased partial pressure of arterial oxygen.

■ Maintain fluid and electrolyte balance. If the patient can take liquids orally, offer them as often as fluid limitations permit. Administer I.V. fluids, as ordered; never give too much too fast because this can increase ICP. Offer the urinal or bedpan every 2 hours. If the patient is incontinent, she may need an indwelling urinary catheter; however, this should be avoided, if possible, because of the risk of infection.

■ Ensure adequate nutrition. Check for gag reflex before offering small oral feedings of semisolid foods. Place the food tray within the patient's visual field because loss of peripheral vision is common. If oral feedings aren't possible, insert a nasogastric tube.

■ Manage GI problems. Be alert for signs that the patient is straining at elimination because this increases ICP. Modify diet, administer stool softeners as ordered, and give laxatives, if necessary. If the patient vomits (usually during the first few days), keep her positioned on her side to prevent aspiration.

■ Provide careful mouth care. Clean and irrigate the patient's mouth to remove food particles. Care for her dentures, if needed.

■ Provide meticulous eye care. Remove secretions with a cotton ball and sterile normal saline solution. Instill eyedrops, as ordered. Patch the patient's affected eye if she can't close the lid.

■ Position the patient and align her extremities correctly. Use high-topped sneakers to prevent footdrop and contracture and convoluted foam, flotation, or pulsating mattress or sheepskin to prevent pressure ulcers. To prevent pneumonia, turn the patient at least every 2 hours. Elevate the affected hand to control dependent edema, and place it in a functional position.

■ Assist the patient with exercise. Perform range-of-motion exercises for both the affected and unaffected sides.

PREVENTION POINTER

Reducing Stroke Risk

Conduct thorough patient teaching to help your patient prevent stroke:

- Stress the need to control such diseases as diabetes and hypertension.
- Teach all patients (especially those at high risk) the importance of following a low-cholesterol, low-salt diet; watching their weight; increasing physical activity; and minimizing stress.
- Discourage women from smoking and explain to them that women taking hormonal contraceptives have an increased risk of stroke if they smoke, especially after age 35.
- Warn women that drinking more than two glasses of alcohol per day increases blood pressure and binge drinking raises their risk of stroke.
- Tell patients to avoid I.V. drug use and cocaine use as these drugs carry a high risk of cerebral embolisms and cardiovascular complications, including strokes and heart attacks, and have been known to occur even with first-time use.

Teach and encourage the patient to use her unaffected side to exercise her affected side.

- Give medications, as ordered, and monitor for and report adverse effects.
- Establish and maintain communication with the patient. If she's aphasic, set up a simple method of communicating basic needs, such as asking simple "yes" or "no" questions. Remember to phrase your questions so she'll be able to answer using this system. If you have to repeat yourself, do so quietly and calmly. (Remember, she doesn't have hearing difficulty.) Also use gestures if necessary to help her understand. Even the unresponsive patient can hear, so don't say anything in her presence that you wouldn't want her to hear and remember.
- Provide psychological support. Set realistic short-term goals. Involve the patient's family in her care whenever possible, and explain her deficits and strengths.
- Begin your rehabilitation of the patient with a stroke on admission. The amount of teaching you'll have to do depends on the extent of neurologic deficit.
- Establish rapport with the patient. Spend time with her, and provide a means of communication. Simplify your language, asking "yes-or-no" questions whenever possible. Don't correct her speech or treat her like a child. Remember that building rapport may be difficult because of the mood changes that may result from brain damage or as a reaction to being dependent.
- If necessary, re-teach the patient to comb her hair, dress, and wash. With the aid of a physical therapist and an occupational therapist, obtain appliances, such as walking frames, hand bars by the toilet, and ramps, as needed. The patient may fail to recognize that she has a paralyzed side (called *unilateral neglect*) and must be taught to inspect that side of her body for injury and to protect it from harm. If speech therapy is indicated, encourage the patient to begin as soon as possi-

ble and follow through with the speech pathologist's suggestions. To reinforce teaching, involve the patient's family in all aspects of rehabilitation. With their cooperation and support, devise a realistic discharge plan, and let them help decide when the patient can return home.

- Before discharge, warn the patient or her family to report any premonitory signs of a stroke, such as severe headache, drowsiness, confusion, and dizziness. Emphasize the importance of regular follow-up visits.
- If aspirin has been prescribed to minimize the risk of embolic stroke, tell the patient to watch for signs of possible GI bleeding. Make sure the patient and her family realize that acetaminophen isn't a substitute for aspirin.
- Emphasize to the patient that, if symptoms develop, she should go to the emergency department immediately.
- Review with the patient ways that she can reduce her risk of having another stroke. (See *Reducing stroke risk.*)

Syphilis

A chronic, infectious, sexually transmitted disease, syphilis begins in the mucous membranes and quickly becomes systemic, spreading to nearby lymph nodes and the bloodstream. This disease, when untreated, is characterized by progressive stages: primary, secondary, latent, and late (formerly called *tertiary*). About 34,000 cases of syphilis, in primary and secondary stages, are reported annually in the United States. Incidence is highest among urban populations, especially in people between ages 15 and 39, drug users, and those infected with the human immunodeficiency virus (HIV). Untreated syphilis leads to crippling or death but the prognosis is excellent with early treatment.

Moreover, women who contract syphilis during pregnancy or who leave their syphilis untreated during pregnancy may infect their infants either during the pregnancy or during delivery, potentially causing the infant to suffer neurologic impairment, seizures, and even death. Prenatal syphilis is 32 times higher in Blacks than in Whites.

Causes

Syphilis is caused by infection with the spirochete *Treponema pallidum.* A spirochete is a wormlike, spiral bacterial organism that infects a person by burrowing into the mucous membranes of the mouth or genitals and causing chancres. Transmission occurs primarily through sexual contact during the primary, secondary, and early latent stages of infection. Prenatal transmission from an infected mother to her fetus via the placenta is also possible. (See *Prenatal syphilis,* page 452.)

Signs and symptoms

Syphilis has three stages: the first stage is the formation of the chancre; the second stage is more severe and may include hair loss; sore throat; skin rash; white patches on the nose,

Prenatal syphilis

A woman can transmit syphilis transplacentally to her unborn child throughout pregnancy. This type of syphilis is commonly called *congenital,* but *prenatal* is a more accurate term. Approximately 50% of infected fetuses die before or shortly after birth. The prognosis is better for infants who develop overt infection after age 2.

Signs and symptoms

The infant with prenatal syphilis may appear healthy at birth, but usually develops characteristic lesions — vesicular, bullous eruptions commonly on the palms and soles — 3 weeks later. Shortly after lesions appear, a maculopapular rash similar to that in secondary syphilis may erupt on the face, mouth, genitalia, palms, or soles. Condylomata lata commonly occur around the anus. Lesions may erupt on the mucous membranes of the mouth, pharynx, and nose. When the infant's larynx is affected, his cry becomes weak and forced. If nasal mucous membranes are involved, he may also develop nasal discharge, which can be slight and mucopurulent or copious with blood-tinged pus. Visceral and bone lesions, liver or spleen enlargement with ascites, and nephrotic syndrome may also occur.

Late prenatal syphilis becomes apparent after age 2; it may be identifiable only through blood studies or may cause unmistakable syphilitic changes, such as screwdriver-shaped central incisors, deformed molars or cusps, thick clavicles, saber shins, bowed tibias, nasal septum perforation, eighth nerve deafness, and neurosyphilis.

Diagnosis and treatment

In the infant with prenatal syphilis, the Venereal Disease Research Laboratory (VDRL) titer, if reactive at birth, stays the same or rises, indicating active disease. The infant's titer drops in 3 months if the mother has received effective prenatal treatment. Absolute diagnosis necessitates dark-field examination of umbilical vein blood or lesion drainage.

An infant with abnormal cerebrospinal fluid (CSF) may be treated with aqueous crystalline penicillin G, I.M. or I.V. (50,000 units/kg of body weight/day divided in two doses for at least 10 days), or aqueous penicillin G procaine I.M. (50,000 units/kg of body weight/day for at least 10 days). An infant with normal CSF may be treated with a single injection of penicillin G benzathine (50,000 units/kg of body weight).

When caring for a child with prenatal syphilis, record the extent of the rash, and watch for signs of systemic involvement, especially laryngeal swelling, jaundice, and decreasing urine output.

mouth, and vagina; fever; headaches; and wartlike lesions. The third stage begins when the disease has progressed so far it involves the brain, heart, and other internal organs.

Primary syphilis develops after an incubation period that generally lasts about 3 weeks. Initially, one or more chancres (small, fluid-filled lesions) erupt on the genitalia; others may erupt on the anus, fingers, lips, tongue, nipples, tonsils, or eyelids. These chancres, which are usually painless, start as papules and then erode; they have indurated, raised edges and clear bases. At the time of their eruption, they are highly contagious. Chancres typically disappear after 3 to 6 weeks, even when untreated. They are usually associated with regional lymphadenopathy (unilateral or bilateral). In females, chancres are commonly overlooked because they usually develop on internal structures — the cervix or the vaginal wall.

Secondary syphilis is characterized by the onset of symmetrical mucocutaneous lesions and general lymphadenopathy, which may develop within a few days or up to 8 weeks after onset of initial chancres. The rash of secondary syphilis can be macular, papular, pustular, or nodular. Lesions are of uniform size, well-defined, and generalized. Macules commonly erupt between rolls of fat on the trunk and, proximally, on the arms, palms, soles, face, and scalp. In warm, moist areas (perineum, scrotum, vulva, and between rolls of fat), the lesions enlarge and erode, producing highly contagious, pink or grayish white lesions (condylomata lata). The rash and the wartlike lesions are highly contagious and may be transmitted by casual contact. This stage may last from 4 to 6 weeks.

Mild constitutional symptoms of syphilis appear in the second stage and may include headache, malaise, anorexia, weight loss, nausea, vomiting, sore throat, and possibly, slight fever. Alopecia may occur, with or without treatment, and is usually temporary. Nails become brittle and pitted.

Latent syphilis is characterized by an absence of clinical symptoms but a reactive serologic test for syphilis. Because infectious mucocutaneous lesions may reappear when infection has lasted less than 4 years, early latent syphilis is considered contagious. Approximately two-thirds of patients remain asymptomatic through the late stage of latent syphilis and death. The rest develop characteristic late-stage symptoms.

Late syphilis is the final, destructive but noninfectious and noncontagious stage of the disease. It has three subtypes, any or all of which may affect the patient: late benign syphilis, cardiovascular syphilis, and neurosyphilis. The lesions of *late benign syphilis* develop between 1 and 10 years after infection on the skin, bones, mucous membranes, upper respiratory tract, liver, or stomach. The typical lesion is a gumma — a chronic, superficial nodule or deep, granulomatous lesion that's solitary, asymmetrical, painless, and indurated. Gummas can be found on any bone — particularly the long bones of the legs — and in any organ. If late syphilis involves the liver, it can cause epigastric pain, tenderness, enlarged spleen, and anemia; if it involves the upper respiratory tract, it may cause perforation of the nasal septum or the palate. In severe cases, late benign syphilis results in destruction of bones or organs, which eventually causes death.

Cardiovascular syphilis develops about 10 years after the initial infection in approximately 10% of patients with late, untreated syphilis. It causes fibrosis of elastic tissue of the aorta

Treponema pallidum

As shown here, dark-field examination revealing spiral-shaped bacterial organisms — *Treponema pallidum* — confirms the diagnosis of syphilis.

and leads to aortitis, most commonly in the ascending and transverse sections of the aortic arch. Cardiovascular syphilis may be asymptomatic or may cause aortic insufficiency or aneurysm.

Symptoms of *neurosyphilis* develop in about 8% of patients with late, untreated syphilis and appear from 5 to 35 years after infection. These clinical effects consist of meningitis and widespread central nervous system damage that may include general paresis, personality changes, and arm and leg weakness.

Diagnosis

Identifying *T. pallidum* from a lesion on dark-field examination confirms the diagnosis of syphilis. This method is most effective when moist lesions are present, as in primary, secondary, and prenatal syphilis. (See Treponema pallidum.)

The fluorescent treponemal antibody-absorption test identifies antigens of *T. pallidum* in tissue, ocular fluid, cerebrospinal fluid (CSF), tracheobronchial secretions, and exudates from lesions. This is the most sensitive test available for detecting syphilis in all stages. Once reactive, it remains so permanently.

Other appropriate procedures include the following:

- *Venereal Disease Research Laboratory* (VDRL) *slide test* and *rapid plasma reagin (RPR) test* detect nonspecific antibodies. Both tests, if positive, become reactive within 1 to 2 weeks after the primary lesion appears or 4 to 5 weeks after the infection begins.
- *CSF examination* identifies neurosyphilis when the total protein level is above 40 mg/dl, the VDRL slide test is reactive, and the cell count exceeds 5 mononuclear cells/µl.

Treatment

Treatment of choice for syphilis is administration of penicillin I.M. For early syphilis, treatment may consist of a single injection of penicillin G benzathine I.M. (2.4 million units). Syphilis of more than 1 year's duration should be treated with penicillin G benzathine I.M. (2.4 million units/week for 3 weeks). Nonpregnant patients who are allergic to penicillin may be treated with oral tetracycline or doxycycline for 15 days for early syphilis; 30 days for late infections. Nonpenicillin therapy for latent or late syphilis should be used only after neurosyphilis has been excluded. Tetracycline is contraindicated in pregnant women because it causes discoloration of the infant's teeth. If a pregnant woman with syphilis is allergic to penicillin, desensitization is recommended to permit the use of penicillin. If syphilis isn't treated in a pregnant patient, it can cause blindness or death of the infant.

Special considerations

- Stress the importance of completing the full course of antibiotic therapy even after symptoms subside.
- Check for a history of drug sensitivity before administering the first dose.
- Practice standard precautions.
- In secondary syphilis, keep lesions clean and dry. If they're draining, dispose of contaminated materials properly.
- In late syphilis, provide symptomatic care during prolonged treatment.
- In cardiovascular syphilis, check for signs of decreased cardiac output (decreased urine output, hypoxia, and decreased sensorium) and pulmonary congestion.
- In neurosyphilis, regularly check level of consciousness, mood, and coherence. Watch for signs of ataxia.
- Urge patients to seek VDRL testing after 3, 6, 12, and 24 months to detect possible relapse. Patients treated for latent or late syphilis should receive blood tests at 6-month intervals for 2 years.
- Be sure to report all cases of syphilis to local public health authorities. Urge the patient to inform sexual partners of her infection so they can also receive treatment.
- Refer the patient and her sexual partners for HIV testing.

Systemic lupus erythematosus

Lupus erythematosus is a chronic inflammatory disorder of the connective tissues that appears in two forms: discoid lupus erythematosus, which affects only the skin, and systemic lupus erythematosus (SLE), which affects multiple organ systems as well as the skin and can be fatal. SLE is characterized by recurring remissions and exacerbations, which are especially common during the spring and summer. The prognosis improves with early detection and treatment but remains poor for patients who develop cardiovascular, renal, or neurologic complications, or severe bacterial infections.

SLE is more common in women than in men. Approximately 90% of SLE cases occur in women. SLE's onset is typically during a woman's reproductive years beginning as early as age 14. Black women are three times more affected than White women. Asian women are also at increased risk.

Causes

Autoimmunity is believed to be the prime mechanism involved in SLE. The body produces antibodies against components of its own cells, such as the antinuclear antibody (ANA), and immune complex disease follows. Women with SLE may produce antibodies against many different tissue

> ### Diagnosing SLE
>
> Diagnosing systemic lupus erythematosus (SLE) is difficult because it commonly mimics other diseases. Symptoms may be vague and vary greatly among patients.
>
> For these reasons, the American Rheumatism Association issued a list of criteria for classifying SLE to be used primarily for consistency in epidemiologic surveys. Usually, four or more of these symptoms are present at some time during the course of the disease:
> - malar or discoid rash
> - photosensitivity
> - oral or nasopharyngeal ulcerations
> - nonerosive arthritis (of two or more peripheral joints)
> - pleuritis or pericarditis
> - profuse proteinuria (more than 0.5 g/day) or excessive cellular casts in urine
> - seizures or psychoses
> - hemolytic anemia, leukopenia, lymphopenia, or thrombocytopenia
> - anti-double-stranded deoxyribonucleic acid or positive findings of antiphospholipid antibodies, including elevated immunoglobulin (Ig) G or IgM anticardiolipin antibodies, positive test result for lupus anticoagulant, or false-positive serologic test results for syphilis
> - abnormal antinuclear antibody titer.

components, such as red blood cells (RBCs), neutrophils, platelets, lymphocytes, or almost any organ or tissue in the body.

Although the exact cause of SLE remains a mystery, available evidence points to interrelated immunologic, environmental, hormonal, and genetic factors, which may include:
- physical or mental stress
- streptococcal or viral infections
- exposure to sunlight or ultraviolet light
- immunization
- pregnancy
- abnormal estrogen metabolism
- treatment with certain drugs, such as procainamide (Pronestyl), hydralazine (Apresoline), anticonvulsants and, less commonly, penicillins, sulfa drugs, and hormonal contraceptives.

Signs and symptoms

The onset of SLE may be acute or insidious and produces no characteristic clinical pattern. (See *Diagnosing SLE.*)

Although SLE may involve any organ system, signs and symptoms all relate to tissue injury and subsequent inflammation and necrosis resulting from the invasion by immune complexes. They commonly include:
- fever
- weight loss
- malaise
- fatigue
- rashes (butterfly pattern)
- polyarthralgia.

Additional signs and symptoms may include:
- joint involvement, similar to rheumatoid arthritis (although the arthritis of lupus is usually nonerosive)
- skin lesions, most commonly an erythematous rash in areas exposed to light (the classic butterfly rash over the nose and cheeks occurs in less than 50% of patients) or a scaly, papu-

lar rash (mimics psoriasis), especially in sun-exposed areas

- vasculitis (especially in the digits), possibly leading to infarctive lesions, necrotic leg ulcers, or digital gangrene
- Raynaud's phenomenon (about 20% of patients)
- patchy alopecia and painless ulcers of the mucous membranes
- pulmonary abnormalities, such as pleurisy, pleural effusions, pneumonitis, pulmonary hypertension and, rarely, pulmonary hemorrhage
- cardiac involvement, such as pericarditis, myocarditis, endocarditis, and early coronary atherosclerosis
- microscopic hematuria, pyuria, and urine sediment with cellular casts due to glomerulonephritis, possibly progressing to kidney failure (particularly when untreated)
- urinary tract infections, possibly due to heightened susceptibility to infection
- seizure disorders and mental dysfunction
- central nervous system (CNS) involvement, such as emotional instability, psychosis, and organic brain syndrome
- headaches, irritability, and depression (common).

Classic symptoms of SLE include:

- aching, malaise, fatigue
- low-grade or spiking fever and chills
- anorexia and weight loss
- lymph node enlargement (diffuse or local; nontender)
- abdominal pain
- nausea, vomiting, diarrhea, constipation
- irregular menstrual periods or amenorrhea during the active phase of SLE.

Possible complications of SLE include concomitant infections, urinary tract infections, renal failure, and osteonecrosis of hip from long-term steroid use.

Diagnosis

Diagnostic test results that may indicate SLE include:

- complete blood count with differential showing anemia and a decreased white blood cell (WBC) count
- decreased platelet count
- elevated erythrocyte sedimentation rate
- serum electrophoresis showing hypergammaglobulinemia.

Other diagnostic tests used to aid diagnosis of SLE include:

- ANA and lupus erythematosus cell tests, which show positive results in active SLE
- anti-double-stranded deoxyribonucleic acid antibody (anti-dsDNA), which is the most specific test for SLE and correlates with disease activity, especially renal involvement, to help monitor response to therapy (possibly low or absent in remission)
- urine studies, which may show RBCs and WBCs, urine casts and sediment, and significant protein loss (more than 0.5 g/24 hours)
- serum complement blood studies, which may show decreased serum complement (C3 and C4) levels indicating active disease
- chest X-ray, which may show pleurisy or lupus pneumonitis

- electrocardiography, which may show a conduction defect with cardiac involvement or pericarditis
- kidney biopsy to determine disease stage and extent of renal involvement
- lupus anticoagulant and anticardiolipin tests, which may be positive in some patients (usually in patients prone to antiphospholipid syndrome of thrombosis, abortion, and thrombocytopenia).

Treatment

Treatment for SLE may include:

- nonsteroidal anti-inflammatory compounds, including aspirin, to control arthritis symptoms
- topical corticosteroid creams such as hydrocortisone buteprate (Acticort) or triamcinolone (Aristocort) for acute skin lesions
- intralesional corticosteroids or antimalarials such as hydroxychloroquine sulfate (Plaquenil) to treat refractory skin lesions
- systemic corticosteroids to reduce systemic symptoms of SLE for acute, generalized exacerbations or for serious disease related to vital organ systems, such as pleuritis, pericarditis, lupus nephritis, vasculitis, and CNS involvement
- high-dose steroids and cytotoxic therapy such as cyclophosphamide (Cytoxan) to treat diffuse proliferative glomerulonephritis
- dialysis or kidney transplant for renal failure
- antihypertensive drugs and dietary changes to minimize effects of renal involvement.

Special considerations

Careful assessment, supportive measures, emotional support, and patient education are all important parts of the care plan for patients with SLE:

- Watch for classic symptoms, such as joint pain or stiffness, weakness, fever, fatigue, and chills. Observe for dyspnea, chest pain, and edema of the extremities. Note the size, type, and location of skin lesions. Check urine for hematuria, scalp for hair loss, and skin and mucous membranes for petechiae, bleeding, ulceration, pallor, and bruising.

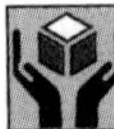

SPECIAL NEEDS

Although pregnancy isn't believed to affect the course of SLE, 20% to 40% of all women with SLE will experience a flare-up during pregnancy. Postpartum flare-ups may be of concern and the patient should be monitored as closely as possible.

- Provide a balanced diet. Renal involvement may mandate a low-sodium, low-protein diet.
- Urge the patient to get plenty of rest. Schedule diagnostic tests and procedures to allow adequate rest. Explain all tests and procedures. Tell the patient that several blood samples are needed initially, then periodically, to monitor progress.
- Apply heat packs to relieve joint pain and stiffness. Encourage regular exercise to maintain full range of motion (ROM) and prevent contractures. Teach ROM exercises as well as body alignment and postural techniques. Arrange for physical therapy and occupational counseling as appropriate.

- Explain the expected benefit of prescribed medications. Watch for adverse effects, especially when the patient is taking high doses of corticosteroids.
- Advise the patient receiving cyclophosphamide to maintain adequate hydration. If prescribed, give mesna to prevent hemorrhagic cystitis and ondansetron to prevent nausea and vomiting.
- Monitor vital signs, intake and output, weight, and laboratory reports. Check pulse rates and observe for orthopnea. Check stools and GI secretions for blood.
- Observe for hypertension, weight gain, and other signs of renal involvement.
- Assess for signs of neurologic damage, such as personality change, paranoid or psychotic behavior, ptosis, and diplopia. Take seizure precautions. If Raynaud's phenomenon is present, warm and protect the patient's hands and feet.
- Offer cosmetic tips, such as suggesting the use of hypoallergenic makeup and referring the patient to a hairdresser who specializes in scalp disorders.
- Advise the patient to purchase medications in quantity, if possible. Warn against "miracle" drugs for relief of arthritis symptoms.
- Refer the patient to the Lupus Foundation of America and the Arthritis Foundation, as necessary.

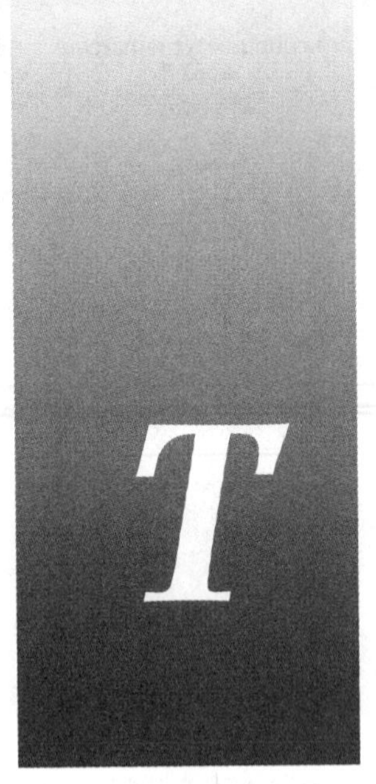

Toxic shock syndrome

Toxic shock syndrome (TSS) is an acute bacterial infection caused by toxin-producing, penicillin-resistant strains of *Staphylococcus aureus*, such as TSS toxin-1 and staphylococcal enterotoxins B and C. The disease primarily affects menstruating women under age 30, especially teenagers, and is associated with continuous use of tampons during menses. Five percent of all cases are fatal.

Causes

TSS has been linked to the use of tampons and intravaginal contraceptive devices, such as the diaphragm and the sponge. Although tampons and intravaginal contraceptive devices are clearly implicated in TSS, their exact role is uncertain. Theoretically, they may contribute to development of TSS by:

- introducing *S. aureus* into the vagina during insertion (insertion with fingers instead of the supplied applicator increases the risk)
- using high-absorbency tampons causes irritation and vaginal dryness, thereby increasing toxin production (occurs especially with rayon tampons)

- traumatizing the vaginal mucosa during insertion, thus leading to infection
- providing a favorable environment for the growth of *S. aureus.*

Although TSS is more closely related to the use of high-absorbency tampons, all tampons are associated with TSS risk. Fortunately, the incidence of TSS has declined significantly since its peak in the mid-1980s, probably due to advances in the way the FDA regulates tampon materials and absorbency as well as withdrawal from the market of those products most associated with TSS. When TSS isn't related to menstruation, it seems to be linked to other *S. aureus* infections, such as from skin abscesses, osteomyelitis, and postsurgical infections.

Signs and symptoms

At first, signs and symptoms of TSS may mimic the signs and symptoms of the flu, making diagnosis difficult. Typically, TSS produces sudden onset of intense muscle pains, fever over 104° F (40° C), chills, vomiting, diarrhea, headache, decreased level of consciousness, rigors, conjunctival hyperemia, and vaginal hyperemia and discharge. These symptoms usually occur during or shortly after menstruation. Severe hypotension occurs with hypovolemic shock. Within a few hours of onset, a deep red rash develops — especially on the palms and soles — and later desquamates. Major complications include persistent neuropsychological abnormalities, mild renal failure, rash, and cyanotic arms and legs. Disseminated intravascular coagulation (DIC) and acute respiratory distress syndrome (ARDS) may also occur.

Diagnosis

Diagnosis is based on clinical findings and the presence of at least three of the following:

- GI effects, including vomiting and profuse diarrhea
- muscular effects, with severe myalgias or a fivefold or greater increase in creatine kinase levels
- mucous membrane effects such as frank hyperemia
- renal involvement with elevated blood urea nitrogen or creatinine levels (at least twice the normal levels)
- liver involvement with elevated bilirubin, aspartate aminotransferase, or alanine aminotransferase levels (at least twice the normal levels)
- blood involvement with signs of thrombocytopenia and a platelet count of less than 100,000/mm^3
- central nervous system effects, such as disorientation without focal signs.

In addition, isolation of *S. aureus* from vaginal discharge or lesions helps support the diagnosis. Negative results on blood tests for Rocky Mountain spotted fever, leptospirosis, and measles help rule out these disorders.

Treatment

Treatment consists of I.V. antistaphylococcal antibiotics that are beta-lactamase resistant, such as oxacillin and nafcillin. To treat shock and prevent organ damage, expect to replace fluids with saline solution and colloids. Pulmonary, cardiac, and renal support may also be required.

Special considerations

- Monitor the patient's vital signs frequently.
- Administer antibiotics slowly and adhere to a strict administration schedule. Be sure to watch for signs of penicillin allergy.
- Obtain specimens of vaginal and cervical secretions for culture of *S. aureus*.
- Remove any tampons from the patient's body immediately.

PREVENTION POINTER

- Tell the woman to avoid tampons if she has had TSS in the past because recurrence is common.
- Provide meticulous wound care.
- Tell the patient to avoid or decrease the use of tampons and other vaginal foreign objects, such as diaphragms and sponges.
- Urge the patient to practice daily feminine hygiene.

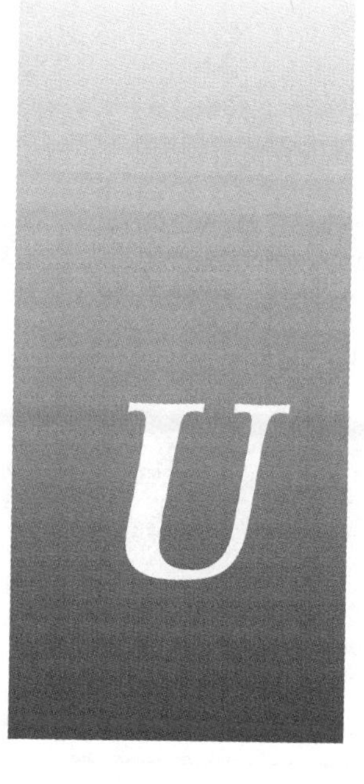

Urinary and stress incontinence

Urinary incontinence is defined as the involuntary loss of urine. It occurs if bladder muscles suddenly contract or muscles around the urethra suddenly relax. Stress incontinence is the loss of urine as a result of physical activity. Urinary incontinence occurs in men and women, but the prevalence in women is two times greater, occurring in 15% to 30% of women. Stress incontinence, the most common form in women, is believed to account for one-half of all cases of urinary incontinence in women. Older women are more likely to suffer from urinary incontinence than younger women. (See *Other forms of urinary incontinence*, page 464.)

Causes

Pregnancy and childbirth, menopause, and the structure of the female urinary tract contribute to the increased incidence of urinary incontinence in women. After pregnancy and childbirth, pelvic floor muscles may weaken. These are the same muscles that squeeze around the urethra to make it close. Decreased levels of estrogen also lead to lower muscular pressure around the urethra. As a result, complete closure of the urethra

Other forms of urinary incontinence

In addition to stress incontinence, women may suffer from other forms of urinary incontinence. These types are listed below along with their major characteristics.

Type	Characteristic
Urge incontinence	▪ Also known as *overactive bladder* ▪ Sudden, strong urge to void ▪ Occurring at unexpected times ▪ Caused by detrusor instability or decreased bladder capacity
Functional incontinence	▪ Related to physical disability, external obstacles, or problems with communication or thinking
Overflow incontinence	▪ Caused by a full bladder ▪ Caused by weak bladder muscles or blocked urethra
Mixed incontinence	▪ When stress incontinence and urge incontinence occur together ▪ Common in women
Transient incontinence	▪ Occurring temporarily (for example, due to infection)

may not occur, or may not be maintained during physical activity. Urinary incontinence has also has been linked to hormone replacement therapy. (See *HRT and urinary incontinence*.)

Other factors that may cause or contribute to urinary incontinence include:

- local causes, such as infection, bladder stones, and pelvic masses
- neurologic causes, such as stroke, multiple sclerosis, birth defects, and spinal injury
- medications, such as diuretics, beta-blockers, and antidepressants
- medical conditions, such as hypothyroidism, diabetes, and depression.

Signs and symptoms

Leakage of urine is the major sign of urinary incontinence. Urinary incontinence is also associated with nocturia, frequent urination (more than 8 times in 24 hours), and the sudden, uncontrollable urge to urinate moderate or large amounts of urine. Stress incontinence is usually associated with loss of small amounts of urine while coughing, laughing, sneezing, jogging, lifting, and other movements that put pressure on the bladder. It may worsen during the week before menses, and commonly increases after menopause. Frequency and nocturia aren't common symptoms of stress incontinence.

Urinary incontinence and stress incontinence have also been associated with:

- disruption of daily activities
- sleep deprivation
- depression

- social isolation
- loss of self-esteem
- altered relationships.

Diagnosis

Diagnostic tests used to evaluate urinary incontinence include:

- The cotton-tipped applicator test can be used to evaluate urethral motility. A sterile cotton swab is inserted 1¼″ (3 cm) into the urethra. When the patient with urinary incontinence coughs, the angle of the cotton swab changes by more than 45 degrees. This is thought to be evidence of poor muscular support.
- Evaluation of the postvoid residual is done by measuring bladder capacity and how much urine remains in the bladder after urination. A postvoid residual of less than 50 ml is considered normal.
- The cough test, which involves having the patient cough as the clinician directly observes for leakage of urine.
- Simple cystometry can evaluate for detrusor instability associated with urge incontinence.
- Urinalysis and culture are typically used to rule out infection as the cause of urinary incontinence.
- Ultrasound is used to visualize the kidneys, ureters, bladder, and urethra.
- Cystoscopy, which involves insertion of a thin tube with a camera into the urethra, allows the clinician to see inside the urethra and bladder.
- Urodynamics measure pressure in the bladder and flow of urine.

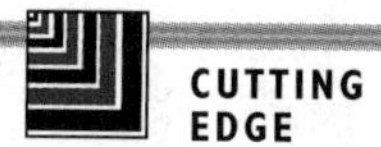

HRT and urinary incontinence

In April of 2003, the results from the Heart and Estrogen/Progestin Replacement Study (HERS) of over 1,200 women revealed that those women who took daily estrogen and progestin replacement therapy were at a greater risk of developing urinary incontinence than those women taking a placebo. After only 1 year, those women taking hormone replacement therapy (HRT) were at one to two times more risk for developing weekly episodes of incontinence. After 4 years, those women were three to five times more likely to become incontinent than those on placebos. Previous data from HERS and other studies have also addressed the possible link between HRT and urinary incontinence.

Treatment

Treatment strategies for urinary incontinence should always begin with the least invasive method. Commonly, a less invasive method is successful and more invasive techniques such as surgery can be avoided. It's important to note that noninvasive techniques require participation and commitment from the patient. These techniques include:

- Kegel exercises, which can be performed by the patient to exercise and strengthen the pelvic floor muscles, can be done with or without insertion of weighted cones into the vagina.

New treatments for stress incontinence

Urinary control devices have recently been developed to treat stress incontinence; many are still in clinical trials. These devices are tiny appliances used to cover or occlude the urethra. The three types of urinary control devices are:
- external occlusive devices
- simple occlusive plugs
- complex valved catheters.

- Electrical stimulation of the pelvic muscles using electrodes in the vagina and rectum can strengthen the muscles similarly to actually exercising them.
- Biofeedback involves the use of a diary or electronic device to document contraction of bladder and urethral muscles. It can help the patient become aware of her body's functioning and allow her to gain control of these muscles.
- Timed voiding and bladder training are techniques that allow the patient to empty her bladder before incontinence occurs. These are effective for overflow and urge incontinence.
- A pessary is a rubber or silicon device inserted into the vagina that exerts pressure on the urethra. The application of a pessary can lead to less stress leakage. (See *New treatments for stress incontinence.*)

Pharmacologic agents can also be used to treat urinary incontinence associated with detrusor instability. Anticholinergics, such as oxybutynin (Ditropan) and tolterodine (Detrol), block involuntary contractions of the bladder. Tricyclic antidepressants, such as imipramine (Tofranil), exert anticholinergic and musculotropic effects. They also increase bladder outlet resistance. Hormones, such as estrogen, help muscles function normally and are effective in treating postmenopausal women with stress incontinence.

In some instances, more invasive treatments may be necessary to relieve the condition. These include:
- implants into the tissue surrounding the urethra
- surgery to pull the bladder up, secure the bladder, or implant an artificial sphincter. (Surgery to treat stress incontinence increased nearly 45% from 1988 to 1998.)

Special considerations

It's important for health care providers to screen patients, especially women, for urinary incontinence. (See *Screening for urinary incontinence.*) Patients may be too embarrassed to admit their symptoms. Reassure patients that it's a common disorder and typically can be treated with fairly conservative measures. In addition:
- Educating women on appropriate hygiene practices is also crucial because genitourinary infections can contribute to or worsen urinary incontinence.
- Sometimes extra weight causes bladder control problems. A good

meal plan and exercise program can lead to weight loss.

- Some drinks and foods may make urine control harder. These include foods with caffeine (coffee, tea, cola, or chocolate) and alcohol.
- Bladder irritants, such as acidic fruits or fruit juices, tomato products, and spicy foods may contribute to urinary incontinence and should be avoided.

Urinary tract infection

The two forms of lower urinary tract infection (UTI) are cystitis (infection of the bladder) and urethritis (infection of the urethra). They're nearly 10 times more common in females than in males (except in elderly males) and affect 10% to 20% of all females at least once.

In males, lower UTIs typically are associated with anatomic or physiologic abnormalities and, therefore, need close evaluation. Most UTIs respond readily to treatment but recurrence and resistant bacterial flare-up during therapy are possible.

Causes

Most lower UTIs result from ascending infection by a single gram-negative, enteric bacterium, such as *Escherichia coli, Klebsiella, Proteus, Enterobacter, Pseudomonas,* and *Serratia.* In a patient with neurogenic bladder, with an indwelling urinary catheter or a fistula between the intestine and bladder, a lower UTI may result from simultaneous infection with multiple pathogens.

Screening for urinary incontinence

Below are questions created by the Association of Women's Health, Obstetric and Neonatal Nurses to effectively screen patients for urinary incontinence. Instruct patients to answer "always," "sometimes," or "never" to the following questions:

1. Do you ever leak urine or water when you don't want to?
2. Do you ever leak urine or water when you cough, laugh, or exercise?
3. Do you ever leak urine or water on the way to use the bathroom?
4. Do you ever use pads, tissue, or cloth in your underwear to catch urine?

Studies suggest that infection results from a breakdown in local defense mechanisms in the bladder that allows bacteria to invade the bladder mucosa and multiply. These bacteria can't be readily eliminated by normal urination.

Bacterial flare-up during treatment is usually caused by the pathogen's resistance to the prescribed antimicrobial therapy. Even a small number of bacteria (fewer than 10,000/ml) in a midstream urine specimen obtained during treatment casts doubt on the effectiveness of treatment.

In almost all patients, recurrent lower UTIs result from reinfection by the same organism or by some new pathogen. In the remaining patients, recurrence reflects persistent infection, usually from renal calculi, chronic bacterial prostatitis, or a

UTI risk factors

Certain factors increase the risk of developing urinary tract infection (UTI), including natural anatomic variations, trauma or invasive procedures, urinary tract obstructions, and urine reflux.

Natural anatomic variations

Females are more prone to UTI than males because the length of the female urethra (about 1″ to 2″ [2.5 to 5 cm]) is shorter than the male urethra (7″ to 8″ [18 to 20.5 cm]). It's also closer to the anus than the male urethra. This proximity facilitates bacterial entry into the urethra from the vagina, perineum, rectum, or a sexual partner.

Pregnant women are especially prone to UTIs because of hormonal changes. In addition, the enlarged uterus exerts greater pressure on the ureters, which restricts urine flow, allowing bacteria to linger longer in the urinary tract.

In men, release of prostatic fluid serves as an antibacterial shield. Men lose this protection around age 50 when the prostate gland begins to enlarge. This enlargement, in turn, may promote urine retention.

Trauma or invasive procedures

Fecal matter, sexual intercourse, and instruments, such as catheters and cystoscopes, can introduce bacteria into the urinary tract to trigger infection.

Obstructions

A narrowed ureter or calculi lodged in the ureters or the bladder can obstruct urine flow. Slowed urine flow allows bacteria to remain and multiply, risking damage to the kidneys.

Reflux

Vesicourethral reflux results when pressure inside the bladder (caused by coughing or sneezing) pushes a small amount of urine from the bladder into the urethra. When the pressure returns to normal, the urine flows back into the bladder, bringing bacteria from the urethra with it.

In vesicoureteral reflux, urine flows from the bladder back into one or both ureters. The vesicoureteral valve normally shuts off reflux. However, damage can prevent the valve from doing its job.

Other risk factors

Urinary stasis can promote infection, which, if undetected, can spread to the entire urinary system. Because urinary tract bacteria thrive on sugars, diabetes is also a risk factor.

structural anomaly that's a source of infection. The high incidence of lower UTI among females probably occurs because natural anatomic features facilitate infection. (See *UTI risk factors.*)

If untreated, chronic UTI can seriously damage the urinary tract lining. Infection of adjacent organs and structures (for example, pyelonephritis) may also occur. In this instance, prognosis is poor unless the patient responds to systemic treatment with multiple I.V. antibiotics.

Signs and symptoms

The patient may complain of urinary urgency and frequency, dysuria, bladder cramps or spasms, itching, a feeling of warmth during urination, nocturia, and urethral discharge (in men). Other complaints include low back pain, malaise, nausea, vomiting, pain or tenderness over the bladder, chills, and flank pain. Inflammation of the bladder wall also causes hematuria and fever.

Diagnosis

Tests used to diagnose lower UTI include:

- Microscopic urinalysis showing red blood cell and white blood cell counts greater than 10 per high-power field suggests lower UTI.
- Clean-catch urinalysis revealing a bacterial count of more than 100,000/ml confirms UTI. Lower counts don't necessarily rule out infection, especially if the patient is urinating frequently, because bacteria require 30 to 45 minutes to reproduce in urine. Clean-catch collection is preferred to catheterization, which can reinfect the bladder with urethral bacteria.
- Sensitivity testing determines the appropriate antimicrobial drug. If the patient history and physical examination warrant, a blood test or a stained smear of urethral discharge can rule out venereal disease.
- Voiding cystoureterography or excretory urography may detect congenital anomalies that predispose the patient to recurrent UTI.

Treatment

Appropriate antimicrobials are the treatment of choice for most initial lower UTIs. A 7- to 10-day course of antibiotics is standard, but studies suggest that a single dose or a 3- to 5-day regimen may be sufficient to render the urine sterile. (Elderly patients may still need 7 to 10 days of antibiotics to fully benefit from treatment.) If a culture shows that urine still isn't sterile after 3 days of antibiotic therapy, bacterial resistance probably has occurred, and a different antibiotic will be prescribed.

A single dose of amoxicillin or co-trimoxazole may be effective for females with acute, uncomplicated UTI. A urine culture taken 1 to 2 weeks later will indicate whether the infection has been eradicated. Recurrent infections from infected renal calculi, chronic prostatitis, or structural abnormalities may necessitate surgery. Prostatitis also requires long-term antibiotic therapy. In patients without these predisposing conditions, long-term, low-dose antibiotic therapy is the treatment of choice.

Special considerations

- If ordered, administer nitrofurantoin macrocrystals with milk or meals to prevent GI distress.
- If sitz baths don't relieve perineal discomfort, apply warm compresses sparingly to the perineum but be careful not to burn the patient. Apply topical antiseptics on the urethral meatus as necessary.
- Collect all urine specimens for culture and sensitivity testing carefully and promptly.
- Monitor the patient for GI disturbances from antimicrobial therapy and for other possible adverse reactions.

PREVENTION POINTER

Preventing UTIs

- To prevent recurrent lower UTIs, teach a female patient to carefully wipe the perineum from front to back and to thoroughly clean it with soap and water after bowel movements. If she's infection-prone, she should urinate immediately after sexual intercourse. Tell her to try not to postpone urination whenever possible and that she should empty her bladder completely.
- Urge the patient to drink about 2 qt (2 L) (at least eight glasses) of fluids per day during treatment. More or less than this amount may alter the antibiotic's effect. Be aware that the elderly patient may resist this suggestion because it causes her to make frequent trips, possibly up and down the stairs, to urinate.
- Explain that fruit juices, especially cranberry juice, and oral doses of vitamin C may help acidify urine and enhance the medication's action.

- Assess the patient for complications of UTI.
- Evaluate the patient's voiding pattern and monitor urine output (volume and characteristics).
- Explain the nature and purpose of antimicrobial therapy. Emphasize the importance of completing the prescribed course of therapy or, with long-term prophylaxis, of strictly adhering to the ordered dosage.
- Familiarize the patient with prescribed medications and their possible adverse effects. If antibiotics cause GI distress, explain that taking nitrofurantoin macrocrystals with milk or a meal can help prevent such problems. If therapy includes phenazopyridine, warn the patient that this drug turns urine red-orange.
- Explain that an uncontaminated midstream urine specimen is essential for accurate diagnosis. Before collection, teach the female patient to clean the perineum properly and to keep the labia separated during urination.
- Suggest warm sitz baths for relief of perineal discomfort.
- Teach the patient ways to prevent future UTIs. (See *Preventing UTIs*.)

Uterine bleeding, abnormal

Abnormal uterine bleeding refers to abnormal endometrial bleeding without recognizable organic lesions. Abnormal uterine bleeding is the indication for almost 25% of gynecologic surgical procedures. Although prognosis varies with the cause, correction of hormonal imbalance or structural abnormality usually corrects the problem.

Causes

Abnormal uterine bleeding usually results from an imbalance in the hormonal-endometrial relationship in which persistent and unopposed stimulation of the endometrium by estrogen occurs. When progesterone secretion is absent but estrogen secretion continues, the endometrium proliferates and become hypervascular. When ovulation doesn't occur, the endometrium is randomly broken down, and exposed vascular channels cause prolonged and excessive bleeding. In most cases of abnormal uterine bleeding, the endometrium shows no pathologic changes. However, in chronic unopposed estrogen stimulation (as from a hormone-producing ovarian tumor), the endometrium may show hyperplastic or malignant changes. Disorders that cause sustained high estrogen levels include:

- polycystic ovary syndrome
- obesity (because enzymes present in peripheral adipose tissue convert the androgen androstenedione to estrogen precursors)
- immaturity of the hypothalamic-pituitary-ovarian mechanism (postpubertal teenagers)
- anovulation (women in their late 30s or early 40s).

Other causes of abnormal uterine bleeding include:

- trauma (foreign object insertion or direct trauma)
- endometriosis
- coagulopathy, such as thrombocytopenia or leukemia (rare)
- drug-induced coagulopathy.

Signs and symptoms

Abnormal uterine bleeding usually occurs as:

- metrorrhagia (episodes of vaginal bleeding between menses)
- hypermenorrhea (heavy or prolonged menses longer than 8 days, also known incorrectly as *menorrhagia*)
- chronic polymenorrhea (menstrual cycle less than 18 days) or oligomenorrhea (infrequent menses)
- fatigue due to anemia
- oligomenorrhea and infertility due to anovulation.

Possible complications of abnormal uterine bleeding include iron deficiency anemia caused by blood loss of more than 1.6 L over a short time, hemorrhagic shock or right-sided heart failure (rare), and endometrial adenocarcinoma due to chronic estrogen stimulation.

Diagnosis

Abnormal uterine bleeding may be caused by anovulation. Diagnosis of anovulation is based on:

- history of abnormal bleeding, bleeding in response to a brief course of progesterone, absence of ovulatory cycle body temperature changes, and low serum progesterone levels
- diagnostic studies ruling out other causes of excessive vaginal bleeding, such as organic, systemic, psychogenic, and endocrine causes, including certain cancers, polyps, pregnancy, and infection
- dilatation and curettage (D&C) or office endometrial biopsy to rule out endometrial hyperplasia and cancer in women over age 35
- hemoglobin levels and hematocrit to determine the need for blood transfusion or iron supplementation.

Treatment

Possible treatment of abnormal uterine bleeding includes:

- high-dose estrogen-progestogen combination therapy (hormonal contraceptives) to control endometrial growth and reestablish a normal cyclic pattern of menstruation (usually given four times daily for 5 to 7 days even though bleeding usually stops in 12 to 24 hours; drug choice and dosage determined by patient's age and cause of bleeding); maintenance therapy with lower dose combination hormonal contraceptives

- endometrial biopsy to rule out endometrial adenocarcinoma (patients age 35 and older)
- progestogen therapy (alternative for many women, such as those susceptible to such adverse effects of estrogen as thrombophlebitis)
- I.V. estrogen followed by progesterone or combination hormonal contraceptives if the patient is young (more likely to be anovulatory) and severely anemic (if oral drug therapy is ineffective)
- D&C (short-lived treatment and not clinically useful, but an important diagnostic tool) with hysteroscopy as a useful adjunct
- iron supplementation or transfusions of packed cells or whole blood, as indicated, due to anemia caused by recurrent or excessive bleeding
- explaining the importance of following the prescribed hormonal therapy and describing the D&C or endometrial biopsy procedure and purpose (if ordered)
- stressing the need for regular checkups to assess the effectiveness of treatment.

Special considerations

- If a patient complains of abnormal bleeding, tell her to record the dates of the bleeding and the number of pads she saturates per day to help assess the pattern and the amount of bleeding. Instruct the patient not to use tampons.
- Instruct the patient to report abnormal bleeding immediately to help rule out major hemorrhagic disorders such as those that occur in abnormal pregnancy.
- To prevent abnormal bleeding due to organic causes and for early detection of malignancy, encourage the patient to have a Papanicolaou test and a pelvic examination annually.
- Offer reassurance and support. The patient may be particularly anxious about excessive or frequent blood loss and passage of clots. Suggest that she minimize blood flow by avoiding strenuous activity and lying down with her feet elevated.

Uterine cancer

The most common gynecologic cancer, uterine cancer (cancer of the endometrium) typically afflicts postmenopausal women between ages 50 and 60. It's uncommon between ages 30 and 40 and rare before age 30. Most premenopausal women who develop uterine cancer have a history of anovulatory menstrual cycles or other hormonal imbalances. About 33,000 new cases of uterine cancer are reported annually; of these, approximately 5,500 are fatal.

Causes

Uterine cancer appears to be linked to several predisposing factors:

- low fertility index and anovulation

- history of infertility or failure of ovulation
- abnormal uterine bleeding
- obesity, hypertension, diabetes, or nulliparity
- familial tendency
- history of uterine polyps or endometrial hyperplasia
- prolonged estrogen therapy without use of progesterone.

In most patients, uterine cancer is an adenocarcinoma that metastasizes late, usually from the endometrium to the cervix, ovaries, fallopian tubes, and other peritoneal structures. It may spread to distant organs, such as the lungs and brain, by way of the blood or the lymphatic system. Lymph node involvement can also occur. Less common uterine tumors include adenoacanthoma, endometrial stromal sarcoma, lymphosarcoma, mixed mesodermal tumors (including carcinosarcoma), and leiomyosarcoma.

Complications of uterine cancer include intestinal obstruction, ascites increasing pain, and hemorrhage.

Signs and symptoms

The patient history may reflect one or more predisposing factors. In the younger patient, it may also reveal spotting and protracted, heavy menstrual periods. The postmenopausal woman may report that bleeding began 12 or more months after menses had stopped. In either case, the patient may describe the discharge as watery at first, then blood-streaked, and gradually becoming bloodier. In more advanced stages, palpation may disclose an enlarged uterus.

Diagnosis

Endometrial, cervical, or endocervical biopsy confirms cancer cells. Fractional dilatation and curettage identifies the problem when the disease is suspected but the endometrial biopsy is negative. Positive diagnosis requires the following tests to provide baseline data and permit staging:

- multiple cervical biopsies and endocervical curettage to pinpoint cervical involvement
- Schiller's test, the staining of the cervix and vagina with an iodine solution that turns healthy tissues brown (cancerous tissues resist the stain)
- computed tomography scan or magnetic resonance imaging to detect metastasis to the myometrium, cervix, lymph nodes, and other organs (see *Staging uterine cancer*, page 474)
- excretory urography and, possibly, cystoscopy to evaluate the urinary system
- proctoscopy or barium enema studies, which may be performed if bowel and rectal involvement are suspected
- blood studies, urinalysis, and cytologic examination of the urine may also help in evaluating the disease and assessing complications of the therapy.

Treatment

Depending on the cancer's extent, treatment may include one or more of the following measures:

- Surgery usually involves total abdominal hysterectomy, bilateral salpingo-oophorectomy or, possibly, omentectomy with or without pelvic or para-aortic lymphadenectomy. To-

Staging uterine cancer

The International Federation of Gynecology and Obstetrics defines uterine (endometrial) cancer in five stages, as outlined below.

Stage 0
Carcinoma in situ

Stage I
Carcinoma confined to the corpus
- *Stage IA*—length of the uterine cavity 8 cm or less
- *Stage IB*—length of the uterine cavity more than 8 cm

Stage I disease is subgrouped by the following histologic grades of the adenocarcinoma:

G1—highly differentiated adenomatous carcinoma
G2—moderately differentiated adenomatous carcinoma with partly solid areas
G3—predominantly solid or entirely undifferentiated carcinoma

Stage II
Carcinoma involving the corpus and the cervix but not extending outside the uterus

Stage III
Carcinoma extending outside the uterus but not outside the true pelvis

Stage IV
Carcinoma extending outside the true pelvis or obviously involving the mucosa of the bladder or rectum
- *Stage IVA*—spread of the growth to adjacent organs
- *Stage IVB*—spread to distant organs

tal pelvic exenteration removes all pelvic organs, including the rectum, bladder, and vagina, and is only performed when the disease is sufficiently contained to allow surgical removal of diseased parts. This surgery seldom is curative, especially in nodal involvement.
- Radiation therapy is used when the tumor isn't well-differentiated. Intracavitary radiation, external radiation, or both may be given 6 weeks before surgery to inhibit recurrence and lengthen survival time.
- Hormonal therapy, using antiestrogenics such as tamoxifen, shows a response rate of 20% to 40%.
- Chemotherapy, including cisplatin and doxorubicin, is usually attempted when other treatments have failed.

Special considerations

- Listen to the patient's fears and concerns. She may be fearful for her survival and concerned that treatment will alter her lifestyle or prevent sexual intimacy. Encourage her to use available support systems to cope with loss of fertility, if applicable. Remain with the patient during periods of severe stress and anxiety.
- Administer pain medications as necessary. Patients who require pain medications for this disease are commonly in the later stages. Encourage the patient to identify actions that

promote comfort and then be sure to perform them as often as possible. Provide distractions and help her perform relaxation techniques that may ease her discomfort.

- Prepare the patient for surgery as indicated.
- Find out whether the patient will have internal or external radiation or both. Usually, internal radiation therapy is used first.
- Provide supportive care for adverse effects of radiation therapy or chemotherapy.
- Depending on the patient's condition and the therapies and treatments selected, she may require a dietitian to help maintain nutritional needs and a physical therapist to help maintain joint mobility and ambulation. In addition, a pain care specialist can help control discomfort and provide options for pain relief. The patient may also benefit from speaking with a spiritual counselor or pastoral care representative. Refer her and her family to the American Cancer Society for support groups.
- Monitor the patient's complete blood count (including differential) regularly for signs of immunosuppression caused by radiation therapy and chemotherapy. Also assess regularly for signs and symptoms of infection, bleeding, and anemia and monitor vital signs.
- Emphasize that prompt treatment significantly improves a patient's likelihood of survival. Discuss tests to diagnose and stage the disease and explain treatments, which may include radiation therapy, surgery, hormonal therapy, chemotherapy, or a combination of these.
- If the patient is premenopausal, explain that removal of her ovaries will induce menopause.
- As appropriate, explain that, except in total pelvic exenteration, the vagina remains intact and that once she recovers, sexual intercourse is possible.
- Describe the procedure for radiation therapy to the patient. Answer the patient's questions and counsel her about radiation's adverse effects. Advise her to rest frequently and maintain a well-balanced diet.
- To minimize skin breakdown and reduce the risk of skin infection, tell the patient to keep the treatment area dry, avoid wearing clothes that rub against the area, and avoid using heating pads, alcohol rubs, or irritating skin creams. Because radiation therapy increases susceptibility to infection (possibly by lowering the white blood cell [WBC] count), encourage her to avoid people with colds or other infections.
- Explain chemotherapy or immunotherapy to the patient and her family and be sure they understand what adverse effects to expect and how to alleviate them. If the patient is receiving a synthetic form of progesterone, such as hydroxyprogesterone, medroxyprogesterone, and megestrol, tell her to watch for depression, dizziness, backache, swelling, breast tenderness, irritability, and abdominal cramps. Instruct her to report signs and symptoms of thrombophlebitis, such as

pain in the calves, numbness, tingling, or loss of leg function.

- Advise the patient receiving chemotherapy that WBC counts must be checked weekly, and reinforce the importance of preventing infection. Assure her that hair loss is temporary, and discuss alternative options such as scarves.
- If the patient is employed and is undergoing chemotherapy, point out that continuing to work during this period may offer an important diversion. Advise her to talk with her employer about a flexible work schedule or working at home as energy permits.

Uterine leiomyomas

Uterine leiomyomas, the most common benign tumors in women, are also known as *myomas*, *fibromyomas*, or *fibroids*. They're tumors composed of smooth muscle that usually occur in the uterine corpus, although they may appear on the cervix or on the round or broad ligament. Uterine leiomyomas occur in 20% to 25% of women of reproductive age and may affect three times as many Blacks as Whites, although the true incidence in either population is unknown.

Leiomyomas are classified according to location. They may be located within the uterine wall (intramural) or protrude into the endometrial cavity (submucous) or from the serosal surface of the uterus (subserous). Of varying size, they're usually firm and surrounded by a pseudocapsule composed of compressed but otherwise normal uterine myometrium. The uterine cavity may become larger, increasing the endometrial surface area. This can cause increased uterine bleeding. (See *Uterine leiomyoma types*.)

Tumors become malignant (leiomyosarcoma) in less than 0.1% of patients, which should serve to comfort women concerned with the possibility of a uterine malignancy in association with a fibroid.

Causes

The cause of uterine leiomyomas is unknown, but some factors implicated as regulators of leiomyoma growth include:

- several growth factors, including epidermal growth factor
- steroid hormones, including estrogen and progesterone (because leiomyomas typically arise after menarche and regress after menopause, which implicates estrogen as a promoter of leiomyoma growth), and growth factors.
- genetic predisposition. (See *Uterine leiomyoma gene*, page 478.)

Signs and symptoms

Approximately one-third of women with uterine leiomyomas experience pain, which may manifest itself as dysmenorrhea, dyspareunia (painful intercourse), or chronic lower abdominal or back pain. Although most uterine leiomyomas are asymptomatic, when present, signs and symptoms include:

Uterine leiomyoma types

There are many types of uterine leiomyomas, as illustrated below.

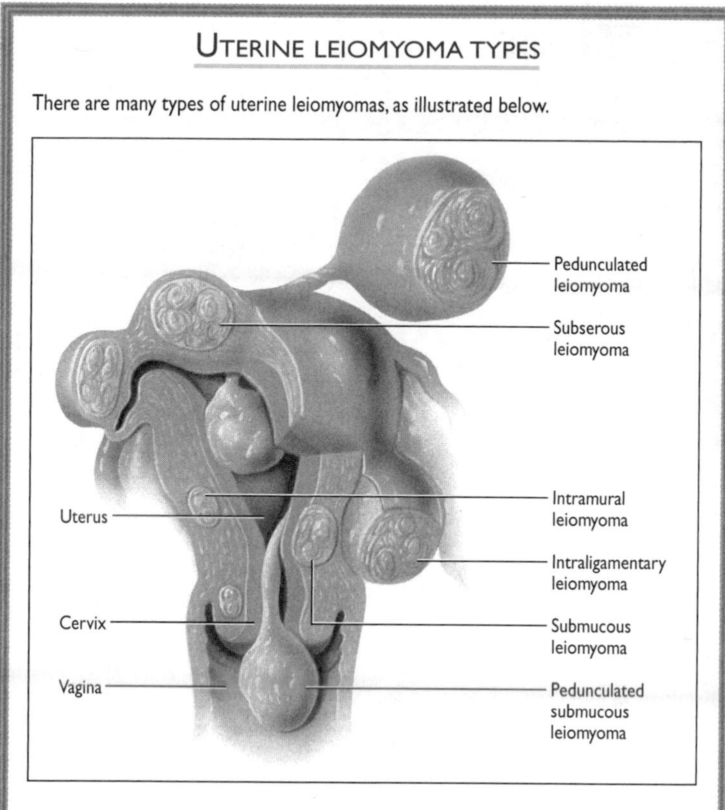

- abnormal bleeding, typically hypermenorrhea with disrupted submucosal vessels (most common symptom)
- pain only associated with torsion of a pedunculated (stemmed) subserous tumor or leiomyomas undergoing degeneration (when the fibroid outgrows its blood supply and shrinks down in size, which can be artificially induced through myolysis, a laparoscopic procedure to shrink fibroids, or uterine artery embolization)
- pelvic pressure and impingement on adjacent viscera (indications for treatment, depending on severity) resulting in mild hydronephrosis (not believed to be an indication for treatment because renal failure rarely, if ever, results)
- urinary frequency, urinary incontinence, or urinary retention due to pelvic pressure on the urinary bladder
- constipation due to pressure on the GI tract.

Various complications and disorders have been attributed to uterine leiomyomas, including recurrent spontaneous abortion, preterm labor, malposition of the fetus, anemia secondary to excessive bleeding, bladder

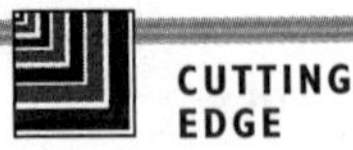

CUTTING EDGE

Uterine leiomyoma gene

Current research suggests that there's a strong genetic component, specifically a mutation in the fumarate hydratase gene, related to the development of uterine leiomyomas. Although more research is necessary, identifying the possible gene is promising for future treatment of uterine leiomyomas.

compression, infection (if tumor protrudes out of the vaginal opening), secondary infertility (rare), and bowel obstruction.

Diagnosis

Diagnosis of leiomyoma may be based on:

- clinical findings (enlarged uterus) and patient history suggesting uterine leiomyomas
- blood studies showing anemia from abnormal bleeding (may support the diagnosis)
- bimanual examination showing enlarged, firm, nontender, and irregularly contoured uterus (also seen with adenomyosis and other pelvic abnormalities)
- ultrasound for accurate assessment of the dimension, number, and location of tumors
- magnetic resonance imaging (especially sensitive to fibroid imaging).

Other diagnostic procedures include:

- hysterosalpingography
- hysteroscopy
- endometrial biopsy (to rule out endometrial cancer in patients over age 35 with abnormal uterine bleeding)
- laparoscopy.

Treatment

Treatment depends on the severity of symptoms, size and location of the tumors, and the patient's age, parity, pregnancy status, desire to have children, and general health. If not severe, treatment may be managed conservatively until the woman reaches menopause, when fibroids most commonly regress.

Treatment options include nonsurgical and surgical procedures. Pharmacologic treatment generally isn't effective in the long term for fibroids. Although usually prescribed by gynecologists, progestational agents are ineffective as primary treatment for fibroids.

In addition to observation, nonsurgical methods include:

- gonadotropin-releasing hormone (GnRH) agonists to rapidly suppress pituitary gonadotropin release, which leads to profound hypoestrogenemia, a 50% reduction in uterine volume (with peak effects occurring in the 12th week of therapy), and consequent benefit of reduction in tumor size before surgery, decreased blood loss during surgery, and increased preoperative hematocrit (best used preoperatively or for up to 6 months in a perimenopausal woman because tumors increase in size after cessation of therapy)

- nonsteroidal anti-inflammatory drugs for dysmenorrhea or pelvic discomfort.

Surgical procedures include:

- abdominal, laparoscopic, or hysteroscopic myomectomy (removal of tumors in the uterine muscle) for patients of any age who want to preserve their uterus
- myolysis (a laparoscopic procedure to treat fibroids without hysterectomy or major surgery, performed on an outpatient basis) to coagulate the fibroids and preserve the uterus and childbearing potential
- uterine artery embolization (radiologic procedure) to block uterine arteries using small pieces of polyvinyl chloride (promising alternative to surgery for many women, but unsupported by long-term studies on success rate, adverse effects, or effects on childbearing and recent anecdotal data suggest decreased time to menopause after embolization)
- hysterectomy (definitive treatment for symptomatic women who have completed childbearing; must involve detailed patient teaching about all available options)
- blood transfusions (with severe anemia due to excessive bleeding).

Special considerations

- Tell the patient to report abnormal bleeding or pelvic pain immediately.
- Reassure the patient that she won't experience premature menopause if her ovaries are left intact.
- In a patient with severe anemia due to excessive bleeding, administer iron supplements and blood transfusions, as ordered.
- Encourage the patient to verbalize her feelings and concerns related to the disease process and its effects on her lifestyle.
- Prior to undergoing surgery, help patients to understand the effects of hysterectomy or oophorectomy, if indicated, on menstruation, menopause, sexual activity, and hormonal balance. Patients should also understand that pregnancy is still possible if multiple myomectomy is necessary, though cesarean delivery may be necessary. Extensive scar tissue may rupture during the contractions of vaginal delivery. (Violation of the endometrial cavity is the classic indication for cesarean delivery in such patients, but it's unclear why a cell layer 1 to 2 cells thick should be protective against uterine dehiscence in subsequent pregnancy.)

Uterine prolapse

Uterine prolapse is the descent of the cervix and uterus into the vagina and beyond. It's caused by relaxation of the uterosacral and cardinal ligaments. Three degrees of uterine prolapse have been described. In first-degree uterine prolapse, the cervix is still within the vagina. In second-degree uterine prolapse, the cervix is at the vaginal introitus. In third-degree uterine prolapse, the cervix and uterus are outside of the vaginal introitus.

Uterine prolapse is more common in older women who have had one or more vaginal births. It's also more common in white women. It may be seen in nulliparous women, children, and infants. In these cases, it's usually due to defects in innervation and the basic uterine supports.

Causes

The most common cause of uterine prolapse is trauma related to childbirth, especially if a woman has delivered large infants or had difficulties with labor and delivery. Genetics may predispose some women to develop uterine prolapse. In addition, advancing age contributes to the loss of muscle tone and the relaxation of the pelvic muscles. The loss of hormonal support with estrogen in postmenopausal women is another contributing factor.

Additional strain on the uterine muscles may be caused by obesity, thereby contributing to uterine prolapse. The same theory applies to patients who suffer from excessive coughing, such as associated with chronic bronchitis and asthma, or straining due to chronic constipation.

Signs and symptoms

Patients with uterine prolapse commonly complain of a bulge or lump in the vagina. Other symptoms may include:

- pain
- pelvic pressure
- backache
- difficulty or pain with sexual intercourse
- disruption of bladder and bowel function
- bleeding if the cervix is ulcerated.

Uterine prolapse may be associated with cystocele and rectocele. Patients with concurrent cystocele may complain of frequent urinary tract infections or other urinary symptoms such as incontinence. Patients with concurrent rectocele may also suffer from hemorrhoids and constipation.

Diagnosis

Uterine prolapse is diagnosed during pelvic examination. The clinician should have the patient bear down and observe for protrusion of the cervix into the vagina or beyond. It may be necessary to examine the woman in the standing position to observe the prolapse. Cystocele and rectocele may also be observed and the ovaries and the bladder may be palpated in lower positions than normal.

Treatment

Usually, uterine prolapse is only treated if a woman is symptomatic. A pessary is inserted into the vagina to hold the uterus in place. Pessaries come in different shapes and sizes and must be fitted to the individual patient. They can be used as a temporary or permanent form of treatment. A pessary requires cleaning by the patient and may irritate the vaginal mucosa. Some patients may complain that it interferes with intercourse because it affects the depth of penetration. Patients must be aware of signs and symptoms of vaginal infections because the presence of a foreign object in the vagina will increase their risk.

Vaginal hysterectomy is the surgical method of choice for effective treatment of uterine prolapse. At the time of hysterectomy, the surgeon can also usually repair sagging vaginal walls, urethra, bladder, or rectum.

Another surgical procedure, laparoscopic suture hysteropexy, may also be used to treat uterine prolapse. It involves plication of the uterosacral ligaments and reattachment of them to the cervix. It's effective and safe, and enables preservation of the uterus.

Special considerations

Nursing care of the patient with uterine prolapse encompasses emotional support and teaching regarding the disorder and treatments:

- Patients may suffer from problems with body image, daily activities, and sexuality.
- Sexual intercourse may produce challenges before and after surgery. The use of lubricants may be suggested.
- The patient should be instructed to avoid lifting or straining, which may worsen the prolapse.
- Give emotional support and guidance to obese patients in their attempt to lose weight.
- Prevention techniques, such as prenatal and postnatal Kegel exercises, can be taught to reduce the risk of uterine prolapse by strengthening the pelvic floor muscles.
- Estrogen replacement therapy in postmenopausal women may be prescribed to help maintain muscle tone; however, the increased risk of endometrial cancer from unopposed estrogen therapy must be discussed with the woman's primary care provider or gynecologist.

V
WX

Vaginal cancer

Vaginal cancer accounts for approximately 2% of all gynecologic cancers. It usually appears as squamous cell carcinoma but occasionally as melanoma, sarcoma, or adenocarcinoma. Primary tumors of the vagina, however, are rare because most vaginal tumors spread from the cervix or the endometrium. This cancer generally occurs in women in their early to mid-50s, particularly when the tumor is squamous cell carcinoma. Some of the rarer types (such as clear cell adenocarcinoma) occur in younger women in their late teens to early 20s and are related to mothers who took diethylstilbestrol during pregnancy. Another type of vaginal cancer, rhabdomyosarcoma, appears in children.

Causes

The exact cause of vaginal cancer remains unknown, but it's thought to be triggered by genital viruses or chronic irritation. Other risk factors include hysterectomy and previous radiation therapy for cancer of the cervix or the rectum.

Vaginal cancer varies in severity according to its location and effect on lymphatic drainage. (The vagina is a thin-walled structure with rich lymphatic drainage.) Similar to cervical cancer, vaginal cancer may progress from an intraepithelial tumor to an invasive cancer. However, it spreads more slowly than cervical cancer.

A lesion in the upper third of the vagina (the most common site) usually metastasizes to the groin nodes; a lesion in the lower third (the second most common site) usually metastasizes to the hypogastric and iliac nodes; but a lesion in the middle third metastasizes erratically. A posterior lesion displaces and distends the vaginal posterior wall before spreading to deep layers. By contrast, an anterior lesion spreads more rapidly into other structures and deep layers because, unlike the posterior wall, the anterior vaginal wall isn't flexible.

Staging vaginal cancer

The International Federation of Gynecology and Obstetrics uses the following staging system to guide prognosis and treatment of vaginal cancer.

Stage 0—carcinoma in situ, intraepithelial carcinoma

Stage I—carcinoma limited to the vaginal wall

Stage II—carcinoma involving the subvaginal tissue but not extending to the pelvic wall

Stage III—carcinoma extending to the pelvic wall

Stage IV—carcinoma extending beyond the true pelvis or involving the mucosa of the bladder or rectum

Signs and symptoms

The most common symptoms of vaginal cancer are abnormal vaginal bleeding and discharge. The patient may also experience bleeding and pelvic or vaginal pain after sexual intercourse. Also, she may have a small or large mass in any part of the vagina. As the cancer progresses, it commonly spreads to the bladder (producing frequent voiding and bladder pain), the rectum (bleeding), vulva (lesion), pubic bone (pain), or other surrounding tissues. Painful urination, constipation, and continuous pain in the pelvis may occur with advanced vaginal cancer.

Diagnosis

The diagnosis of vaginal cancer is based on the presence of abnormal cells on a vaginal Papanicolaou smear. Careful examination and a biopsy rule out the cervix and vulva as primary sites of the lesion. In many cases, however, the cervix contains the primary lesion that has metastasized to the vagina. Then any visible lesion is biopsied and evaluated histologically. Visualization of the entire vagina is sometimes difficult because the speculum blades may hide a lesion or the patient may be uncooperative because of discomfort. When lesions aren't visible, colposcopy is used to identify abnormalities. Painting the suspected vaginal area with Lugol's solution also helps identify malignant areas by staining glycogen-containing normal tissue, while leaving abnormal tissue unstained. (See *Staging vaginal cancer.*)

Treatment

In early stages, treatment aims to preserve the normal parts of the vagina. Topical chemotherapy with 5-fluorouracil and laser surgery can be used for stages 0 and I. Radiation or surgery varies with the size, depth, and location of the lesion and the patient's desire to maintain a functional vagina. Preservation of a functional vagina is generally possible only in the early stages. Survival rates are the same for patients treated with radiation and those treated with surgery.

Surgery is usually recommended only when the tumor is so extensive that exenteration is needed because close proximity to the bladder and rectum permits only minimal tissue margins around resected vaginal tissue.

Radiation therapy is the preferred treatment of advanced vaginal cancer. Most patients need preliminary external radiation treatment to shrink the tumor before internal radiation can begin. Then, if the tumor is localized to the vault and the cervix is present, radiation (using radium or cesium) can be given with an intrauterine tandem or ovoids; if the cervix is absent, a specially designed vaginal applicator is used instead.

To minimize complications, radioactive sources and filters are carefully placed away from radiosensitive tissues, such as the bladder and rectum. Internal radiation lasts 48 to 72 hours, depending on the dosage. (See *Safe time for a radiation implant.*)

Special considerations

For internal radiation:

- Explain the internal radiation procedure, answer the patient's questions, and encourage her to express her fears and concerns.
- Because the effects of radiation are cumulative, wear a radiosensitive badge and a lead shield (if available) when you enter the patient's room, and adhere to internal radiation safety precautions.
- Check with the radiation therapist concerning the maximum recommended time that you can safely spend with the patient when giving direct care.
- While the radiation source is in place, the patient must lie flat on her back. Insert an indwelling urinary catheter (usually done in the operating room), and don't change the patient's linens unless they're soiled. Give only partial bed baths, and make sure the patient has a call bell, phone, water, or anything else she needs within easy reach. The physician will order a clear-liquid or low-residue diet and an antidiarrheal drug to prevent bowel movements.
- To compensate for immobility, encourage the patient to do active range-of-motion exercises with both arms.
- Before radiation treatment, explain the necessity of immobilization, and tell the patient what it entails (such as no linen changes and the use of an indwelling urinary catheter). Throughout therapy, encourage her to express her anxieties.
- Instruct the patient to use a stent or perform prescribed exercises to pre-

Safe time for a radiation implant

Internal radiation with cesium or radium can be administered if the cancer is localized to the vault. Distance defines safe exposure to the radioactive implant (cesium, in the case illustrated below).

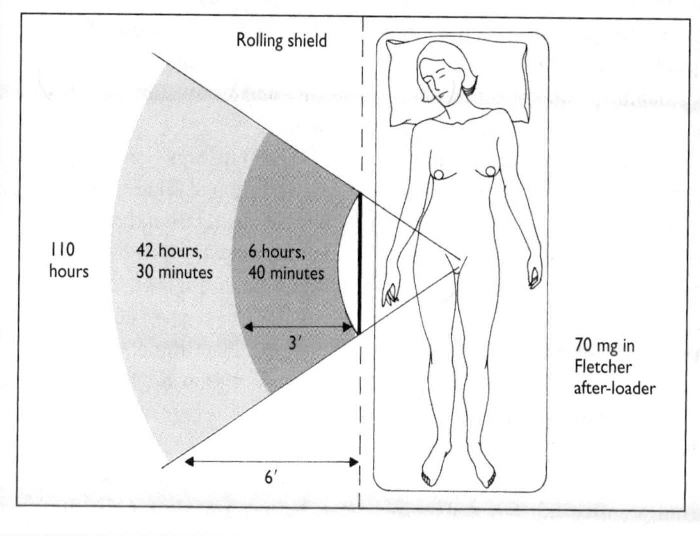

vent vaginal stenosis. Sexual intercourse is also helpful in preventing stenosis.

Vaginismus

Vaginismus is involuntary spastic constriction of the lower vaginal muscles, usually from fear of vaginal penetration. This disorder may coexist with dyspareunia and, if severe, may prevent intercourse (a common cause of unconsummated marriages). Vaginismus affects females of all ages and backgrounds. The prognosis is excellent for a motivated patient who doesn't have untreatable organic abnormalities.

Causes

Vaginismus may be physical or psychological in origin. It may occur spontaneously as a protective reflex to pain or result from organic causes, such as hymenal abnormalities, genital herpes, obstetric trauma, and atrophic vaginitis.

Psychological causes may include:

- childhood and adolescent exposure to rigid, punitive, and guilt-ridden attitudes toward sex
- fears resulting from painful or traumatic sexual experiences, such as incest or rape
- early traumatic experience with pelvic examinations

- fear of pregnancy, sexually transmitted disease, or cancer.

Signs and symptoms

The female with vaginismus typically experiences muscle spasm with constriction and pain on insertion of any object into the vagina, such as a tampon, diaphragm, or speculum. She may profess a lack of sexual interest or a normal level of sexual desire.

Diagnosis

Diagnosis depends on the sexual history and pelvic examination to rule out physical disorders. The sexual history must include:

- early childhood experiences and family attitudes toward sex
- previous and current sexual responses
- contraceptive practices and reproductive goals
- feelings about her sexual partner
- specific details about pain on insertion of any object into the vagina.

A carefully performed pelvic examination confirms the diagnosis by showing involuntary constriction of the musculature surrounding the outer portion of the vagina. When the disorder causes marked distress or interpersonal difficulty, it may fulfill the *DSM-IV-TR* diagnostic criteria.

Treatment

Treatment is designed to eliminate maladaptive muscle constriction and underlying psychological problems. In Masters and Johnson therapy, the patient uses a graduated series of dilators, which she inserts into her vagina while tensing and relaxing her pelvic muscles. The patient controls the amount of time that the dilator is left in place and the movement of the dilator. Together with her sexual partner, she begins sensate focus and counseling therapy to increase sexual responsiveness, improve communication skills, and resolve any underlying conflicts.

Kaplan therapy also uses progressive insertion of dilators or fingers (in vivo/desensitization therapy), with behavior therapy (imagining vaginal penetration until it can be tolerated) and, if necessary, psychoanalysis and hypnosis. Practitioners of both Masters and Johnson and Kaplan therapies claim a 100% cure rate.

Special considerations

- Because a pelvic examination may be painful for the patient with vaginismus, proceed gradually at the patient's own pace. Support the patient throughout the pelvic examination, explaining each step before it's done. Encourage her to verbalize her feelings, and take plenty of time to answer her questions.
- Teach the patient about the anatomy and physiology of the reproductive system, contraception, and human sexual response. This can be done quite naturally during the pelvic examination.
- Ask if the patient is taking any medications that may affect her sexual response, such as antihypertensives, tranquilizers, or steroids. If she has insufficient lubrication for intercourse, tell her about different types

of lubricating gels and creams that are available over-the-counter.

Varicose veins

Varicose veins are dilated, tortuous veins engorged with blood that results from improper venous valve function. They can be primary, originating in the superficial veins, or secondary, occurring in the deep veins.

About 10% to 20% of Americans have primary varicose veins, which account for approximately 90% of varicose veins. They're twice as common in women as in men. Primary varicose veins also tend to be familial and affect both legs. Usually, secondary varicose veins occur in one leg. Both types are more common in middle adulthood.

Without treatment, varicose veins continue to enlarge. And, although there's no cure, certain measures, such as walking and using compression stockings, can reduce symptoms. Surgery may remove varicose veins; however, the condition can occur in other veins.

Causes

Veins are thin-walled, distensible vessels with valves that keep blood flowing in one direction. Any condition that weakens, destroys, or distends these valves allows blood backflow to the previous valve. If a valve can't hold the pooling blood, it may become incompetent, allowing even more blood to flow backward. As the volume of venous blood builds, pressure in the vein increases and the vein becomes distended. As the vein is stretched, its wall weakens and it loses its elasticity. As the vein enlarges, it becomes lumpy and tortuous. As hydrostatic pressure increases, plasma is forced out of the vein and into the surrounding tissue, resulting in edema.

Primary varicose veins can result from:

- congenital weakness of the valves or venous wall
- conditions that produce prolonged venous stasis or increased intra-abdominal pressure, such as pregnancy, obesity, constipation, wearing tight clothes, or standing for prolonged periods
- occupations that necessitate standing for an extended period
- family history of varicose veins.

Secondary varicose veins can result from:

- deep vein thrombosis
- venous malformation
- arteriovenous fistulas
- trauma to the venous system
- occlusion.

Signs and symptoms

Signs and symptoms of varicose veins may include:

- dilated, tortuous, purplish, ropelike veins, particularly in the calves, due to venous pooling
- edema of the calves and ankles due to deep vein incompetence
- leg heaviness that worsens in the evening and in warm weather (caused by venous pooling)
- dull aching in the legs after prolonged standing or walking, which may be due to tissue breakdown

- aching during menses as a result of increased fluid retention.

Possible complications of varicose veins include blood clots secondary to venous stasis, venous stasis ulcers, and chronic venous insufficiency.

SPECIAL NEEDS

As a person ages, veins dilate and stretch, increasing susceptibility to varicose veins and chronic venous insufficiency. Because the skin is friable and can easily break down, venous stasis ulcers in an older adult caused by chronic venous insufficiency may take longer to heal.

Diagnosis

Tests used to help diagnose varicose veins include:

- manual compression test to detect a palpable impulse when the vein is firmly occluded at least 8″ (20 cm) above the point of palpation, indicating incompetent valves in the vein
- Trendelenburg's test (retrograde filling test) to detect incompetent valves in deep and superficial veins
- photoplethysmography to characterize venous blood flow by noting changes in the skin's circulation
- Doppler ultrasonography to detect the presence or absence of venous backflow in deep or superficial veins
- venous outflow and reflux plethysmography to detect deep venous occlusion (invasive; not routinely used)
- ascending and descending venography to demonstrate venous occlusion and patterns of collateral flow.

Treatment

Correction of varicose veins typically involves:

- treatment of the underlying cause, such as abdominal tumor and obesity, if possible
- antiembolism stockings or elastic bandages to counteract swelling by supporting the veins and improving circulation
- regular exercise program that promotes muscular contraction to force blood through the veins and reduce venous pooling
- injection of a sclerosing agent into small to medium-sized varicosities
- surgical stripping and ligation of severe varicose veins
- phlebectomy (removing varicose vein through small incisions in the skin), which may be performed in an outpatient setting.

Additional treatment measures include:

- discouraging the patient from wearing constrictive clothing that interferes with venous return
- encouraging the obese patient to lose weight to reduce increased intra-abdominal pressure
- telling the patient to elevate her legs above her heart whenever possible to promote venous return
- instructing the patient to avoid prolonged standing or sitting because these actions enhance venous pooling.

Special considerations

- After stripping and ligation or after injection of a sclerosing agent, administer analgesics, as ordered, to relieve pain.

- Frequently check circulation in toes (color and temperature), and observe elastic bandages for bleeding. When ordered, rewrap bandages at least once per shift, wrapping from toe to thigh with the leg elevated.
- Watch for signs and symptoms of complications, such as sensory loss in the leg (which could indicate saphenous nerve damage), calf pain (which could indicate thrombophlebitis), and fever (a sign of infection).
- Encourage the patient to ambulate after surgery and elevate her legs whenever possible to reduce swelling.

Vulval cancer

Cancer of the vulva accounts for approximately 4% of all gynecologic malignancies. It can occur at any age, even in infants, but its peak incidence is in the mid-60s. The most common vulval cancer is squamous cell carcinoma. Early diagnosis increases the chance of effective treatment and survival. Lymph node dissection demonstrates a 5-year survival rate in 85% of patients if it reveals no positive nodes; otherwise, the survival rate falls to less than 75%.

Causes

Although the cause of vulval cancer is unknown, several factors seem to predispose women to this disease:

- leukoplakia (white epithelial hyperplasia) — in about 25% of patients
- chronic vulval granulomatous disease
- chronic pruritus of the vulva with friction, swelling, and dryness
- pigmented moles that are constantly irritated by clothing or perineal pads
- irradiation of the skin such as nonspecific treatment for pelvic cancer
- sexually transmitted diseases, such as herpes simplex and condyloma acuminatum caused by human papilloma virus (HPV)
- obesity
- hypertension
- diabetes.

Signs and symptoms

In 50% of patients, cancer of the vulva begins with vulval pruritus, bleeding, or a small vulval mass (which may start as a small ulcer on the surface that, eventually, becomes infected and painful). These symptoms call for immediate diagnostic evaluation. Less common indications include a mass in the groin or abnormal urination or defecation. (See *Carcinoma of the vulva*, page 490.)

Diagnosis

Pruritus, bleeding, small vulval mass, or a Papanicolaou smear that reveals abnormal cells strongly suggests vulval cancer. Firm diagnosis requires histologic examination. Abnormal tissues for biopsy are identified by colposcopic examination to pinpoint vulval lesions or abnormal skin changes and by staining with toluidine blue dye, which, after rinsing with dilute acetic acid, is retained by diseased tissues.

Other diagnostic measures include complete blood count, X-ray, electrocardiogram, and thorough physical (including pelvic) examination. Occa-

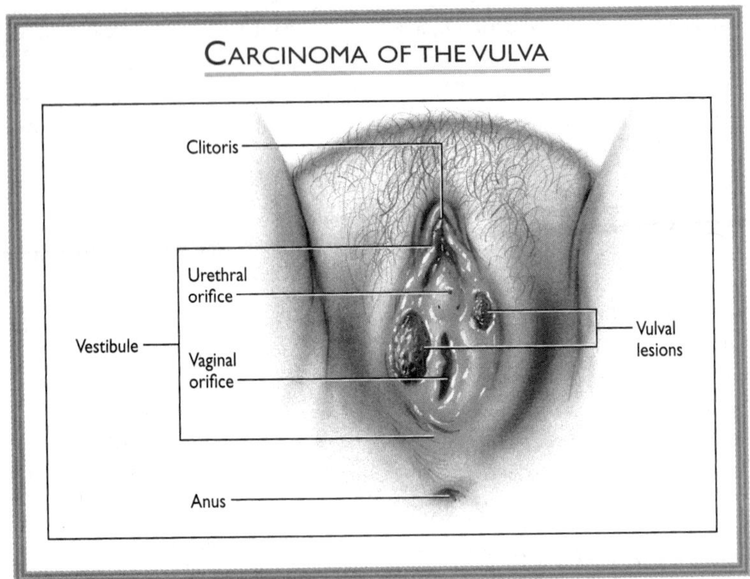

sionally, a CT scan may pinpoint lymph node involvement. (See *Staging vulval cancer.*)

Treatment

Depending on the stage of the disease, cancer of the vulva usually calls for radical or simple vulvectomy (or laser therapy for some small lesions). Radical vulvectomy requires bilateral dissection of superficial and deep inguinal lymph nodes. Depending on the extent of metastasis, resection may include the urethra, vagina, and bowel, leaving an open perineal wound until healing — about 2 to 3 months. Plastic surgery, including mucocutaneous graft to reconstruct pelvic structures, may be done later.

Small, confined lesions with no lymph node involvement may require a simple vulvectomy or hemivulvectomy (without pelvic node dissection). Personal considerations (young age of patient, active sexual life) may also mandate such conservative management. However, a simple vulvectomy requires careful postoperative surveillance because it leaves the patient at higher risk for developing a new lesion.

If extensive metastasis, advanced age, or fragile health rules out surgery, irradiation of the primary lesion offers palliative treatment.

Special considerations

Patient teaching, preoperative and postoperative care, and psychological support can help prevent complications and speed recovery.

Before surgery:

- Supplement and reinforce what the physician has told the patient about the surgery and postoperative procedures, such as the use of an indwelling urinary catheter, preventive respiratory care, and exercises to prevent venous stasis.

- Encourage the patient to ask questions, and answer them honestly.

After surgery:

- Provide scrupulous routine gynecologic care and special care to reduce pressure at the operative site, reduce tension on suture lines, and promote healing through better air circulation.
- Place the patient on an air mattress or convoluted foam mattress, and use a cradle to support the top covers.
- Periodically reposition the patient with pillows. Make sure her bed has a half-frame trapeze bar to help her move.
- For several days after surgery, the patient will be maintained on I.V. fluids or a clear liquid diet. As ordered, give her an antidiarrheal drug three times daily to reduce the discomfort and possible infection caused by defecation. Later, as ordered, give stool softeners and a low-residue diet to combat constipation.
- Teach the patient how to clean the surgical tube thoroughly.
- Check the operative site regularly for bleeding, foul-smelling discharge, or other signs of infection. The wound area will look lumpy, bruised, and battered, making it difficult to detect occult bleeding. This situation calls for a physician or a primary nurse who can more easily detect subtle changes in appearance.
- Within 5 to 10 days after surgery, as ordered, help the patient to walk. Encourage and assist her in coughing and range-of-motion exercises.

Staging vulval cancer

The International Federation of Gynecology and Obstetrics and the American Joint Committee on Cancer defines vulval cancer in five stages as outlined below.

- *Stage 0*—carcinoma in situ
- *Stage I*—tumor confined to skin surface of vulva, 2 cm or less in greatest dimension
  - *Stage IA*—invasion of underlying connective tissue less than 1 mm
  - *Stage IB*—invasion of underlying connective tissue greater than 1 mm
- *Stage II*—tumor confined to the vulva, perineum, or both; more than 2 cm in greatest dimension
- *Stage III*—tumor of any size with contiguous spread to the lower urethra and any or all of the vagina, the perineum, and the anus
- *Stage IV*—tumor of any size that infiltrates the bladder or rectal mucosa or both (including the upper part of the urethral mucosa or is fixed to the pubic bone and any other distant metastases)

- To prevent urine contamination, the patient will have an indwelling urinary catheter in place for about 2 weeks. Record fluid intake and output, and provide standard catheter care.
- Counsel the patient and her partner about resumption of sexual activity. Explain that sensation in the vulva will eventually return after the nerve endings heal, and they'll probably be able to have sexual intercourse 6 to 8 weeks following surgery. Explain that they may want to try different sexual

techniques, especially if surgery has removed the clitoris. Help the patient adjust to the drastic change in her body image.

Vulvovaginitis

Vulvovaginitis is inflammation of the vulva (vulvitis) and vagina (vaginitis). Because of the proximity of these two structures, inflammation of one occasionally causes inflammation of the other. Vulvovaginitis may occur at any age and affects most females at some point in their lives. The prognosis is excellent with treatment.

Causes

Common causes of vaginitis (with or without consequent vulvitis) include:

- infection with *Trichomonas vaginalis*, a protozoan flagellate, usually transmitted through sexual intercourse
- infection with *Candida albicans* (a fungus that requires glucose for growth), with an increase in incidence during the secretory phase of the menstrual cycle (commonly affecting hormonal contraceptive users, diabetics, and up to 75% of patients receiving systemic antibiotics and occurring twice as often in pregnant females as nonpregnant females)
- infection with *Gardnerella vaginalis*, a gram-negative bacillus.

Common causes of vulvitis include:

- parasitic infection with *Phthirus pubis* (crab louse)
- trauma (skin breakdown, which may lead to secondary infection)
- poor personal hygiene
- chemical irritations or allergic reactions to hygiene sprays, douches, detergents, clothing, or toilet paper
- vulval atrophy in menopausal women due to decreasing estrogen levels
- retention of a foreign body, such as a tampon or a diaphragm.

Signs and symptoms

In trichomonal vaginitis, vaginal discharge is thin, bubbly, green-tinged, and malodorous. This infection causes marked irritation and itching, and urinary symptoms, such as burning and frequency. Candidal vaginitis produces a thick, white, cottage-cheese-like discharge and red, edematous mucous membranes with white flecks adhering to the vaginal wall. It's commonly accompanied by intense itching. *G. vaginalis* produces a gray, foul, "fishy" smelling discharge.

Acute vulvitis causes a mild to severe inflammatory reaction, including edema, erythema, burning, and pruritus. Severe pain on urination and dyspareunia may necessitate immediate treatment. Herpes infection may cause painful ulceration or vesicle formation during the active phase. Chronic vulvitis generally causes relatively mild inflammation, possibly associated with severe edema that may involve the entire perineum.

Diagnosis

Diagnosis of vaginitis requires identification of the infectious organism during microscopic examination of vaginal exudate on a wet slide preparation (a drop of vaginal exudate placed in normal saline solution):

- In trichomonal infections, the presence of motile, flagellated trichomonads confirms the diagnosis.
- In candidal vaginitis, 10% potassium hydroxide is added to the slide; diagnosis requires identification of *C. albicans* fungi.
- In *Gardnerella*, the presence of clue cells (epithelial cells with obscured borders) is revealed.

Diagnosis of vulvitis or suspected venereal disease may require complete blood count, urinalysis, cytology screening, biopsy of chronic lesions to rule out malignancy, culture of exudate from acute lesions, and possible human immunodeficiency virus testing.

Treatment

Common therapeutic measures for vulvovaginitis include:

- metronidazole (Flagyl) orally for the patient with trichomonal vaginitis and for all sexual partners
- topical miconazole 2% (Monistat 7) or clotrimazole 1% (Gyne-Lotrimin 7) for candidal infection
- oral or vaginal metronidazole for *Gardnerella*
- oral fluconazole (Diflucan) as a single dose for *Candida*
- doxycycline (Adoxa) for 1 week combined with a single dose of erythromycin (Erythrocin) for chlamydial infections.

Cold compresses or cool sitz baths may provide relief from pruritus in acute vulvitis; severe inflammation may require warm compresses. Other therapy includes avoiding drying soaps, wearing loose clothing to promote air circulation, and applying topical corticosteroids to reduce inflammation. Chronic vulvitis may respond to topical hydrocortisone or antipruritics and good hygiene (especially in elderly or incontinent patients). Topical estrogen ointments may be used to treat atrophic vulvovaginitis. No cure currently exists for herpesvirus infections; however, oral and topical acyclovir decreases the duration and symptoms of active lesions.

Special considerations

- Ask the patient if she has any drug allergies. Stress the importance of taking the medication for the length of time prescribed, even if symptoms subside.
- Teach the patient how to insert vaginal ointments and suppositories. Tell her to remain prone for at least 30 minutes after insertion to promote absorption (insertion at bedtime is ideal). Suggest she wear a pad to prevent staining her underclothing.
- Encourage good hygiene. Advise the patient with a history of recurrent vulvovaginitis to wear all-cotton underpants. Advise her to avoid wearing tight-fitting pants and panty hose, which encourage the growth of the infecting organisms.
- Report notifiable cases of sexually transmitted diseases to local public health authorities.
- Tell the patient that persistent, recurring candidiasis may suggest diabetes or undiagnosed pregnancy.

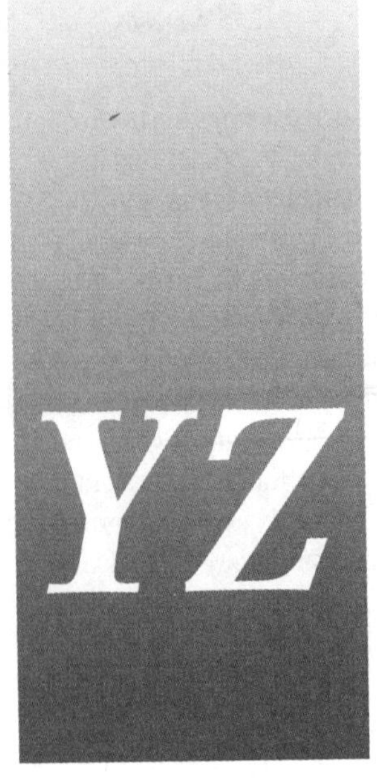

Yeast infection

Vaginitis is the most common gynecologic problem seen in primary care and gynecology settings. A vaginal yeast infection, also called *vulvovaginal candidiasis*, is one of three types of vaginitis. The other types are bacterial vaginosis and trichomoniasis. Yeasts are always present in the vagina in small numbers; however, symptoms only appear when overgrowth occurs. As with the other forms of vaginitis, a yeast infection is triggered by changes in the vaginal ecosystem. It's estimated that 75% of all women will have a vaginal yeast infection at some point in their lives.

Causes

The most common cause (about 90%) of a vaginal yeast infection is a fungus called *Candida albicans*. Other fungi that may also be responsible include:

- *C. glabrata*
- *C. parapsilosis*
- *C. tropicalis*
- *Saccharomyces cerevisiae.*

It's unknown exactly why some women are more prone to yeast infections. Even so, some predisposing factors have been identified, including:

- antibiotic use
- hormonal contraceptives (oral and topical)

- corticosteroid therapy
- douching
- human immunodeficiency virus infection or other immunosuppressed states
- hormones
- increased frequency of sexual intercourse
- multiple sex partners
- oral or anal sexual intercourse
- obesity
- pregnancy
- sexually transmitted diseases
- stress
- tissue abrasion that allows yeast to infiltrate the vaginal epithelium
- uncontrolled diabetes mellitus
- vaginal medications.

Characteristic yeast infection

Yeast infections in women are common. Characteristic signs include vulvovaginal edema, redness, white flecks adhering to the vaginal wall, and a thick, white, nonmalodorous discharge.

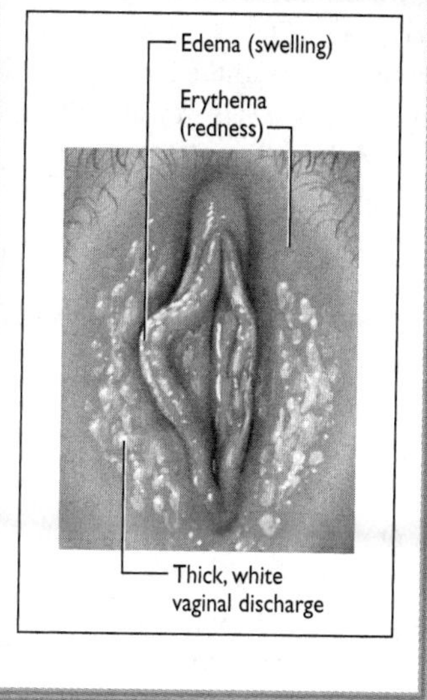

Signs and symptoms

The most common complaint of women with yeast infections is vulval and vaginal itching. They may also experience irritation and inflammation. Other symptoms may include:

- dyspareunia (painful intercourse)
- external dysuria as urine passes over the inflamed labia
- burning sensation during urination
- cottage cheese-like discharge.

Women may notice a worsening of symptoms during the week before the onset of menses, with relief during and after menses, due to the hormonal changes that occur during the menstrual cycle. On physical examination, the clinician may note vulvovaginal edema and erythema. A thick, white, usually nonmalodorous discharge may be present. White flecks may be noted adhering to the vaginal wall. Excoriations may be observed due to scratching or irritation, and the vagina may look and feel dry. (See *Characteristic yeast infection.*)

Diagnosis

To diagnose a yeast infection, the clinician must:

- assess the color and consistency of any discharge
- check the pH of vaginal fluid
- assess for the presence of amines by performing a whiff test
- prepare wet mount slides with saline and potassium hydroxide (KOH).

Vaginal pH is normal (greater than 4.5) in clients with yeast infection. A whiff test is performed by mixing the vaginal discharge with one or two drops of 10% to 20% KOH and assessing for odor. An odor shouldn't be present in patients with yeast infection; this is called a *negative whiff test.* A positive whiff test is associated with bacterial vaginosis. Microscopic evaluation of the saline slide and KOH wet mounts usually reveal budding yeast cells and pseudohyphae, although they aren't always seen.

Further testing with fungal cultures is indicated in patients with recurrent yeast infections or infections refractory to treatment.

Treatment

Yeast infections can be treated topically or orally. Topical treatments are generally more effective and may be given as creams, suppositories, or a combination of both. Doses are given each night for 3 to 7 days, depending on the agent and concentration. Recurrent or refractory infections warrant longer therapy. Topical medications include:

- clotrimazole (Mycelex)
- miconazole (Monistat)
- butoconazole (Femstat)
- terconazole (Terazol).

Oral treatment is commonly preferred because it isn't as messy and patients are more likely to comply. However, the adverse effect of hepatotoxicity must be kept in mind. One oral dose of fluconazole (Diflucan) can be given. For those with vulvar itching and burning, a topical antifungal may be prescribed to relieve the discomfort when applied externally.

Several over-the-counter treatments are available and can be recommended for clients with previously diagnosed yeast infections who have recurrence of the same symptoms.

Special considerations

Care of the patient with a yeast infection includes teaching about treatment and prevention. Self-diagnosis, treatment, and prevention must also be addressed.

- For the patient who is self-treating, if symptoms persist or if they recur within 2 months, medical care should be sought.
- Intercourse should be avoided until treatment is complete.
- Partner treatment isn't necessary unless symptoms appear, then topical treatment can be given.
- Patients who are pregnant should be treated for 7 days with a topical medication.
- Patients should be taught about vaginal hygiene, including the following:
  - Avoid tight-fitting clothes.
  - Wear cotton underwear.
  - Dry the vaginal area well after bathing.
  - Wipe from front to back after using the toilet.
  - Change out of wet swimsuits or damp clothes promptly.
  - Avoid deodorant sanitary pads, tampons, and toilet paper.
  - Discourage douching or using feminine hygiene sprays.
  - Decrease intake of sugar and yeast-containing foods and beverages.

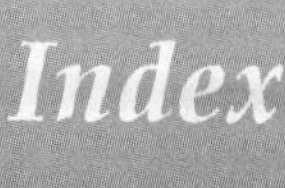

Index

Index

i refers to an illustration; t refers to a table.

i refers to an illustration; t refers to a table.

---

i refers to an illustration; t refers to a table.

I

J

K

L

M

i refers to an illustration; t refers to a table.

i refers to an illustration; t refers to a table.

i refers to an illustration; t refers to a table.

i refers to an illustration; t refers to a table.